Genotoxicity and Mutagenicity - Mechanisms and Test Methods

Edited by Sonia Soloneski and Marcelo L. Larramendy

Published in London, United Kingdom

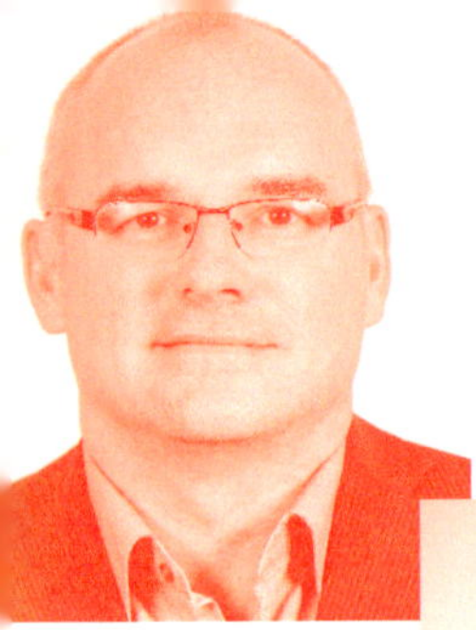
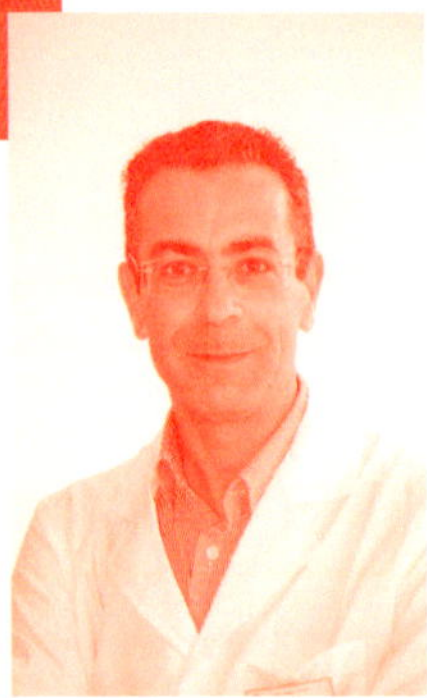
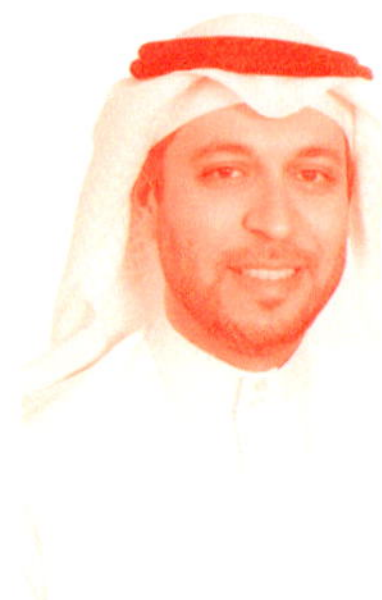
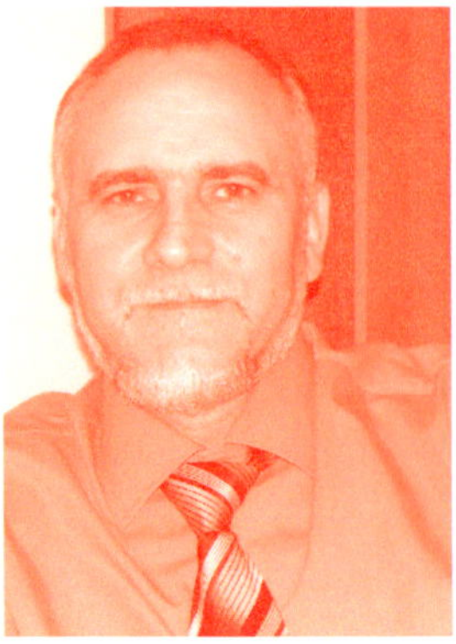
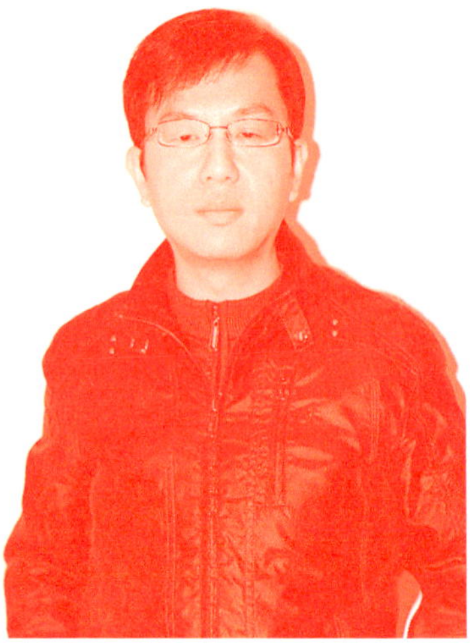
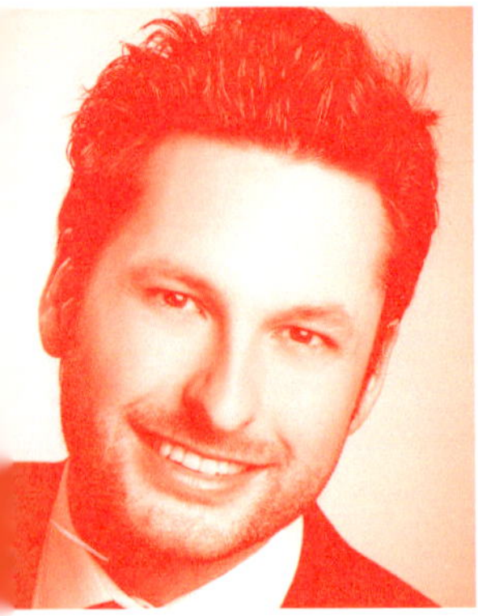
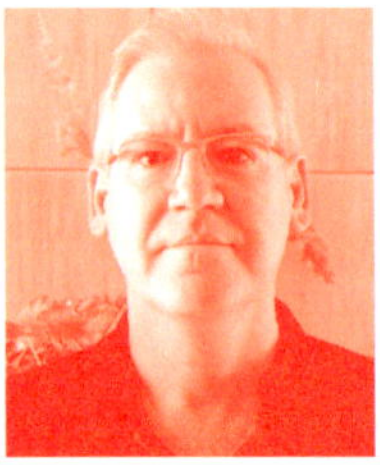

IntechOpen

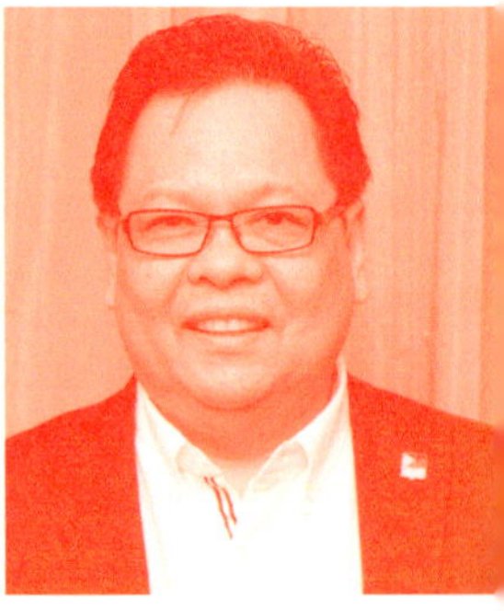
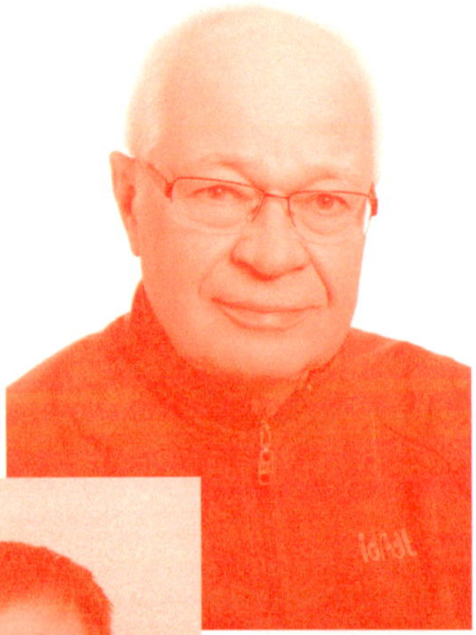
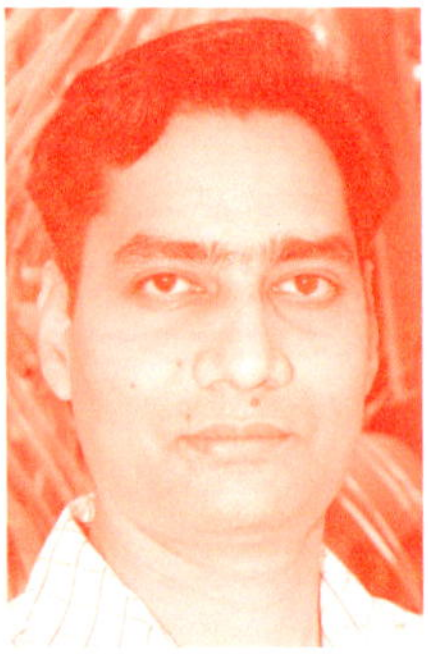
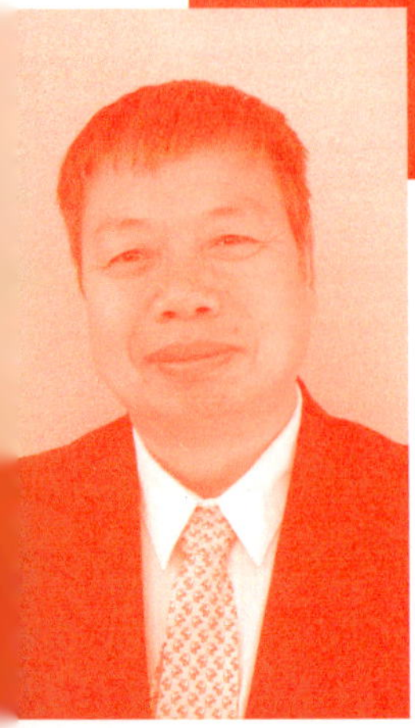
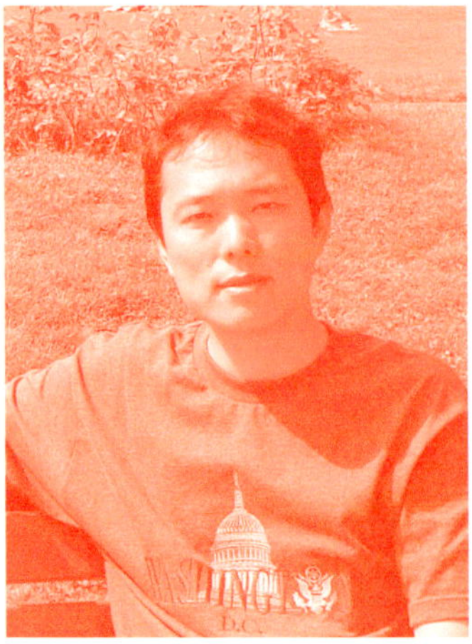
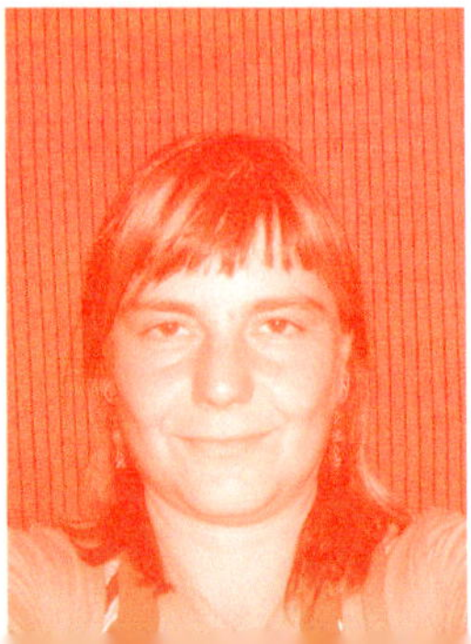

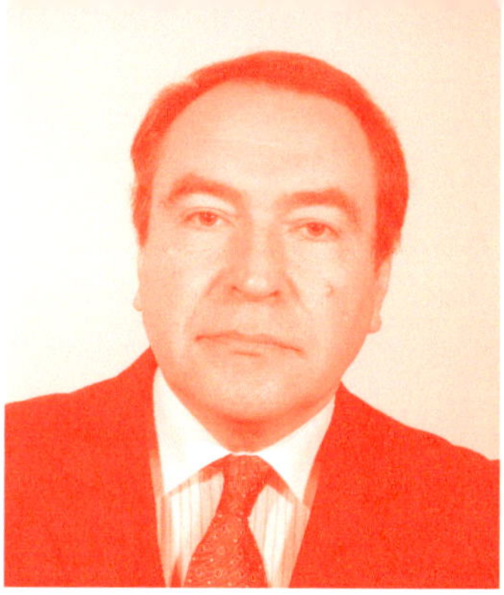

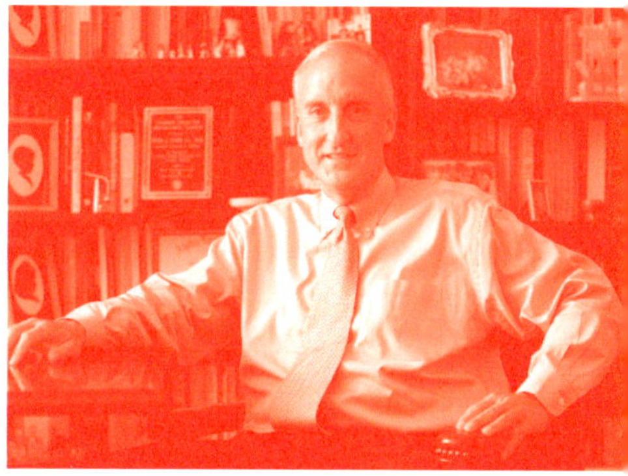

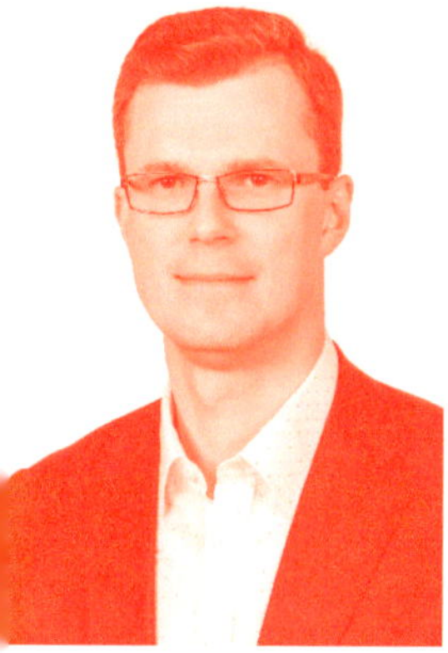

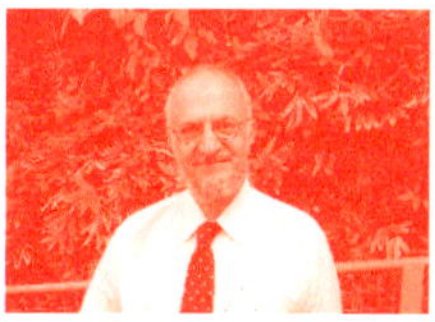

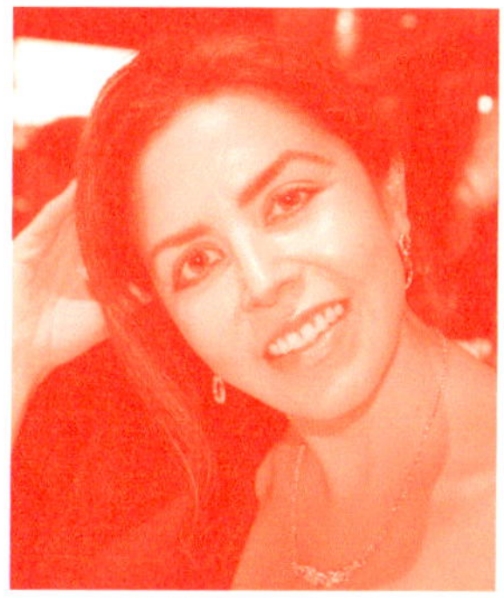

Supporting open minds since 2005

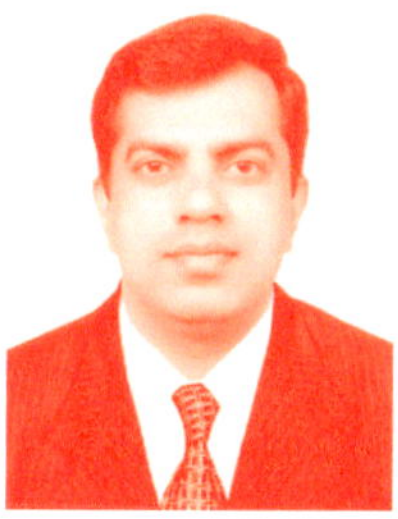

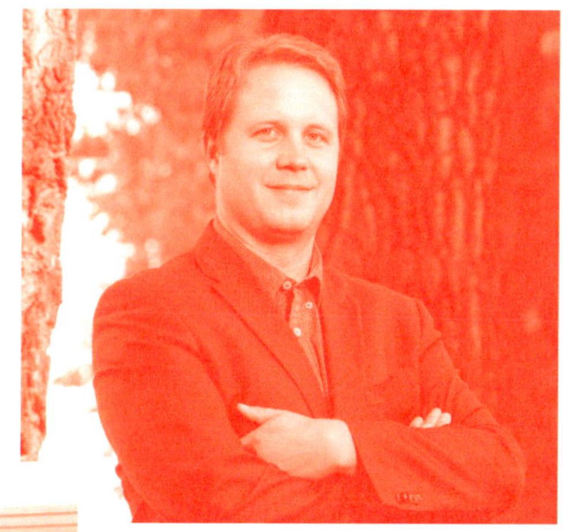

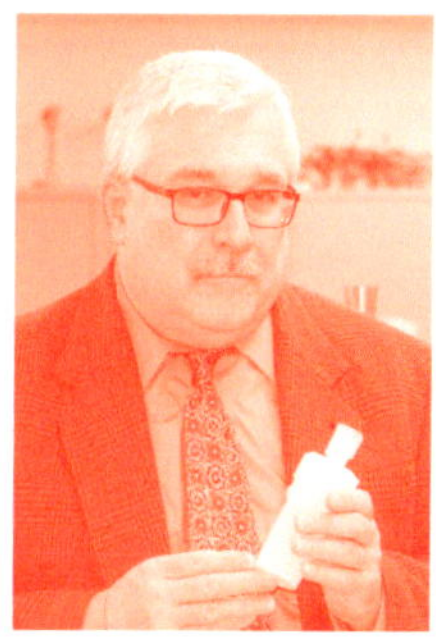

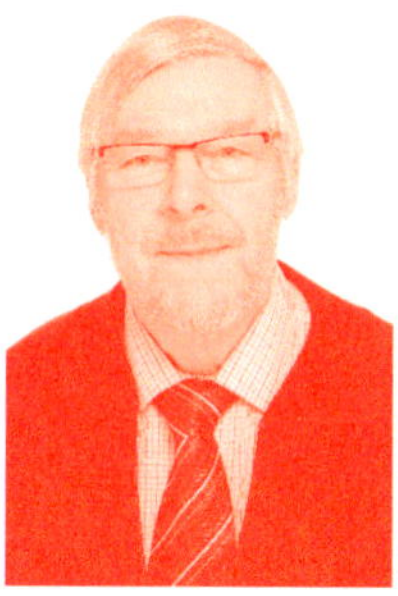

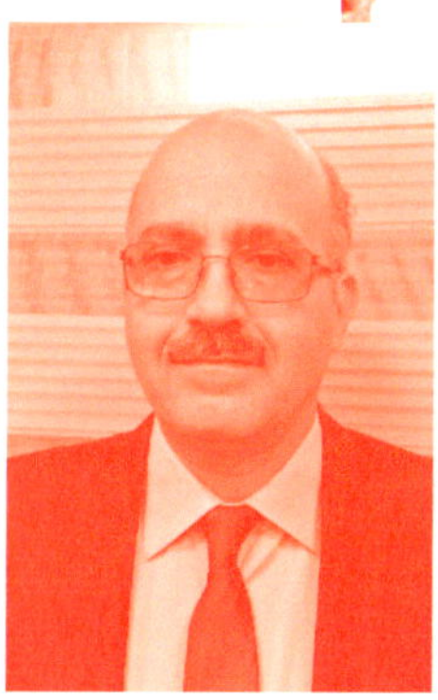

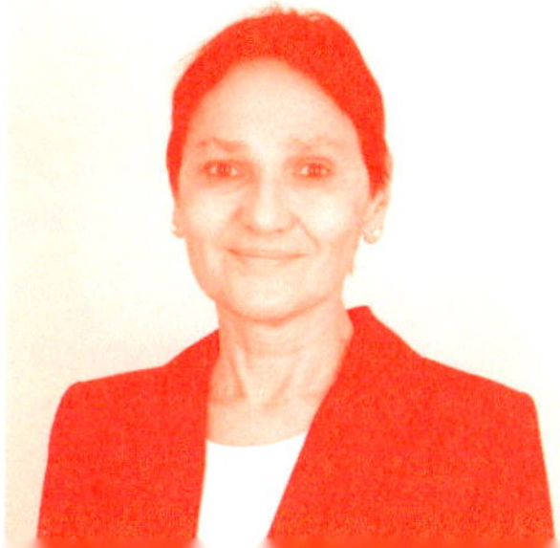

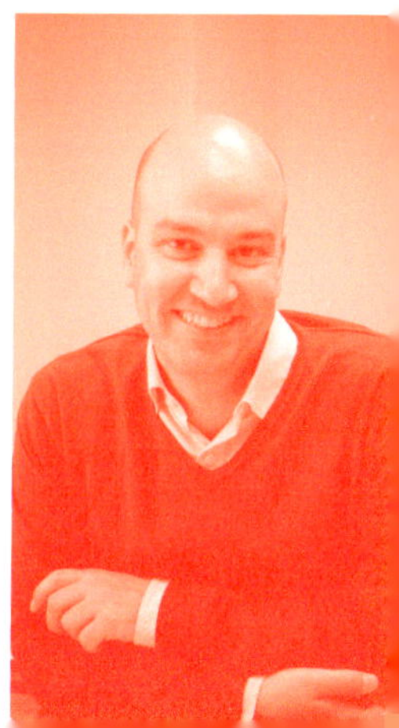

Genotoxicity and Mutagenicity - Mechanisms and Test Methods
http://dx.doi.org/10.5772/intechopen.84992
Edited by Sonia Soloneski and Marcelo L. Larramendy

Contributors
Viktoria Mykhailenko, Viktor Kyrychenko, Oleksandr Bragin, Dmytro Chuiko, Peter Ostoich, Michaela Beltcheva, Roumiana Metcheva, Michael Thomas Fasullo, Alexander A. A. Zhgun, Adel Abelhakeem, El-Shimaa Mohamed Naguib Abdel-Hafez, Isabel Gaivão, Maria Sierra, João Ferreira, Teresa Fortoul-van der Goes, Marcela Rojas-Lemus, Gabriela Guerrero-Palomo, Patricia Bizarro-Nevares, Adriana Gonzalez-Villalva, Martha Ustarroz-Cano, Nelly Lopez-Valdez, Brenda Casarrubias-Tabarez, Norma Rivera-Fernandez, Otto Tavera-Cabrera, Armando Rodríguez-Zepeda, Francisco Pasos-Nájera, Parthasarathy Chandrakesan, Janani Panneerselvam, Dongfeng Qu, Courtney Houchen, Michael Bronze, María Eugenia Cervantes-Valencia

First published in London, United Kingdom, 2021 by IntechOpen
IntechOpen is the global imprint of INTECHOPEN LIMITED, registered in England and Wales, registration number: 11086078, 5 Princes Gate Court, London, SW7 2QJ, United Kingdom
Printed in Croatia

British Library Cataloguing-in-Publication Data
A catalogue record for this book is available from the British Library

Additional hard and PDF copies can be obtained from orders@intechopen.com

Genotoxicity and Mutagenicity - Mechanisms and Test Methods
Edited by Sonia Soloneski and Marcelo L. Larramendy
p. cm.
Print ISBN 978-1-83880-041-3
Online ISBN 978-1-83880-042-0
eBook (PDF) ISBN 978-1-83962-167-3

For EU product safety concerns:
IN TECH d.o.o., Prolaz Marije Krucifikse Kozulić 3, 51000 Rijeka, Croatia, info@intechopen.com or visit our website at intechopen.com.

Meet the editors

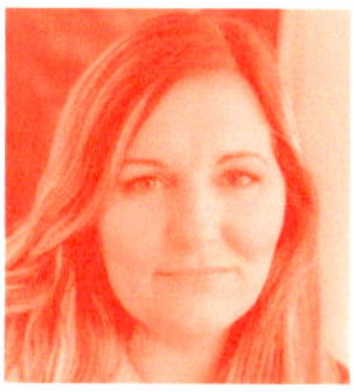

Sonia Soloneski has a Ph.D. in Natural Sciences and is an Assistant Professor of Molecular Cell Biology at the School of Natural Sciences and Museum of La Plata, National University of La Plata, Argentina. She is a member of the National Scientific and Technological Research Council (CONICET) of Argentina in the genetic toxicology field, the Latin American Association of Environmental Mutagenesis, Teratogenesis, and Carcinogenesis (ALAMCTA), the Argentinean Society of Toxicology (ATA), the Argentinean Society of Genetics (SAG), the Argentinean Society of Biology (SAB), and the Society of Environmental Toxicology and Chemistry (SETAC). She has authored more than 380 contributions in the field, including scientific publications in peer-reviewed journals and research communications. She has served as a review member for more than 30 scientific international journals. She has been a plenary speaker in scientific conferences and a member of scientific committees. She is a specialist in issues related to genetic toxicology, mutagenesis, and ecotoxicology.

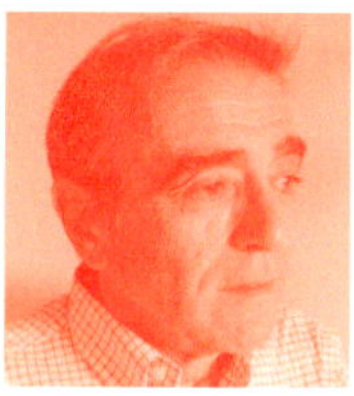

Marcelo L. Larramendy, Ph.D., serves as a Professor of Molecular Cell Biology at the School of Natural Sciences and Museum (National University of La Plata, Argentina). He was appointed as Senior Researcher of the National Scientific and Technological Research Council of Argentina. He is a former member of the Executive Committee of the Latin American Association of Environmental Mutagenesis, Teratogenesis, and Carcinogenesis. He is the author of more than 450 contributions, including scientific publications, research communications, and conferences worldwide. He is the recipient of several national and international awards. Prof. Larramendy is a regular lecturer at the international A. Hollaender courses organized by the IAEMS and a former guest scientist at NIH (USA) and the University of Helsinki, (Finland). He is an expert in genetic toxicology and is, or has been, a referee for more than 20 international scientific journals. He was a member of the International Panel of Experts at the International Agency for Research on Cancer (IARC, WHO, Lyon, France) in 2015 for the evaluation of DDT, 2,4-D, and Lindane. Presently, Prof. Dr. Larramendy is Head of the Laboratory of Molecular Cytogenetics and Genotoxicology at the UNLP.

Contents

Preface

Organisms living in the real world are inevitably exposed to many chemical, physical, and biological agents that are harmful: food additives, natural toxins, pesticides, nanomaterials, metals, radiation, and viruses, among others. However, most of these agents, if not all, may have unexpected consequences on the biota. Organisms are continuously exposed to heterogeneous xenobiotics released into different habitats either deliberately, inadvertently, or through non-regulated industrial discharges. Understanding how these agents can produce genetic alterations in DNA and what their role is in different biological systems continue to receive intense attention in fields such as health, pharmaceutical, environment, industry, agriculture, and food sectors.

Mutagenicity denotes the generation of stable changes in the DNA molecule that differ from the normal sequence of an organism, which may result in a transmissible change in the genotype of living organisms. Any damaged genetic material could result in mutations, thus stimulating carcinogenic progression or establishing a framework for hereditary disorders. Whereas mutations are generated mainly by exogenous agents, named mutagens, the term genotoxic describes the capability of those chemical, physical, and biological agents to directly affect the structure of DNA, the cellular spindle apparatus, and/or the topoisomerase enzymes that modulate DNA topology during DNA replication as well as chromosome segregation, which are, finally, responsible for the fidelity of the genome. However, genotoxic damage to DNA is not always associated with mutations. Spontaneous mutations arise from a variety of sources due to errors in DNA replication, repair, and recombination, and the presence of transposable genetic elements. Many agents can produce chemically reactive species during their metabolism, or are themselves reactive and may, therefore, cause irreversible changes to DNA.

Heritable changes are the origin of innate metabolic deficiencies in cellular systems, generating morbidity and mortality in organisms. Genetic disorders can be produced by a mutation in only one or in multiple genes, through a combination of gene mutations and environmental factors or by damage at the chromosomal level that affects the number and/or structure of entire chromosome(s), or parts thereof. Mutations in cells are not only involved in the initiation and promotion of several human diseases, including cancer, but are also implicated in several genetic disorders, like anaemia, diabetes, cardiovascular alterations, obesity, atherosclerosis, and numerous other degenerative disorders. Currently, scientists recognize more than 4,000 human diseases that are produced by mutations as a result of a combinatorial failure of more than one of these processes.

As indicated in a book we published some years ago, entitled "Genotoxicity-A Predictable Risk To Our Actual World", without knowledge of the mutagenic and genotoxic properties of chemical, physical, and biological agents, the evaluation of responses in living organisms, including humans, is difficult, and consequently the regulation of genotoxicants is a complex and difficult process. Accurate identification of the different classes of environmental genotoxicants and mutagens would permit international regulatory scientific agencies to use this information in a variety of legislative decisions to establish priorities of public and scientific concern.

We have attempted to compile information from different fields, highlighting the detrimental influence that mutagenic and genotoxic agents inflict on DNA and how antimutagenic and anticarcinogenic modulators are able to reduce the negative impact of such toxic agents on living species. Antimutagens and anticarcinogens are agents that decrease the number of mutations in cells, modulating host defence mechanisms. Therefore, knowledge regarding the mechanism of action of potentially mutagenic and/or carcinogenic agents provides the basis for elucidation of how these protective chemicals exert a response. Antimutagens are employed as one of the key methods to increase cellular resistance to mutagens. They are able to reduce or even remove the mutagenic effects exerted by toxic xenobiotics, stimulating compensatory repair and tolerance pathways in the DNA. In regard to their mode of action, antimutagens can act by influencing different targets, such as cellular membranes, DNA damage repair, replication, chromatin organization, and cell signalling.

This book opens with an interesting discussion about the use of yeast as a model organism for studying the biological effects of the P450-mediated metabolism of xenobiotics. This chapter also focuses on strategies for employing multiple genetic endpoints in screening chemicals, yeast strains that facilitate phenotyping cytochrome P450 polymorphisms to test the safety of thousands of chemicals, the limitations of animal systems, the advantages of model organisms, and the humanization of yeast cells by expressing human cytochrome P450 genes. The second chapter describes a possible molecular mechanism for how the addition of exogenous polyamines may increase the production of improved strains of filamentous fungi and the biotechnological applications of this phenomenon. The third chapter provides information on chemical and physical mutagenesis in breeding, exemplified by new modern homozygous self-pollinated sunflower lines, as well as additional recommendations on the use of methods to induce mutagenesis, including methods of generation, investigation, and subsequent use of mutations. The fourth chapter comprises an excellent review comparing the specific toxicity and genotoxicity exerted by heavy metals such as lead and cadmium using mammalian cells as a biological matrix in the context of ecotoxicology. The fifth chapter describes the importance of doublecortin-like kinase 1 (DCLK1), a member of the protein kinase superfamily and the doublecortin family, and its role in DNA damage response and repair, via direct and indirect mechanisms. It is well known that DCLK1 is expressed in cancer stem cells, and is implicated in initiating tumours. The sixth chapter reviews the role of oxidative stress induced by vanadium (a common mechanism of action of metal pollutants), observed in in vivo and in vitro systems, highlighting the way the production of free radicals inflicts damage in biomolecules including DNA, proteins, lipids, and carbohydrates. In addition, the chapter emphasizes the protective role of two water-soluble antioxidants, namely carnosine and ascorbate, present in biological systems. The seventh chapter constitutes an update on how the w-/w+ somatic mutation and recombination test of Drosophila melanogaster are employed extensively for antigenotoxicity analysis, focusing on actual published results to aid in the development of a reliable protocol in antigenotoxicity. Finally, this book comprises a chapter discussing the properties of antimutagenic substances with multiple mechanisms of action, in addition to introducing different aspects of natural and synthetic antimutagens.

Further, the chapter includes a brief compilation of scientific findings, either from dietary sources or synthetic agents, with potential to combat the disorders caused by the mutagenic agents, noting possible future perspectives and mechanisms of antimutagenics.

The editors of Genotoxicity and Mutagenicity - Mechanisms and Test Methods are enormously grateful to all contributing authors for sharing their knowledge and insights in this book. They have made an extensive effort to gather the information included in every chapter. Readers are challenged to interpret the significance of various mechanisms and tested methodologies for detecting the causes and consequences of mutagenic and genotoxic agents. We hope that the topics discussed here encourage all those interested to explore new aspects of the fields of mutagenesis and genotoxicity by stimulating scientific dialogue. The publication of this book is of great importance to scientists, biologists, pharmacologists, physicians, and veterinarians, as well as engineers, teachers, graduate students, and administrators of environmental programmes, who can make use of these investigations to understand some aspects of mutagenic and genotoxic issues, making this volume a valuable reference in the future.

Sonia Soloneski Ph.D. and Marcelo L. Larramendy Ph.D.
School of Natural Sciences and Museum,
National University of La Plata,
La Plata, Argentina

Chapter 1

Genotoxic Assays for Measuring P450 Activation of Chemical Mutagens

Michael Fasullo

Abstract

This review discusses using yeast as a model organism for studying the biological effects of P450-mediated metabolism of xenobiotics. We discuss the challenges of testing the safety of thousands of chemicals currently introduced into the market place, the limitations of the animal systems, the advantages of model organisms, and the humanization of the yeast cells by expressing human cytochrome P450 (CYP) genes. We discuss strategies in utilizing multiple genetic endpoints in screening chemicals and yeast strains that facilitate phenotyping CYP polymorphisms. In particular, we discuss yeast mutants that facilitate xenobiotic import and retention and particular DNA repair mutants that can facilitate in measuring genotoxic endpoints and elucidating genotoxic mechanisms. New directions in toxicogenetics suggest that particular DNA damaging agents may interact with chromatin and perturb gene silencing, which may also generate genetic instabilities. By introducing human CYP genes into yeast strains, new strategies can be explored for high-throughput testing of xenobiotics and identifying potent DNA damaging agents.

Keywords: cytochrome P450 polymorphisms, genotoxins, budding yeast, recombination assays

1. Introduction

Genotoxins are generally referred to as chemical agents that cause DNA damage, which, in turn, can initiate recombination or mutation events or chromosome loss [1]. While mutagens and recombinagens are genotoxic, not all genotoxins are directly mutagenic [2]. Genotoxic exposure has been correlated to birth defects [3], cardiovascular disease [4], carcinogenesis [5], and accelerated aging [6]. Public health depends on minimizing exposure to genotoxic chemicals. Nonetheless, thousands of chemicals have yet to be tested, and new chemicals are annually synthesized. Federal agencies mandate that all chemicals be tested for safety before being introduced into the marketplace [7]. Generally, this testing has involved rapid screens for bacterial mutagenesis, micronuclei assays or comet assays for testing DNA fragmentation, and animal testing for determining carcinogenicity. Animal testing is often expensive and time-consuming and has increasingly raised ethical concerns. While microbial plate assays, such as the Ames test [8], have been standard in identifying chemical mutagens, some chemicals that test negative in the Ames assays are carcinogenic, while others that test positive in the Ames assays are not carcinogens [8, 9]. Many chemicals are not genotoxic per se but require metabolic bioactivation [10]. The bioactivated compound is generally a highly reactive intermediate in a pathway which renders hydrophobic compounds more hydrophilic to facilitate excretion. While bioactivation does occur in specific animal models, toxicity outcomes differ depending on the species [11]. Thus, there is a need for metabolic competent cell-based assays that can measure multiple genotoxic endpoints.

Bioactivation occurs by phase I and phase II enzymes; phase I enzymes generally hydroxylate compounds so that phase II enzymes can conjugate larger molecules, facilitating the export and excretion of the modified compound. Phase I enzymes include cytochrome P450 monooxygenases (CYPs), which compose a superfamily of over 50 genes, and catalyze the formation of highly reactive electrophiles and epoxides, as intermediates in xenobiotic metabolism [12, 13]. Up to 80% of all bioactivations require CYPs [14]. For catalytic efficiency, the CYP proteins must be reduced by oxidoreductases, which are colocalized with CYPs in the endoplasmic reticulum (ER [15]).

Saccharomyces cerevisiae (budding yeast) is an excellent eukaryotic model organism for studying the genotoxicity of xenobiotics, including pharmaceuticals, pesticides, insecticides, and suspected carcinogens. Similar to bacterial organisms, yeast strains are easy to culture, grow rapidly, and can be manipulated genetically, rendering it possible to perform high-throughput analysis [16]. Many yeast genes are similar to human genes, and approximately 30% of can be functionally replaced by the human orthologue [17, 18]. DNA repair pathways and genes are also similar [17, 16]. Mitochondrial genotoxicity can also be measured [19]. Thus, identifying genotoxins and understanding their mechanisms in budding yeast can elucidate whether similar mechanisms occur in human cells.

However, yeasts also have some disadvantages. First, yeast cells contain a cell wall that blocks entry to carcinogens, and higher chemical concentrations are required in yeast than in mammalian organisms to observe similar genotoxic endpoints [1, 20]. Second, yeast lacks some functions of mammalian cells; while there are many yeast genes that have human homologs, other human DNA repair genes, such as p53, BRCA1, and BRCA2, have no corresponding yeast homologs. Nonetheless, the ability to modify the yeast genome has enabled yeast biologists to enhance carcinogen uptake and retention in cells [20, 21].

Engineered yeast strains enable high-throughput screens for identifying genotoxins among the thousands of novel synthetic chemicals, circumventing the limitations and reducing the escalating costs of animal tests. By expressing specific human cytochrome P450 genes in the engineered strains, tissue-specific metabolic activation can be simulated. Besides identifying genotoxins, engineered yeast strains can elucidate genotoxic mechanisms by measuring multiple genetic alterations, as well as DNA and organelle damage. Future engineering of yeast strains may identify additional human metabolic genes that can confer resistance to P450-activated genotoxins.

This review will address (1) characterization of human CYPs that activate the majority of carcinogens, (2) yeast vectors that have been engineered to express these CYPs, (3) plate and reporter assays that have been used to detect CYP-dependent activated compounds in yeast, (4) chemicals which have been identified and mechanistic insights that have been garnered by utilizing yeast genetics, (5) studies that have phenotypes P450 polymorphisms, (6) comparisons with other model eukaryotes, and (7) future directions in guiding genotoxic assays.

2. Phase I and phase II enzymes that bioactivate xenobiotics

While 57 CYPs have been identified, approximately 80% of all bioactivation is mediated by just 7 CYPs: CYP1A1, 1A2, 1B1, 2A13, 2A6, 2E1, and 3A4 [22]. Xenobiotic chemicals that are activated by these CYPs include polycyclic aromatic hydrocarbons (PAHs), aryl- and heterocyclic amines (HAAs), and nitrosamines, as well as small molecules such as benzene, naphthalene, and furans [22]. Examples of CYP-activated xenobiotics include tobacco carcinogens, industrial solvents, and food carcinogens, including the most potent liver carcinogen, aflatoxin B1 (AFB1). The importance of individual CYPs is underscored by observations that particular knockout mice are more resistant to environmental carcinogens, for example, fewer tumors arise in *Cyp1b1*$^{-/-}$ and *Cyp2a5* $^{-/-}$ knockout mice after exposure to 7,12-dimethylbenz[a]anthracene [23] and 4-(methylnitrosamino)-1-(3-pyridyl)-1-butanone (NNK) [24], respectively.

Phase II enzymes include glutathione S-transferases, N-acetyl transferases, epoxide hydrolases, glucuronidases, and sulfotransferases. They serve to both inactivate highly reactive intermediates that are formed by phase I enzymes and conjugate larger molecules onto the products of phase I reactions to facilitate export and excretion [25]. While some phase II enzymes, such as glutathione S-transferases (GSTs), may inactivate epoxide intermediates, other phase II enzymes, such as N-acetyl transferases (NATs), may facilitate the conversion of hydroxylated heterocyclic aromatic amines to highly nitrenium ions (**Figure 1** [25]). For example, 2-amino-3-methylimidazo[4,5-*f*]quinoline (IQ) is hydroxylated by CYP1A2 in the liver [26]. Further modification by NAT2 acetylates the hydroxylated product, resulting in an unstable intermediate yielding a reactive nitrenium ion; this nitrenium ion reacts with DNA yielding deoxyguanine DNA adducts [25, 26]. Pathways by which activated HAAs drive colon carcinogenesis are unclear. One notion is that reactive IQ metabolites can also be glucuronidated in the liver and excreted into

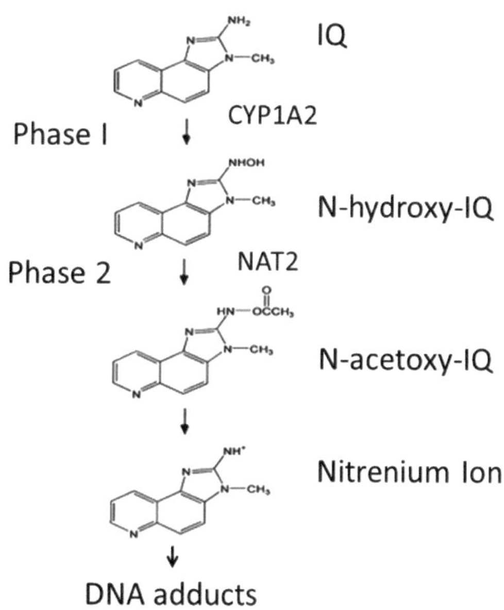

Figure 1.
Phase 1 and phase 2 metabolism of IQ. CYP1A2 generates the formation of N-hydroxy IQ. NAT2 generates an unstable molecule, N-acetoxy-IQ, which then generates a reactive nitrenium ion. The reactive nitrenium ion interacts with DNA to form adducts, particularly at the C8 and C2 positions of guanine. Figure was adapted from Kim and Guengerich [25].

the colon. Gut microbial glucuronidases then cleave the glucose and reactivate the compound leading to genotoxicity in the colon [27]. An alternative notion is that IQ is bioactivated to a mutagen in situ in the colon. Expression of multiple mammalian phase I and phase II enzymes may be important in rendering some compounds genotoxic; examples include CYP1A1 and epoxide hydrolase in the activation of benzo[a]pyrene and CYP2E1 and SULT1A1 for the activation of 2,5-dimethylfuran (DMF) and furfuryl alcohol (FFA) [5, 22].

When compounds are substrates for multiple CYPs or phase II enzymes, products of varying toxicity can be generated; examples of substrates include estradiol, N-acetyl-p-aminophenol (APAP or acetaminophen), and AFB1. In the case of estradiol, CYP1A2 and CYP3A4 predominately hydroxylate estradiol in the 2′ position generating 2′ hydroxyestradiol [28, 29], while CYP1B1 hydroxylates estradiol in the 4′ position generating 4′ hydroxyestradiol; further modification of 4′-hydroxyestradiol by peroxidases generates a highly reactive form that generates DNA adducts, while 2′ hydroxylestradiol can be detoxified [29]. In the case of acetaminophen, most acetaminophen is converted to nontoxic forms by sulfotransferases and glucuronidases; CYP2E1 converts acetaminophen to N-acetyl-*p*-benzoquinone imine (NAPQI), which depletes glutathione levels, causes oxidative stress, and is highly toxic in the liver [30]. Since CYP2E1 is induced by alcohol, the combination of alcohol and acetaminophen can be lethal [29]. Regarding AFB1, AFB1 is metabolized by CYP1A2 and CYP3A4 into a toxic epoxide intermediate, while the extrahepatic CYP1A1 can also convert AFB1 to AFM, which is still genotoxic but not as carcinogenic [31]. Because expression and inducibility of CYPs vary among individuals and multiple CYPs are expressed in tissues, it can be difficult to identify which CYP(s) generates the activated genotoxin.

Yeast presents advantages in deciphering which human CYPs can metabolize genotoxins. First, the three endogenous yeast CYPs largely function to synthesize ergosterol or dityrosine synthesis [32, 33]. Second, expression of CYPs in yeast can be regulated by inducible promoters or by copy number, mitigating potential toxic effects of their expression [34, 35]. Considering that CYP proteins locate to the yeast ER, the entire CYP cDNA can be expressed without truncating the sequence that encodes the N-terminus, as it is necessary for efficient CYP expression in *Escherichia coli* [36]. Third, although CYPs are differentially degraded [37], they are sufficiently stable to activate carcinogens for extended time duration, circumventing problems of transient or variable expression observed in cultures derived from cryopreserved hepatocytes. Based on genotoxic endpoints that can be easily scored, it is possible to phenotype CYP polymorphisms and to determine whether their substrate specificities are altered.

2.1 Mammalian CYP expression in budding yeast

Yeast has been an attractive organism for the expression of heterologous proteins and useful for characterizing biochemical properties of mammalian cytochrome P450 properties. Its success at producing large quantities of human proteins, such as human insulin [38], has largely been due to an advanced understanding of both the transcriptional and translational machinery of eukaryotic gene expression, including well-characterized transcriptional promoters and terminators [39]. Constitutive promoters for expression include *ADH1*, *GAPDH*, *PGK1*, *TPI*, *ENO*, *PYK1*, and *TEF*, while inducible promoters include *GAL1–10*, *CUP1*, *PHO5*, and *ADH* [40]. Expression can be further amplified by high-copy-number vectors or modulated by single-copy vectors, which have been well-described in the literature [34]. Oeda et al. [41] expressed rat CYP2E1cDNA using the constitutive *ADH1* promoter and the phosphoglycerol kinase (pGK) terminator using a high-copy-number vector.

The ability to bind carbon monoxide (CO) confirmed the presence of the recombinant protein. Characterization of human CYP3A4 produced in yeast underscored its broad substrate specificity [42, 43]. Additional in vitro studies involved expressing either human or rat cDNAs of CYP1A1, CYP2E1, CYP1A2, and CYP1B1 and confirming their biochemical properties [43]. A list of CYPs that have been expressed in yeast is shown in **Table 1**.

While inserting mammalian cDNA into expression vector by standard molecular techniques of subcloning can be tedious, many mammalian CYP cDNAs are now commercially available in gateway compatible DNA vectors. Gateway compatible vectors contain small segments of DNA, referred to as attP and attB sites, which

CYP gene	Expression vector	Enzymatic assays	Carcinogen activation	Genotoxic assays/ biosensor reporter	References
CYP1A1	pSB229, pRS424 CYP1A1	EROD[1]	BaP-DHD[4]	HR[9], mutation, growth curves	[46, 50, 51]
			AFB1[5]	HR, mutation, growth curves Yfp-Rad51 foci	[46, 50, 51]
			IQ[6]	Growth curves	[51]
CYP1A2	pCS316, pAAH5N	EROD,MROD[2], LND[3]	AFB1	HR, mutation Yfp-Rad51 foci	[43, 50]
			MeIQx[7]	HR	[87]
			IQ	HR	[87]
CYP1A2/ NAT2	pGP100	MROD, SMZ assay	IQ, MeIQx, MeIQ	HR	[87]
CYP1B1	pYES2, pAG24	EROD	AFB1, BaP-DHD		[111]
CYP2A6	pAAH5N	LND			[43]
CYP2B6	pAAH5N, pESC-URA3	LND, 7-ethoxycoumarin-3-carbonitrile deethylation	N-nitrodimethyl amine		[43]
			AFB1	RAD54-GFP	[71]
CYP2C8	pAAH5N	LND			[43]
CYP2C9	pAAH5N	Lauric acid (omega-1)-hydroxylation			[43]
CYP2C18	pAAH5N	LND			[43]
CYP2D6	pAAH5N, pESC-URA3	LND, debrisoquine 4-hydroxylation, ethoxycoumarin-3-carbonitrile deethylation		RAD54-GFP	[71]

CYP gene	Expression vector	Enzymatic assays	Carcinogen activation	Genotoxic assays/ biosensor reporter	References
CYP2E1	pAAH5N	Lauric acid (omega-1)-hydroxylation			[43]
CYP3A4	pAAH5N, pMA34, pESC-URA3	Diclorofenac, testosterone 6β-hydroxylation, ethoxycoumarin-3-carbonitrile deethylation	AFB1	HR, growth curves RAD54-GFP, RNR3-GFP	[67, 71]
			IQ		[67]
			BaP[8]	RAD54-GFP	[71]

[1]*Ethoxyresorufin deethylase (EROD).*
[2]*Methyoxyresorufin demethylase (MROD).*
[3]*Lidocaine N-deethylation (LND).*
[4]*Benzo[a]pyrene 7,8, dihydrodiol (BaP-DHD).*
[5]*Aflatoxin B1 (AFB1).*
[6]*2-Amino-3-methylimidazo-[4,5-f]quinoline (IQ).*
[7]*2-Amino-3,8-dimethylimidazo-[4,5-f]quinoxaline (MeIQx).*
[8]*Benzo[a]pyrene,*
[9]*homologous recombination (HR).*

Table 1.
Human P450 genes that have been expressed in yeast.

flank the insert and are substrates for site-specific recombinases [44]. CYP cDNAs inserted into donor vectors can then be transferred into recipient yeast expression vectors by mixing the appropriate DNAs with recombinases; these reagents are commercially available and eliminate protocols using restriction enzymes and ligase. Recipient yeast expression vectors include multi-copied vectors as well as inducible and constitutive promoters [44]. An additional mechanism to increase CYP expression is to enhance translation of mRNA; Kozak sequences can be inserted into DNA sequences that encode mRNA upstream untranslated regions (UTR) [45].

2.2 Assays for detecting CYP expression

Enzymatic assays to measure CYP activity have often relied on converting non-fluorescent substrates into fluorescent products or measuring products by high-performance liquid chromatography (HPLC). Fluorescent products can be measured in a 96-well plate on a plate reader. The assay mix involves NADPH or a NADPH-regenerating system, such as glucose dehydrogenase; the pH is critical so the assay mix must be carefully buffered [46]. Microsome preparations of cytochrome P450s from yeast involve lysing cells using glass beads, centrifugation to remove debris, and precipitating microsomes using NaCL and polyethylene glycol [47]. These microsome fractions can be further concentrated by ultracentrifugation and stored at −80°C for extended time periods. Activity measurements are expressed as picomole of product per minute per mg protein; more precise measurements of CYP protein concentration can be obtained by measuring absorbance at a 450nm wavelength after the sample has been exposed to CO.

To optimize mammalian enzyme activity in yeast cells, it is necessary to co-express the CYP, human oxidoreductase (hOR), and cytochrome B (cytB) oxidoreductase [48]. Because yeasts contain endogenous oxidoreductases [49], the overexpression of the hOR is not a requirement for expression of all CYPs but generally does enhance CYP activity. For example, expression of hOR is required to measure CYP1A1 but not CYP1A2 activity [49, 50]. Other investigators have shown that the insertion of hOR directly in the genome is sufficient to obtain extracts to monitor the activity of CYP1A1 and CYP3A4 [51, 52].

3. Genotoxic assays

To be proven positive, the genotoxic effects must be dose dependent and reproducible. Examples of genotoxic agents include those that directly bind to or modify DNA, induce reactive oxygen species (ROS), and inhibit topoisomerases and other proteins involved in DNA metabolism. These genotoxic agents can cause a multiplicity of DNA insults, including DNA base modifications, DNA adducts, cross-links, and single- and double-strand breaks. Different DNA damage insults can quantitatively result in different biological endpoints. For example, a single double-strand break is sufficient to initiate genome rearrangements and trigger cell cycle arrest [53], while other types of DNA damage, such as particular cross-links and abasic sites, are effectively tolerated by DNA replication bypass pathways (for reviews, [54]). These replication bypass pathways include template switching and error-free polymerase switch mechanisms that may not trigger cell cycle arrest or a DNA damage response [54]. Thus, there is a need for measurements of multiple genotoxic endpoints to accurately assess the biological effect of any genotoxin.

Genotoxic endpoints include direct measurements of DNA damage and DNA adducts, reporter assays that detect transcriptional induction of DNA damage-inducible genes, growth assays for monitoring fitness [55], and plate assays for detecting recombination and mutations. Reporter assays involve yeast strains that contain a DNA damage-inducible promoter linked to a protein tag whose fluorescence or activity can be readily detected. Examples of proteins whose activity can be readily measured include lacZ, encoding β-galactoside, and GUS encoding β-glucuronidase (reviewed in [1]). Signaling assays have been successfully employed for high-throughput analysis using 96-well plate platforms and flow cytometry. The plate assays can elucidate endpoints of genotoxicity, while reporter assays can identify a chemical as a genotoxic assay and establish minimum concentrations in which a chemical may have an effect. Plate assays have been successful in measuring multiple genotoxic endpoints, including mutation [56, 57], homologous recombination [2], retrotransposition [58], and gross chromosomal rearrangements [59]. Plate assays involve inoculating engineered yeast strains on selective media, and after an incubation period, selected colonies can be counted and viability can be measured on nonselective media.

Direct assays to measure DNA strand breaks include chromosomal DNA integrity by pulse-field electrophoresis [60] and by single-cell comet assays [61]. Pulse-field electrophoresis has been successfully used to monitor repair of radiation-induced double-stranded DNA and the integrity of rDNA. Single-cell comet assays involve exposing cells to chemical agents, embedding them in agarose, subjecting them to an electric field, and staining for DNA [61]. Fragmented DNA migrates faster in an electric field, and the fragmented DNA appears as a "tail" [62]. Chemical DNA adducts, such as AFB1-N7-guanine adducts, can be detected using high-performance liquid chromatography, mass spectrometry (LC/MS–MS) after cells have been lysed and DNA has been extracted and acid hydrolyzed [63, 64].

3.1 Reporter assays

Reporter assays with fluorescent readouts are useful in detecting cells that have been exposed to genotoxins that induce DNA damage. Fluorescence can be monitored using 96-well plates, rendering it possible to perform high-throughput analysis. Fluorescent cells can also be imaged using flow cytometry platforms, such as the Amnis Image Stream [65], which can also measure cell type, DNA content, and cell cycle stages. DNA damage reporters include *RAD54*-GFP [66], *RNR3*-GFP [67], and *HUG1*-GFP [68]. These fusions have been widely used because signal-to-noise ratio is very low. *RAD54* is a DNA repair gene that functions in recombinational repair of double-strand breaks; GreenScreen assay (GSA) utilizes the *RAD54*-GFP reporter in high-throughput screens [69]. The RadarScreen assay uses a *RAD54* β-galactosidase reporter construct in which β-galactosidase cleaves the substrate into galactose and luciferin [70]. *HUG1* encodes an inhibitor of ribonucleotide reductase, while *RNR3* encodes the large subunit of ribonucleotide reductase that is specifically induced because of DNA damage [71]. The fluorescent markers can be enhanced using yEGFP, engineered for yeast codon bias. While *RNR3* and *RAD54* promoters have been extensively used, promoters for *PLM2,* encoding a putative transcription factor, and for *DIN7*, encoding a mitochondrial nuclease, have been recently reported to be more inducible for detection of genotoxins [1]. These studies indicate that there are robust reporters with sensitive readouts for screening genotoxins.

Genotoxins that inhibit histone deacetylases, such as Sir2, can be detected using reporters that detect expression of the silent mating-type locus (*HML*). In a strain containing one such fluorescent reporter, the cre recombinase gene was placed within the *HML* locus, while loxP recombination sequences were positioned flanking an intervening sequence that occluded a promoter from transcribing the GFP reporter [72]. Transient expression of cre triggers recombination at the loxP sites and excision of the intervening sequence, thus allowing the promoter to transcribe GFP. While this assay does not directly measure genotoxicity, inhibition of Sir2 can trigger rDNA instability [73].

3.2 Plate assays for detecting recombination, mutation, and microsatellite instabilities

Plate assays that detect mutation and recombination endpoints consist of selections or screens for prototrophic or drug resistance markers. Several genotoxic endpoints can be determined by color phenotypes. For example, Ade^{+} colonies are white, while *ade2* and *ade3* colonies are red. Recombination between two non-revertible *ade2* and *ade3* alleles can be observed by visualizing colony sectors [74]. A similar scheme can also be employed for detecting mutations that affect the *SUP4-o* function in suppressing *ade2* nonsense alleles [75]. By choosing different prototrophic selections for individual assays, combinations of these assays in a single strain can facilitate measurements for multiple genotoxic endpoints, including mutation and recombination. Typically, the strains are diploids. Prototype strains included D7, which allows for measuring multiple number of mutation event [57]. For designing strains to detect DNA damage-associated homologous recombination between heteroalleles or between repeated sequences (ectopic recombination), gene editing and one-step gene replacement [76] rendered it possible to position non-revertible markers in tandem, on homologs or on nonhomologous chromosomes. For example, *ade2-a* and *ade2-n* alleles can be used for measuring intrachromatid gene conversion and recombination between homologs [74]. By deleting the entire wild-type gene, and positioning overlapping gene fragments at preselected positions in the yeast genome, frequencies of rare recombinants can be selected. For example, *his3* gene fragments, *his3-Δ3'* and *his3-Δ5'*, can be positioned at predetermined positions in the genome and His^+ recombinants for measuring frequencies of unequal sister chromatid exchange (SCE), translocations, and intrachromatid deletions [77]. Schiestl et al. [2] used a diploid strain that contained a *his3* deletion on one chromosome and a disrupted *HIS3* gene to measure intrachromatid recombination; this strain has also been referred to as the "DEL" assay. The complete deletion of *HIS3*, *his3-Δ200*, also enabled a selection for monitoring Ty1 transposition. Boeke et al. [78] inserted an artificial intron in an inverted orientation within *HIS3* contained within Ty1 so that His^+ cells could only result when retrotransposition of Ty1 occurred. Transposition of *HIS3*, as well as chromosomal rearrangements generated by recombination between *his3* fragments, can be physically characterized by pulse-field gel electrophoresis (**Figure 2**).

A plate assay that detects gross chromosomal rearrangements was devised in haploid strains. This assay involved two drug selection markers, *CAN1* and *URA3*, where the *URA3* gene was inserted near *CAN1* on the right arm of chromosome V at the *HXT13* locus; the right arm of chromosome V is not required for viability [79]. *CAN1* encodes the arginine permease gene and confers sensitivity to the arginine analog, canavanine, while *URA3* confers sensitivity to the drug 5-fluoro-orotic acid (FOA). Since the frequencies of spontaneous Can^R FOA^R is extremely low, 3.5×10^{-10} [79], most Can^R FOA^R selected colonies contain gross chromosomal rearrangements, in which deletions, translocations, or multiple rearrangements have

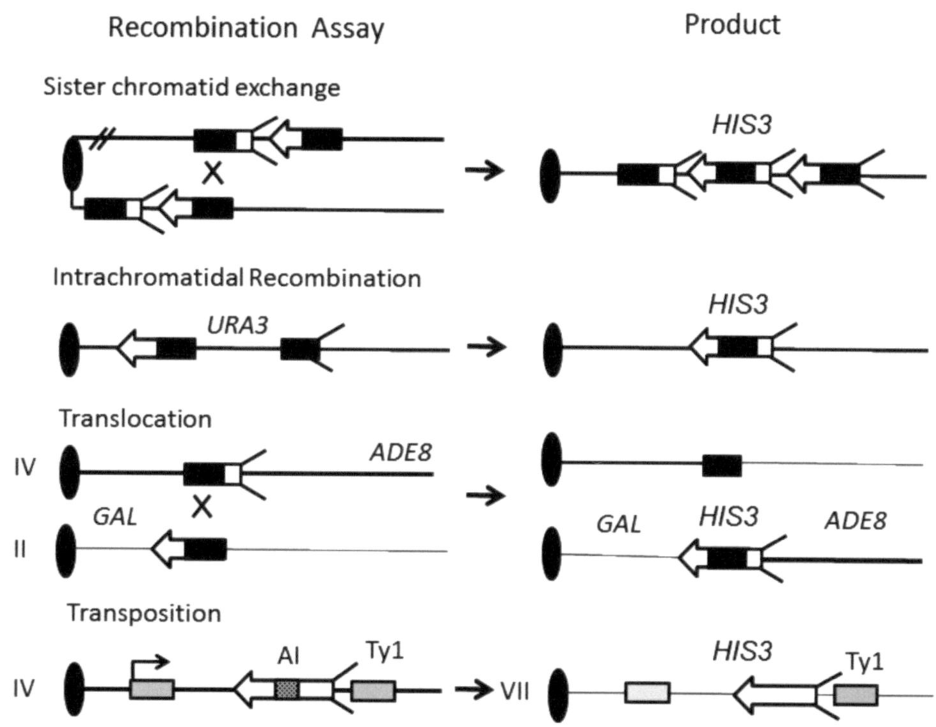

Figure 2.
Recombination assays that are used in detecting DNA damage-associated recombination. The HIS3 *gene is shown with an arrow and feathers. The fragment that lacks the 3' end is shown without the arrow; the fragment that lacks the 5' end is shown without the arrow. The two fragments share approximately 300 bp of homology. The Roman numerals represent different chromosomes. The oval represents the centromere. For simplicity, the left arm of the chromosomes is not shown. In the transposition assay, an artificial intron (AI) is inserted in the* HIS3 *so that it is in the opposite orientation as the* HIS3 *promoter. For* HIS3 *to be expressed, the Ty1 element must first be transcribed, the AI spliced from the mRNA, and the mRNA reverse transcribed and integrated into the chromosome.*

occurred that conferred resistance to both drugs. However, because drug sensitivity is dominant, Can^R FOA^R recombinants are detected in haploid strains.

By combining different gene fragments and alleles, as well as drug-resistant markers, multiple genotoxic endpoints, including heteroallelic recombination, unequal SCE, translocations, and mutation, can be measured within a single strain. As an example, Fasullo et al. [64] designed a haploid strain useful in measuring frequencies of DNA damage-associated mutations and unequal SCE after exposure to AFB1. A useful diploid strain was also engineered for measuring frequencies of DNA damage-associated homolog recombination between heteroalleles and ectopic recombination between gene fragments on nonhomologous chromosomes [64]. While these plate assays can elucidate genotoxic endpoints, their noise-to-signal ratio can vary, depending on the frequencies of spontaneous events. While frequencies of spontaneous mutations at *CAN1* are relatively low, 10^{-6}, the frequencies of spontaneous recombinants can vary from 10^{-4} to 10^{-10} [79]. Higher frequencies of spontaneous recombination are generally associated with intrachromosomal events, while lower frequencies of spontaneous recombination are associated with ectopic recombination between gene fragments on nonhomologous chromosomes. The lower the spontaneous frequency infers the higher the signal-to-noise ratio; thus, DNA damage-associated recombinants may be identified at exposures to lower concentrations of genotoxins.

While there are a multitude of plate assays for detecting nuclear genotoxic stress, there are fewer assays for detecting mitochondrial genotoxic stress. In part this is due to few auxotrophic markers, the high copy number (50–100) of mitochondrial DNA, and random segregation of mitochondria in mitosis [80]. Nonetheless, mitochondrial deficient yeast can be detected by the petite colony phenotype and the color phenotype of Ade^- mutants that appear pink or white in contrast to red on YPD media that is limiting in adenine [81]. In addition, Sia et al. [82] constructed a mitochondrial reporter gene arg8(m). This reporter has poly(AT) or poly(GT) out-of-frame insertions within the coding sequence so that Arg^+ prototrophs can be selected resulting from microsatellite instability.

While the plate and reporter assays are useful for detecting genotoxins and elucidating their mechanisms, yeast lacks many metabolic activities found in metabolically competent mammalian cells. Some protocols to activate carcinogens use rat S9 fractions, which may produce more metabolites than human CYPs, [83–85]. To mitigate this deficiency, human CYPs have been introduced into the strains for both plate assays and reporter assays. For example, Bui et al. [71] expressed CYP1A2, CYP2C9, CYP3A4, and CYP2D6 in a strain that monitors RAD54-GFP. Sengstag et al. [50] and Fasullo et al. [64, 67] have expressed CYP1A1, CYP1A2, and CYP3A4 in strains that monitor translocations, mutations, and unequal SCE. Guo et al. [86] have introduced CYP1A2 into multiple yeast mutants to determine AFB1 resistance. Paladino et al. [87] have expressed CYP1A2 and NAT2 to activate a variety of heterocyclic aromatic amine in strains to measure homology-directed translocations. Both CYP-containing reporter strains and plate assay strains expand the repertoire of chemicals that can be tested by high-throughput analysis.

4. Chemicals that test positive in the yeast strains

Overall, thousands of chemicals have been tested using either one or both plate and reporter-based assays [1]. Van Gompel et al. [69] report on the screening of 2698 proprietary compounds and pharmaceuticals using the GreenScreen assay; of these compounds, approximately 7% of those 164 that test positive are also positive in the Ames assays, demonstrating that agents that test positive represent overlapping groups. Screens of industrial, environmental, and food carcinogens have used multitude tester strains, including the "DEL" and transposition assays [88]. Chemical agents include those that directly inflict DNA damage, induce ROS, inhibit DNA metabolic function, and alter histone modification. Metallic nanoparticles also test positive in several assays although their mechanism of action has yet to be determined [89]. Whereas almost all chemicals that test positive in plate assays will also test positive in reporter assays, the converse is not necessarily true. These results demonstrate that several reporter assays are capable of high-throughput screening and can identify multiple compounds that test positive in additional genotoxic assays.

Several agents that cause direct DNA damage, such as base pair damage, cross-links, DNA adducts, or DNA strand breaks, test positive in reporter assays and may test positive in one or more of the plate assays [90]. For example, alkylating agents, such as methyl methane sulfonate (MMS), increase frequencies of mutations, recombination, gross chromosomal rearrangements (GCRs), and retrotransposition. Interestingly, alkylating agents also test positive in enhancing expression of the silent mating-type locus *HML* [91]. Other types of alkylating agents, such as 1-methyl-3-nitro-1-nitrosoguanidine (MNNG) and ethyl methane sulfonate (EMS), test positive in reporter and mutation assays; however, frequencies of DNA damage-associated sister chromatid exchange events are only modestly increased [58, 64, 67]. Cross-linking agents, such as cis-platinum and other UV-mimetic agents, also tend to be positive in a broad range of reporter assays, including those for retrotransposition and homologous recombination [90]. Finally, radiomimetic agents that cause strand breaks, such as zeocin and bleomycin, test positive in many reporter assays as well as assays for gross chromosomal rearrangements and translocations [59]. These studies demonstrate that while a subset of alkylating agents manifest broad genotoxicity, frequencies of DNA damage associated with GCRs and translocations manifest the highest increase after exposure to agents that cause double-strand breaks.

Chemical agents that inhibit DNA metabolic and repair functions are often genotoxic. These include camptothecin, which inhibits topoisomerase I and causes single-strand breaks and replication fork collapse, and hydroxyurea, which blocks DNA replication by inhibiting ribonucleotide reductase and thus depleting deoxynucleotides [92, 93]. Other metabolic inhibitors include those that inhibit dihydrofolate reductase, and result in uracil incorporation also tests positive in a broad range of plate assays, including those for sister chromatid recombination, heteroallelic recombination, and translocations. Cd^{2+} exposure inhibits mismatch repair [94] and is also genotoxic [95]. These studies indicate that genotoxins include chemicals that may directly inhibit critical enzymes in DNA metabolism.

While chemicals are individually screened in many plate and reporter assays, combination of chemicals can also enhance DNA damage or enhance mutagenesis. An example includes intercalating agents, such as acridine and bleomycin; the insertion of acridine in the DNA helix facilitates bleomycin access to the minor groove and subsequent strand breakage [96]. In addition, by inhibiting mismatch repair, Cd^{2+} exposure facilitates the mutagenesis by alkylating agents [94]. These studies indicate that combinations of genotoxins can accelerate genome instability.

Mitochondria are particularly prone to DNA intercalating agents, and agents that cause oxidative damage, and reduce or cause imbalance to deoxynucleotide pools [97]. ROS-associated damage in the mitochondrial genome, associated with oxidative phosphorylation, is not repaired by nucleotide excision repair (NER) but by base excision repair (BER) [1]. In addition, mitochondrial DNA is circular and therefore is more prone to DNA intercalating agents that can cause topological stress, such as ethidium bromide and acridine compounds [98]. Several fluorescent

CYP allele	Amino acid substitution	Enzyme assay	Disease association	Genotoxic endpoints	Reference
CYP1A1*2C	1462V (near heme binding site)	EROD[1]	Lung, prostate and breast cancer	Rad51 foci, growth curves, HR[4]	[51]
CYP1A1*4	T461N (near heme binding site)	EROD	Endometrial and lung cancer	Rad51 foci, growth curves, HR	[51]
CYP1A2*5	C406Y	MROD[2]	ND	Rad51 foci, growth curves, HR	[63]
CYP1A2*3	D348N	MROD	ND	Rad51 foci, growth curves, HR	[63]
CYP1A2*4	I386F	MROD	ND	Rad51 foci, growth curves, HR	[63]
CYP1B1*7	R48G; A119S; L432V; A443G	BaP-DHD epoxidation[3]	L432V has an increased risk for prostate and lung	NT	[110]
CYP1B1*12	G61E	BaP-DHD epoxidation	Glaucoma	NT	[110]
CYP1B1*18	G365W	BaP-DHD epoxidation	Glaucoma	NT	[110]
CYP1B1*23	P437L	BaP-DHD epoxidation	Glaucoma	NT	[110]
CYP2E1		Benzene hydroxylation		NT	[111, 112]
CYP2E1*2	**R76H**	Benzene hydroxylation	Bladder cancer (reduced risk in Asian population)	NT	[111, 112]
CYP2E1*3	V389I	Benzene hydroxylation	Bladder cancer (reduced risk in Asian population)	NT	[111, 112]
CYP2E1*4	V179I	Benzene hydroxylation	Bladder cancer	NT	[111, 112]

[1]Ethoxyresorufin deethylase (EROD).
[2]Methyoxyresorufin demethylase (MROD).
[3]Benzo[a]pyrene 7,8, dihydrodiol (BaP-DHD).
[4]Homologous recombination (HR).
ND = not determined, NT = not tested.

Table 2.
Cytochrome P450 polymorphisms expressed in yeast.

dyes can also induce mitochondrial DNA damage [1]. Replication of mitochondrial DNA depends on a single polymerase, DNA polymerase γ [99]. Therefore, chemicals that inhibit mitochondrial DNA polymerase, such as dideoxynucleoside antiretrovirals, are often genotoxic [100]. Thus, yeast screens that detect mitochondrial DNA damage are useful in screening off-target effects on antiretroviral agents.

While many carcinogens are directly genotoxic, others require metabolic activation. The list of CYPs expressed in yeast and chemical agents that are activated are listed in **Table 2**. The agents tested include polyaromatic hydrocarbons (BaP-DHD), mycotoxins (AFB1), and heterocyclic aromatic amines (2-amino-3,8-dimethylimidazo-[4,5-f]quinoxaline (MeIQx), 2-amino-3, 4-dimethylimidazo-[4,5-f] quinoline (MeIQ), and 2-amino-3-methylimidazo-[4,5-f]quinoline (IQ)). Bui et al. [71] introduced human CYPs into strains to measure induction of GFP using the reporter *RAD54*-GFP. Li et al. [52] used a sensitive fluorimetric assay to measure inhibition of secreted dextranase; the assay consists of strains expressing *Lipomyces kononenkoae* amylase, CYP3A4, and hOR [52]. The amylase-expressing strain detected AFB1 at 2 ng/ml and the T-2 mycotoxin [52].

Activation of these compounds has also been determined by measuring DNA recombination and mutation; DNA adducts have been detected after AFB1 and BaP-DHD exposure. Frequencies of mutations and recombination may be differentially elevated by CYP-activated genotoxins. For example, CYP1A1 and CYP1A2 activation of AFB1 in yeast results in a 20–50-fold increase in the stimulation of recombination but only a fivefold increase in mutation frequency [50]. However, CYP1A1-mediated activation of BaP-DHD results in a higher activation of mutation but somewhat diminished activation of recombination [50]. Because the background frequency is so low, the CYP1A2-expressing strains containing the translocation assay have been particularly useful in detecting the DNA damage-associated recombinants [50].

5. Yeast mutants that exhibit enhanced phenotypes after genotoxin exposure

Various gene mutations can increase the signal-to-noise ratio. Typically, these mutations are encoded in cells lacking cell wall components, nucleotide or base excision repair genes, and xenobiotic transporters. Strains that lack cell wall components and xenobiotic transporters include *pdr5*, *snq2*, *cwp1*, *cwp2* [1]. Strains that lack NER and BER genes include those mutated in *rad1* and *mag1*, respectively. Several strains also contain deletions in *yap1* [101], a gene that encodes a transcription factor that confers transcriptional induction among antioxidant genes, such as *TRX2*, and is required for H_2O_2 and Cd resistance [102]. Several strains have been designed so that multiple genes are mutated to enhance the genotoxic signal. Wei et al. [103] have used a septuplet deletion mutant (*snq2*, *prd5*, *cwp1*, *cwp2*, *yap1*, *rad1*, *mag1*) in combination with an integrated HUG1-yEGFP reporter as a very sensitive detection for multiple chemicals. Deletion of NER genes has been successful in enhancing DNA damage-associated recombination after exposure to BaP-DHD and AFB1 [104].

While deleting DNA repair genes may enhance signal-to-noise ratios for reporter assays and some recombination and mutation assays, particular DNA repair defects may decrease frequencies of DNA damage-associated recombination in particular plate assays. For example, blocking nonhomologous end joining (NHEJ) may increase homologous recombination initiated by double-strand breaks in haploid strains, while decreasing DSB-associated translocations [105]; the likely explanation is that competing DNA repair pathways for recombination are differentially favored for homologous vs. NHEJ. *Rad1* mutations may confer lower DNA damage-associated recombination in assays, such as the "DEL" assay [106]. The *rad1* mutants are defective in the Rad1/Rad10 nuclease; this nuclease cleaves 3′ blocked termini and is important in single-strand annealing mechanisms. However, other *rad* mutants that are deficient in NER, such as *rad4*, may be suitable for observing both enhanced DNA damage-associated recombination and mutations [67].

One strategy has been to use DNA repair mutants that are knocked out in multiple DNA repair pathways to assess the genotoxicity of chemicals. For example, *rad4 rad51* double mutants, which are deficient in both NER and in recombinational repair, are synergistically more sensitive to UV and many chemical UV-mimetic agents. By introducing CYP genes into the *rad4rad51*, the strain also becomes synergistically more sensitive to AFB1 as well as extremely sensitive to other PAHs and HAAs [51, 67].

Mechanistic insights into how genotoxic agents stimulate chromosomal instability are also gained from studies of checkpoint genes. For example, deleting the *RAD9*-mediated checkpoint which triggers G2 arrest confers higher levels of DNA damage-associated recombination (translocations) after cells are exposed to X-rays and radiomimetic agents that cause breaks such as MMS and bleomycin. Enhanced translocation frequencies are also observed after *rad9* cells are exposed to camptothecin, an inhibitor of topoisomerase I. On the other hand, *rad9* deletion does not confer higher levels of recombination associated with agents, such as 4-nitroquinoline oxide (4-NQO), that cause bulky DNA damage [107]. These observations suggest that agents that stimulate DNA break formation may be identified if they enhance recombination in *rad9* mutants.

6. Phenotyping CYP polymorphisms in budding yeast

The CYP genes are highly polymorphic, and particular polymorphisms have been identified as risk factors for cancer [13, 22, 108] and glaucoma [109]. While yeast strains are useful in elucidating the genotoxicity of P450-activated carcinogens, yeast strains are also useful in characterizing human CYP polymorphisms. CYP1A1, CYP1A2, CYP1B1, and CYP2E1 polymorphisms have been studied in yeast [51, 63, 110–112]. The polymorphisms can be characterized in a number of ways: (1) substrate specificity, (2) activity with a defined substrate, (3) genotoxic endpoints, and (4) DNA adducts. For example, CYP1A2 polymorphisms have different affinities for heterocyclic aromatic amines; these polymorphisms have been also characterized by their ability to bioactivate aflatoxin B1. Activity assays have been performed for polymorphisms in CYP2E1, CYP1B1, CYP1A1, and CYP1A2 [51, 63, 110, 111]. In general activity assays agree with those performed when assays are performed in other model systems, such as *E. coli* [113].

Several CYP1A1 polymorphisms are present in a significant percentage of the population and may be risk factors for lung and breast cancer. For example, CYP1A1 I462V and CYP1A1 T461N have been correlated to have higher incidence of lung, breast, and endometrial cancer [114, 115]. A plausible hypothesis is that CYP1A1 I462V and CYP1A1 T461N are more active in converting breast- and lung-associated carcinogens into genotoxins. However, another model suggests that CYP1A1 is protective, since CYP1A1 knockout mice actually have a higher incidence of carcinogen-associated cancer [10]. Freedland et al. [51] measured multiple genotoxic endpoints in yeast strains expressing CYP1A1 I462V after exposure to multiple carcinogens and interestingly found a reduced level of bioactivation. This is consistent with a model that CYP1A1 may actually be protective and compete with other CYPs that convert carcinogens into active genotoxins [10].

7. Implications for higher eukaryotes

The ability to perform high-throughput screening to identify genotoxins using yeast strains containing sensitive reporter facilitates the identification of chemicals that merit more detailed and expensive studies. While yeast reporter strains can be useful for high-throughput identification of genotoxins, yeast plate assays and genetics can elucidate mechanisms. Genotoxins that stimulate recombination and retrotransposition in yeast are likely to stimulate genetic instability in higher eukaryotes. Indeed, many recombinagens that have tested positive in yeast also test positive in higher eukaryotes. An excellent example is AFB1, which is also a recombinagen in human cell lines [116].

8. Conclusions and future directions

Yeast assays for detecting genotoxins and identifying genotoxic mechanisms are urgently needed to screen a multitude of industrial chemicals, pesticides, and pharmaceuticals. These assays have already been successful in screening thousands of chemicals, aiding in our understanding of genotoxic mechanisms. These assays have been further empowered by the technology to introduce human phase I and phase II metabolism in yeast cells. While the reporter assays enable high-throughput studies for rapid identification of genotoxins, the multitude of plate assays enables mechanistic studies to elucidate genotoxic mechanisms. The future challenge is to combine many of the reporters and plate assays so that both the screening and the mechanistic studies can be expedited.

Currently, the mechanisms of many chemical agents, which increase cancer risk, are unknown. Of particular interests are many small-molecule toxicants present in industrial workplace or which are extensively used in agriculture. How exposure to mixtures of these chemicals increases genotoxicity will be important in assessing risk factors to human health.

Acknowledgements

The author was supported by NIH grants R21ES015954, F33ES021133, and R15E023685.

Conflict of interest

The author declares no conflict of interest.

Author details

Michael Fasullo
State University of New York Polytechnic Institute, Albany, New York, United States

*Address all correspondence to: mfasullo@sunypoly.edu

References

[1] Eki T. Yeast-based genotoxicity tests for assessing DNA alterations and DNA stress responses: A 40-year overview. Applied Microbiology and Biotechnology. 2018;**102**:2493-2507. DOI: 10.1007/s00253-018-8783-1

[2] Schiestl RH. Nonmutagenic carcinogens induce intrachromosomal recombination in yeast. Nature. 1989;**337**:285-288. DOI: 10.1038/337285a0

[3] Keshava N, Ong TM. Occupational exposure to genotoxic agents. Mutation Research. 1999;**437**:175-194. DOI: 10.1016/s1383-5742(99)00083-6

[4] Shukla PC, Singh KK, Yanagawa B, Teoh H, Verma S. DNA damage repair and cardiovascular diseases. The Canadian Journal of Cardiology. 2010;**26**:13A-16A. DOI: 10.1016/s0828-282x(10)71055-2

[5] Barnes JL, Zubair M, John K, Poirier MC, Martin FL. Carcinogens and DNA damage. Biochemical Society Transactions. 2018;**46**:1213-1224. DOI: 10.1042/BST20180519

[6] Vijg J, Suh Y. Genome instability and aging. Annual Review of Physiology. 2013;**75**:645-668. DOI: 10.1146/annurev-physiol-030212-183715

[7] Food and Drug Administration, HHS. International Conference on Harmonisation; Guidance on S2(R1) genotoxicity testing and data interpretation for pharmaceuticals intended for human use; availability. Notice. Federal Register. 2012;**77**:33748-33749

[8] Ames BN, Durston WE, Yamasaki E, Lee FD. Carcinogens are mutagens: A simple test system combining liver homogenates for activation and bacteria for detection. Proceedings of the National Academy of Sciences of the United States of America. 1973;**70**:2281-22855. DOI: 10.1073/pnas.70.8.2281

[9] Mortelmans K, Zeiger E. The Ames Salmonella/microsome mutagenicity assay. Mutation Research. 2000;**455**:29-60. DOI: 10.1016/s0027-5107(00)00064-6

[10] Nebert DW, Dalton TP. The role of cytochrome P450 enzymes in endogenous signalling pathways and environmental carcinogenesis. Nature Reviews. Cancer. 2006;**6**:947-960. DOI: 10.1038/nrc2015

[11] Baillie TA, Rettie AE. Role of biotransformation in drug-induced toxicity: Influence of intra- and inter-species differences in drug metabolism. Drug Metabolism and Pharmacokinetics. 2011;**26**:15-29. DOI: 10.2133/dmpk.DMPK-10-RV-089

[12] Omura T. Forty years of cytochrome P450. Biochemical and Biophysical Research Communications. 1999;**266**:690-698. DOI: 10.1006/bbrc.1999.1887

[13] Guengerich FP, Waterman MR, Egli M. Recent structural insights into cytochrome P450 function. Trends in Pharmacological Sciences. 2016;**37**:625-640. DOI: 10.1016/j.tips.2016.05.006

[14] Zanger UM, Schwab M. Cytochrome P450 enzymes in drug metabolism: Regulation of gene expression, enzyme activities, and impact of genetic variation. Pharmacology & Therapeutics. 2013;**138**:103-141. DOI: 10.1016/j.pharmthera.2012.12.007

[15] Ding X, Kaminsky LS. Human extrahepatic cytochromes P450: Function in xenobiotic metabolism and tissue-selective chemical toxicity in the respiratory and gastrointestinal tracts. Annual Review

of Pharmacology and Toxicology. 2003;**43**:149-173. DOI: 10.1146/annurev.pharmtox.43.100901.140251

[16] Botstein D, Chervitz SA, Cherry JM. Yeast as a model organism. Science. 1997;**277**:1259-1260. DOI: 10.1126/science.277.5330.1259

[17] Cherry JM, Hong EL, Amundsen C, Balakrishnan R, Binkley G, Chan ET, et al. Saccharomyces genome database: The genomics resource of budding yeast. Nucleic Acids Research. 2012;**40**:D700-D705. DOI: 10.1093/nar/gkr1029

[18] Kachroo AH, Laurent JM, Yellman CM, Meyer AG, Wilke CO, Marcotte EM. Systematic humanization of yeast genes reveals conserved functions and genetic modularity. Science. 2015;**348**:921-925. DOI: 10.1126/science.aaa0769

[19] Ferguson LR, von Borstel RC. Induction of the cytoplasmic 'petite' mutation by chemical and physical agents in *Saccharomyces cerevisiae*. Mutation Research. 1992;**265**:103-148. DOI: 10.1016/0027-5107(92)90042-z

[20] van Leeuwen JS, Vermeulen NP, Chris Vos J. Yeast as a humanized model organism for biotransformation-related toxicity. Current Drug Metabolism. 2012;**13**:1464-1475. DOI: 10.2174/138920012803762783

[21] Paget V, Lechevrel M, André V, Goff JL, Pottier D, Billet S, et al. Benzo[a]pyrene, aflatoxine B_1 and acetaldehyde mutational patterns in TP53 gene using a functional assay: Relevance to human cancer aetiology. PLoS One. 2012;**7**:e30921. DOI: 10.1371/journal.pone.0030921

[22] Rendic S, Guengerich FP. Contributions of human enzymes in carcinogen metabolism. Chemical Research in Toxicology. 2012;**25**:1316-1383. DOI: 10.1021/tx300132k

[23] Buters JT, Sakai S, Richter T, Pineau T, Alexander DL, Savas U, et al. Cytochrome P450 CYP1B1 determines susceptibility to 7,12-dimethylbenz[a]anthracene-induced lymphomas. Proceedings of the National Academy of Sciences of the United States of America. 1999;**96**:1977-1982. DOI: 10.1073/pnas.96.5.1977

[24] Zhou X, D'Agostino J, Xie F, Ding X. Role of CYP2A5 in the bioactivation of the lung carcinogen 4-(methylnitrosamino)-1-(3-pyridyl)-1-butanone in mice. The Journal of Pharmacology and Experimental Therapeutics. 2012;**341**:233-241. DOI: 10.1124/jpet.111.190173

[25] Kim D, Guengerich FP. Cytochrome P450 activation of arylamines and heterocyclic amines. Annual Review of Pharmacology and Toxicology. 2005;**45**:27-49. DOI: 10.1146/annurev.pharmtox.45.120403.100010

[26] Turesky RJ, Le Marchand L. Metabolism and biomarkers of heterocyclic aromatic amines in molecular epidemiology studies: Lessons learned from aromatic amines. Chemical Research in Toxicology. 2011;**24**:1169-1214. DOI: 10.1021/tx200135s

[27] Zhang J, Lacroix C, Wortmann E, Ruscheweyh HJ, Sunagawa S, Sturla SJ, et al. Gut microbial beta-glucuronidase and glycerol/diol dehydratase activity contribute to dietary heterocyclic amine biotransformation. BMC Microbiology. 2019;**19**:99. DOI: 10.1186/s12866-019-1483-x

[28] Tsuchiya Y, Nakajima M, Yokoi T. Cytochrome P450-mediated metabolism of estrogens and its regulation in human. Cancer Letters. 2005;**227**:115-124. DOI: 10.1016/j.canlet.2004.10.007

[29] Hayes CL, Spink DC, Spink BC, Cao JQ, Walker NJ, Sutter TR. 17

beta-estradiol hydroxylation catalyzed by human cytochrome P450 1B1. Proceedings of the National Academy of Sciences of the United States of America. 1996;**93**:9776-9781. DOI: 10.1073/pnas.93.18.9776

[30] McGill MR, Jaeschke H. Metabolism and disposition of acetaminophen: recent advances in relation to hepatotoxicity and diagnosis. Pharmaceutical Research. 2013;**30**:2174-2187. DOI: 10.1007/s11095-013-1007-6

[31] Gross-Steinmeyer K, Eaton DL. Dietary modulation of the biotransformation and genotoxicity of aflatoxin B(1). Toxicology. 2012;**28**(299):69-79. DOI: 10.1016/j.tox.2012.05.016

[32] Kelly SL, Lamb DC, Baldwin BC, Corran AJ, Kelly DE. Characterization of *Saccharomyces cerevisiae* CYP61, sterol delta22-desaturase, and inhibition by azole antifungal agents. The Journal of Biological Chemistry. 1997;**272**:9986-9988. DOI: 10.1074/jbc.272.15.9986

[33] Briza P, Eckerstorfer M, Breitenbach M. The sporulation-specific enzymes encoded by the DIT1 and DIT2 genes catalyze a two-step reaction leading to a soluble LL-dityrosine-containing precursor of the yeast spore wall. Proceedings of the National Academy of Sciences of the United States of America. 1994;**91**:4524-4528. DOI: 10.1073/pnas.91.10.4524

[34] Sikorski RS, Hieter P. A system of shuttle vectors and yeast host strains designed for efficient manipulation of DNA in *Saccharomyces cerevisiae*. Genetics. 1989;**122**:19-27

[35] Mumberg D, Müller R, Funk M. Yeast vectors for the controlled expression of heterologous proteins in different genetic backgrounds. Gene. 1995;**156**:119-122. DOI: 10.1016/0378-1119(95)00037-7

[36] Zelasko S, Palaria A, Das A. Optimizations to achieve high-level expression of cytochrome P450 proteins using *Escherichia coli* expression systems. Protein Expression and Purification. 2013;**92**:77-87. DOI: 10.1016/j.pep.2013.07.017

[37] Liao M, Faouzi S, Karyakin A, Correia MA. Endoplasmic reticulum-associated degradation of cytochrome P450 CYP3A4 in *Saccharomyces cerevisiae*: Further characterization of cellular participants and structural determinants. Molecular Pharmacology. 2006;**69**:1897-1904. DOI: 10.1124/mol.105.021816

[38] Thim L, Hansen MT, Norris K, Hoegh I, Boel E, Forstrom J, et al. Secretion and processing of insulin precursors in yeast. Proceedings of the National Academy of Sciences of the United States of America. 1986;**83**:6766-6770. DOI: 10.1073/pnas.83.18.6766

[39] Cigan AM, Donahue TF. Sequence and structural features associated with translational initiator regions in yeast—A review. Gene. 1987;**59**:1-18. DOI: 10.1016/0378-1119(87)90261-7

[40] Hamann T, Møller BL. Improved cloning and expression of cytochrome P450s and cytochrome P450 reductase in yeast. Protein Expression and Purification. 2007;**56**:121-127. DOI: 10.1016/j.pep.2007.06.007

[41] Oeda K, Sakaki T, Ohkawa H. Expression of rat liver cytochrome P-450MC cDNA in *Saccharomyces cerevisiae*. DNA. 1985;**4**:203-210. DOI: 10.1089/dna.1985.4.203

[42] Renaud JP, Cullin C, Pompon D, Beaune P, Mansuy D. Expression of human liver cytochrome P450 IIIA4 in yeast. A functional model for the hepatic enzyme. European Journal of Biochemistry. 1990;**194**:889-896. DOI: 10.1111/j.1432-1033.1990.tb19483.x

[43] Imaoka S, Yamada T, Hiroi T, Hayashi K, Sakaki T, Yabusaki Y, et al. Multiple forms of human P450 expressed in *Saccharomyces cerevisiae*. Systematic characterization and comparison with those of the rat. Biochemical Pharmacology. 1996;**51**:1041-1050. DOI: 10.1016/0006-2952(96)00052-4

[44] Alberti S, Gitler AD, Lindquist S. A suite of Gateway cloning vectors for high-throughput genetic analysis in *Saccharomyces cerevisiae*. Yeast. 2007;**24**:913-919. DOI: 10.1002/yea.1502

[45] Kozak M. Initiation of translation in prokaryotes and eukaryotes. Gene. 1999;**234**:187-208. DOI: 10.1016/s0378-1119(99)00210-3

[46] Eugster HP, Bärtsch S, Würgler FE, Sengstag C. Functional co-expression of human oxidoreductase and cytochrome P450 1A1 in *Saccharomyces cerevisiae* results in increased EROD activity. Biochemical and Biophysical Research Communications. 1992;**185**(2):641-647. DOI: 10.1016/0006-291x(92)91673-e

[47] Pompon D, Louerat B, Bronine A, Urban P. Yeast expression of animal and plant P450s in optimized redox environments. Methods in Enzymology. 1996;**272**:51-64. DOI: 10.1016/s0076-6879(96)72008-6

[48] Peyronneau MA, Renaud JP, Truan G, Urban P, Pompon D, Mansuy D. Optimization of yeast-expressed human liver cytochrome P450 3A4 catalytic activities by coexpressing NADPH-cytochrome P450 reductase and cytochrome b5. European Journal of Biochemistry. 1992;**207**(1):109-116. DOI: 10.1111/j.1432-1033.1992.tb17027.x

[49] Murakami H, Yabusaki Y, Sakaki T, Shibata M, Ohkawa H. Expression of cloned yeast NADPH-cytochrome P450 reductase gene in *Saccharomyces cerevisiae*. Journal of Biochemistry. 1990;**108**:859-865. DOI: 10.1093/oxfordjournals.jbchem.a123293

[50] Sengstag C, Weibel B, Fasullo M. Genotoxicity of aflatoxin B1: Evidence for a recombination-mediated mechanism in *Saccharomyces cerevisiae*. Cancer Research. 1996;**56**:5457-5465

[51] Freedland J, Cera C, Fasullo M. CYP1A1 I462V polymorphism is associated with reduced genotoxicity in yeast despite positive association with increased cancer risk. Mutation Research. 2017;**815**:35-43. DOI: 10.1016/j.mrgentox.2017.02.002

[52] Li X, Millson S, Coker R, Evans I. A sensitive bioassay for the mycotoxin aflatoxin B(1), which also responds to the mycotoxins aflatoxin G(1) and T-2 toxin, using engineered baker's yeast. Journal of Microbiological Methods. 2009;**77**:285-291. DOI: 10.1016/j.mimet.2009.03.003

[53] Lee SE, Pellicioli A, Demeter J, Vaze MP, Gasch AP, Malkova A, et al. Arrest, adaptation, and recovery following a chromosome double-strand break in *Saccharomyces cerevisiae*. Cold Spring Harbor Symposia on Quantitative Biology. 2000;**65**:303-314. DOI: 10.1101/sqb.2000.65.303

[54] Chang DJ, Cimprich KA. DNA damage tolerance: When it's OK to make mistakes. Nature Chemical Biology. 2009;**5**:82-90. DOI: 10.1038/nchembio.139

[55] Toussaint M, Levasseur G, Gervais-Bird J, Wellinger RJ, Elela SA, Conconi A. A high-throughput method to measure the sensitivity of yeast cells to genotoxic agents in liquid cultures. Mutation Research. 2006;**606**(1-2):92-105. DOI: 10.1016/j.mrgentox.2006.03.006

[56] Moustacchi E. Mutagenicity testing with eukaryotic microorganisms.

Archives of Toxicology. 1980;**46**:99-110. DOI: 10.1007/bf00361249

[57] Zimmermann FK, Kern R, Rasenberger H. A yeast strain for simultaneous detection of induced mitotic crossing over, mitotic gene conversion and reverse mutation. Mutation Research/Fundamental and Molecular Mechanisms of Mutagenesis. 1975;**28**:381-388. DOI: 10.1016/0027-5107(75)90232-8

[58] Fasullo M, Dave P, Rothstein R. DNA-damaging agents stimulate the formation of directed reciprocal translocations in *Saccharomyces cerevisiae*. Mutation Research. 1994;**314**(2):121-133. DOI: 10.1016/0921-8777(94)90076-0

[59] Myung K, Kolodner RD. Induction of genome instability by DNA damage in *Saccharomyces cerevisiae*. DNA Repair (Amst). 2003;**2**:243-258. DOI: 10.1016/S1568-7864(02)00216-1

[60] Geigl EM, Eckardt-Schupp F. Chromosome-specific identification and quantification of S1 nuclease-sensitive sites in yeast chromatin by pulsed-field gel electrophoresis. Molecular Microbiology. 1990;**4**:801-810. DOI: 10.1111/j.1365-2958.1990.tb00650.x

[61] Miloshev G, Mihaylov I, Anachkova B. Application of the single cell gel electrophoresis on yeast cells. Mutation Research. 2002;**513**:69-74. DOI: 10.1016/s1383-5718(01)00286-8

[62] Zhang M, Cao G, Guo X, Gao Y, Li W, Lu D. A comet assay for DNA damage and repair after exposure to carbon-ion beams or X-rays in *Saccharomyces cerevisiae*. Dose Response. 2018;**16**(3):1559325818792467. DOI: 10.1177/1559325818792467

[63] Fasullo M, Smith A, Egner P, Cera C. Activation of Aflatoxin B_1 by expression of CYP1A2 polymorphisms in *Saccharomyces cerevisiae*. Mutation Research. 2014;**761**:18-26. DOI: 10.1016/j.mrgentox.2014.01.009

[64] Fasullo M, Sun M, Egner P. Stimulation of sister chromatid exchanges and mutation by aflatoxin B1-DNA adducts in *Saccharomyces cerevisiae* requires MEC1 ATR, RAD53, and DUN1. Molecular Carcinogenesis. 2008;**47**(8):608-615. DOI: 10.1002/mc.20417

[65] Basiji DA. Principles of Amnis imaging flow cytometry. Methods in Molecular Biology. 2016;**1389**:13-21. DOI: 10.1007/978-1-4939-3302-0_2

[66] Westerink WM, Stevenson JC, Lauwers A, Griffioen G, Horbach GJ, Schoonen WG. Evaluation of the Vitotox and RadarScreen assays for the rapid assessment of genotoxicity in the early research phase of drug development. Mutation Research. 2009;**676**:113-130. DOI: 10.1016/j.mrgentox.2009.04.008

[67] Fasullo M, Freedland J, Cera C, Egner P, Hartog M, Ding X. An in vitro system for measuring genotoxicity mediated by human CYP3A4. Environmental and Molecular Mutagenesis. 2017;**58**:217-227. DOI: 10.1002/em.22093

[68] Benton MG, Glasser NR, Palecek SP. The utilization of a *Saccharomyces cerevisiae* HUG1P-GFP promoter-reporter construct for the selective detection of DNA damage. Mutation Research. 2007;**633**(1):21-34. DOI: 10.1016/j.mrgentox.2007.05.002

[69] van Gompel J, Woestenborghs F, Beerens D, Mackie C, Cahill PA, Knight AW, et al. An assessment of the utility of the yeast GreenScreen assay in pharmaceutical screening. Mutagenesis. 2005;**20**:449-454. DOI: 10.1093/mutage/gei062

[70] Tian Y, Lu Y, Xu X, Wang C, Zhou T, Li X. Construction and comparison of yeast whole-cell biosensors

regulated by two RAD54 promoters capable of detecting genotoxic compounds. Toxicology Mechanisms and Methods. 2017;**27**:115-120. DOI: 10.1080/15376516.2016.1266540

[71] Bui VN, Nguyen TT, Mai CT, Bettarel Y, Hoang TY, Trinh TT, et al. Procarcinogens—Determination and evaluation by yeast-based biosensor transformed with plasmids incorporating RAD54 reporter construct and cytochrome P450 genes. PLoS One. 2016;**11**(12):e0168721. DOI: 10.1371/journal.pone.0168721

[72] Dodson AE, Rine J. Heritable capture of heterochromatin dynamics in *Saccharomyces cerevisiae*. eLife. 2015;**12**(4):e05007. DOI: 10.7554/eLife.05007

[73] Eot-Houllier G, Fulcrand G, Magnaghi-Jaulin L, Jaulin C. Histone deacetylase inhibitors and genomic instability. Cancer Letters. 2009;**274**(2):169-176. DOI: 10.1016/j.canlet.2008.06.005

[74] Huang KN, Symington LS. Mutation of the gene encoding protein kinase C 1 stimulates mitotic recombination in *Saccharomyces cerevisiae*. Molecular and Cellular Biology. 1994;**14**(9):6039-6045. DOI: 10.1128/MCB.14.9.6039

[75] Shaaban SA, Krupp BM, Hall BD. Termination-altering mutations in the second-largest subunit of yeast RNA polymerase III. Molecular and Cellular Biology. 1995;**15**:1467-1478. DOI: 10.1128/mcb.15.3.1467

[76] Rothstein R. Targeting, disruption, replacement, and allele rescue: integrative DNA transformation in yeast. Methods in Enzymology. 1991;**194**:281-301. DOI: 10.1016/0076-6879(91)94022-5

[77] Fasullo MT, Davis RW. Recombinational substrates designed to study recombination between unique and repetitive sequences in vivo. Proceedings of the National Academy of Sciences of the United States of America. 1987;**84**:6215-6219. DOI: 10.1073/pnas.84.17.6215

[78] Boeke JD, Garfinkel DJ, Styles CA, Fink GR. Ty elements transpose through an RNA intermediate. Cell. 1985;**40**:491-500. DOI: 10.1016/0092-8674(85)90197-7

[79] Myung K, Datta A, Kolodner RD. Suppression of spontaneous chromosomal rearrangements by S phase checkpoint functions in *Saccharomyces cerevisiae*. Cell. 2001;**104**:397-408. DOI: 10.1016/s0092-8674(01)00227-6

[80] Dujon B, Slonimski PP. Mechanisms and rules for transmission, recombination and segregation of mitochondria genes in *Saccharomyces cerevisiae*. In: Bücher T, Neupert W, Sebald W, Werner S, editors. Genetics and Biogenesis of Chloroplasts and Mitochondria. Amsterdam: North-Holland Biomedical Press; 1976. pp. 405-414

[81] Ferguson LR, Denny WA. Genotoxicity of non-covalent interactions: DNA intercalators. Mutation Research. 2007;**623**(1-2):14-23. DOI: 10.1016/j.mrfmmm.2007.03.014

[82] Sia EA, Butler CA, Dominska M, Greenwell P, Fox TD, Petes TD. Analysis of microsatellite mutations in the mitochondrial DNA of *Saccharomyces cerevisiae*. Proceedings of the National Academy of Sciences of the United States of America. 2000;**97**:250-255. DOI: 10.1073/pnas.97.1.250

[83] Obach RS, Dobo KL. Comparison of metabolite profiles generated in Aroclor-induced rat liver and human liver subcellular fractions: Considerations for in vitro genotoxicity hazard assessment. Environmental and Molecular Mutagenesis.

2008;**49**:631-641. DOI: 10.1002/em.20416

[84] Johnson TE, Umbenhauer DR, Galloway SM. Human liver S-9 metabolic activation: proficiency in cytogenetic assays and comparison with phenobarbital/beta-naphthoflavone or aroclor 1254 induced rat S-9. Environmental and Molecular Mutagenesis. 1996;**28**:51-59. DOI: 10.1002/(SICI)1098-2280(1996)28:1<51:AID-EM8>3.0.CO;2-H

[85] Golizeh M, Sleno L. Optimized proteomic analysis of rat liver microsomes using dual enzyme digestion with 2D-LC-MS/MS. Journal of Proteomics. 2013;**82**:166-178. DOI: 10.1016/j.jprot.2013.02.001

[86] Guo Y, Breeden LL, Zarbl H, Preston BD, Eaton DL. Expression of a human cytochrome p450 in yeast permits analysis of pathways for response to and repair of aflatoxin-induced DNA damage. Molecular and Cellular Biology. 2005;**25**:5823-5833. DOI: 10.1128/MCB.25.14.5823-5833.2005

[87] Paladino G, Weibel B, Sengstag C. Heterocyclic aromatic amines efficiently induce mitotic recombination in metabolically competent *Saccharomyces cerevisiae* strains. Carcinogenesis. 1999;**20**:2143-2152. DOI: 10.1093/carcin/20.11.2143

[88] Pesheva M, Krastanova O, Stamenova R, Kantardjiev D, Venkov P. The response of Ty1 test to genotoxins. Archives of Toxicology. 2008;**82**:779-785. DOI: 10.1007/s00204-008-0299-5

[89] Lan J, Gou N, Gao C, He M, Gu AZ. Comparative and mechanistic genotoxicity assessment of nanomaterials via a quantitative toxicogenomics approach across multiple species. Environmental Science & Technology. 2014;**48**(21):12937-12945. DOI: 10.1021/es503065q

[90] Kupiec M. Damage-induced recombination in the yeast *Saccharomyces cerevisiae*. Mutation Research. 2000;**451**(1-2):91-105. DOI: 10.1016/s0027-5107(00)00042-7

[91] Derevensky M, Fasullo M. DNA damaging agents trigger the expression of the HML silent mating type locus in *Saccharomyces cerevisiae*. Mutation Research, Genetic Toxicology and Environmental Mutagenesis. 2018;**835**:16-20. DOI: 10.1016/j.mrgentox.2018.08.007

[92] Galli A, Schiestl RH. Hydroxyurea induces recombination in dividing but not in G1 or G2 cell cycle arrested yeast cells. Mutation Research. 1996;**354**:69-75. DOI: 10.1016/0027-5107(96)00037-1

[93] Fasullo M. Thymidylate depletion stimulates homologous recombination by *UNG1*-dependent and *UNG1*-independent mechanisms in *Saccharomyces cerevisiae*. Annals of Mutagenesis. 2017;**1**:1005

[94] Jin YH, Clark AB, Slebos RJ, et al. Cadmium is a mutagen that acts by inhibiting mismatch repair. Nature Genetics. 2003;**34**(3):326-329. DOI: 10.1038/ng1172

[95] Brennan RJ, Schiestl RH. Cadmium is an inducer of oxidative stress in yeast. Mutation Research. 1996;**356**(2):171-178. DOI: 10.1016/0027-5107(96)00051-6

[96] Hoffmann GR, Ronan MV, Sylvia KE, Tartaglione JP. Enhancement of the recombinagenic and mutagenic activities of bleomycin in yeast by intercalation of acridine compounds into DNA. Mutagenesis. 2009;**24**(4):317-329. DOI: 10.1093/mutage/gep012

[97] Berglund AK, Navarrete C, Engqvist MK, Hoberg E, Szilagyi Z, Taylor RW, et al. Nucleotide pools dictate the identity and frequency of ribonucleotide incorporation in

mitochondrial DNA. PLoS Genetics. 2011;**13**(2):e1006628. DOI: 10.1371/journal.pgen.1006628

[98] Dujardin G, Robert B, Clavilier L. Effect of hydroxyurea treatment on transmission and recombination of mitochondrial genes in *Saccharomyces cerevisiae*: A new method to modify the input of mitochondrial genes in crosses. Molecular & General Genetics. 1978;**160**(1):101-110. DOI: 10.1007/bf00275125

[99] Foury F. Cloning and sequencing of the nuclear gene MIP1 encoding the catalytic subunit of the yeast mitochondrial DNA polymerase. The Journal of Biological Chemistry. 1989;**264**:20552-20560. DOI: 10.1007/bf00275125

[100] Baruffini E, Lodi T. Construction and validation of a yeast model system for studying in vivo the susceptibility to nucleoside analogues of DNA polymerase gamma allelic variants. Mitochondrion. 2010;**10**:183-187. DOI: 10.1016/j.mito.2009.10.002

[101] Gounalaki N, Thireos G. Yap1p, a yeast transcriptional activator that mediates multidrug resistance, regulates the metabolic stress response. The EMBO Journal. 1994;**13**:4036-4041. DOI: 10.1002/j.1460-2075.1994.tb06720.x

[102] Kuge S, Jones N. YAP1 dependent activation of TRX2 is essential for the response of *Saccharomyces cerevisiae* to oxidative stress by hydroperoxides. The EMBO Journal. 1994;**13**(3):655-664. DOI: 10.1002/j.1460-2075.1994.tb06304.x

[103] Wei T, Zhang C, Xu X, Hanna M, Zhang X, Wang Y, et al. Construction and evaluation of two biosensors based on yeast transcriptional response to genotoxic chemicals. Biosensors & Bioelectronics. 2013;**44**:138-145. DOI: 10.1016/j.bios.2013.01.029

[104] Keller-Seitz M, Certa U, Sengstag C, Wurgler F, Sun M, Fasullo M. Transcriptional response of the yeast to the carcinogen Aflatoxin B1: Recombinational repair involving RAD51 and RAD1. Mol. Biol. Cell. 2004;**15**:4321-4336. DOI: 10.1091/mbc.e04-05-0375

[105] Fasullo M, Bennett T, Dave P. Expression of *Saccharomyces cerevisiae* MATa and MAT alpha enhances the HO endonuclease-stimulation of chromosomal rearrangements directed by his3 recombinational substrates. Mutation Research. 1999;**433**(1):33-44. DOI: 10.1016/s0921-8777(98)00059-7

[106] Schiestl RH, Prakash S. RAD1, an excision repair gene of *Saccharomyces cerevisiae*, is also involved in recombination. Molecular and Cellular Biology. 1988;**8**:3619-3626. DOI: 10.1128/mcb.8.9.3619

[107] Fasullo M, Zeng L, Giallanza P. Enhanced stimulation of chromosomal translocations by radiomimetic DNA damaging agents and camptothecin in *Saccharomyces cerevisiae* rad9 checkpoint mutants. Mutation Research. 2004;**547**(1-2):123-132. DOI: 10.1016/j.mrfmmm.2003.12.010

[108] He X, Feng S. Role of metabolic enzymes P450 (CYP) on activating procarcinogen and their polymorphisms on the risk of cancers. Current Drug Metabolism. 2015;**16**:850-863. DOI: 10.2174/138920021610151210164501

[109] Stoilov I, Akarsu AN, Alozie I, Child A, Barsoum-Homsy M, Turacli ME, et al. Sequence analysis and homology modeling suggest that primary congenital glaucoma on 2p21 results from mutations disrupting either the hinge region or the conserved core structures of cytochrome P4501B1. American Journal of Human Genetics. 1998;**62**:573-584. DOI: 10.1086/301764

[110] Mammen JS, Pittman GS, Li Y, Abou-Zahr F, Bejjani BA, Bell DA, et al. Single amino acid mutations, but not common polymorphisms, decrease the activity of CYP1B1 against benzo[a] pyrene-7R-trans-7,8-dihydrodiol. Carcinogenesis. 2003;**24**:1247-1255. DOI: 10.1093/carcin/bgg088

[111] Hanioka N, Yamamoto M, Tanaka-Kagawa T, Jinno H, Narimatsu S. Functional characterization of human cytochrome P4502E1 allelic variants: In vitro metabolism of benzene and toluene by recombinant enzymes expressed in yeast cells. Archives of Toxicology. 2010;**84**:363-371. DOI: 10.1007/s00204-009-0504-1

[112] Yin X, Xiong W, Wang Y, Tang W, Xi W, Qian S, et al. Association of CYP2E1 gene polymorphisms with bladder cancer risk: A systematic review and meta-analysis. Medicine (Baltimore). 2018;**97**(39):e11910. DOI: 10.1097/MD.0000000000011910

[113] Guengerich FP, Parikh A, Turesky RJ, Josephy PD. Inter-individual differences in the metabolism of environmental toxicants: Cytochrome P450 1A2 as a prototype. Mutation Research. 1999;**16**(428):115-124. DOI: 10.1016/s1383-5742(99)00039-3

[114] Cascorbi I, Brockmöller J, Roots I. A C4887A polymorphism in exon 7 of human CYP1A1: Population frequency, mutation linkages, and impact on lung cancer susceptibility. Cancer Research. 1996;**56**:4965-4969

[115] Esteller M, Garcia A, Martinez-Palones JM, Xercavins J, Reventos J. Germline polymorphisms in cytochrome-P450 1A1 (C4887 CYP1A1) and methylenetetrahydrofolate reductase (MTHFR) genes and endometrial cancer susceptibility. Carcinogenesis. 1997;**18**:2307-2311. DOI: 10.1093/carcin/18.12.2307

[116] Stettler PM, Sengstag C. Liver carcinogen aflatoxin B1 as an inducer of mitotic recombination in a human cell line. Molecular Carcinogenesis. 2001;**31**:125-138. DOI: 10.1002/mc.1047

Chapter 2

Random Mutagenesis of Filamentous Fungi Strains for High-Yield Production of Secondary Metabolites: The Role of Polyamines

Alexander A. Zhgun

Abstract

A filamentous fungus (also called molds or moldy fungus) is a taxonomically diverse organism from phylum *Zygomycota* and *Ascomycota* with filamentous hyphae and has the ability to produce airborne spores or conidia. Currently, more than 70,000 molds are known, and some of them contain unique and unusual biochemical pathways. A number of products from such pathways, especially, the secondary metabolite (SM) pathways are used as important pharmaceuticals, including antibiotics, statins, and immunodepresants. Under different conditions, the individual species can produce more than 100 SM. The strain improvement programs lead to high yielding in target SM and significant reduction of spin-off products. The main tool for the strain improvement of filamentous fungi is random mutagenesis and screening. The majority of industrial overproducing SM strains were developed with the help of such technique over the past 50–70 years; the yield of the target SM increased by 100- to 1000-fold or more. Moreover, most of the strains have reached their technological limit of improvement. A new round of mutagenesis has not increased overproduction. Recently, it was shown that that the addition of exogenous polyamines may increase the production of such improved strains of filamentous fungi. The possible molecular mechanism of this phenomenon and its biotechnological applications are discussed.

Keywords: filamentous fungi, random mutagenesis and screening, strain improvement, secondary metabolites, polyamines

1. Introduction

Improved strains of filamentous fungi are widely used in the biotechnology industry for recycling of secondary raw materials [1–3] as biosorbents [4], in fermentation of cheese [5], wine [6, 7], and other food products [8, 9], as well as for the production of enzymes [10–13], organic acids [14, 15], secondary metabolites (SMs) [16, 17], or for steroid transformation [18, 19]. There are four main tools for fungal strain improvement: (1) sexual crossing [20, 21], (2) somatic crossing (including parasexual recombination [22]), (3) random mutagenesis by physical or/and chemical

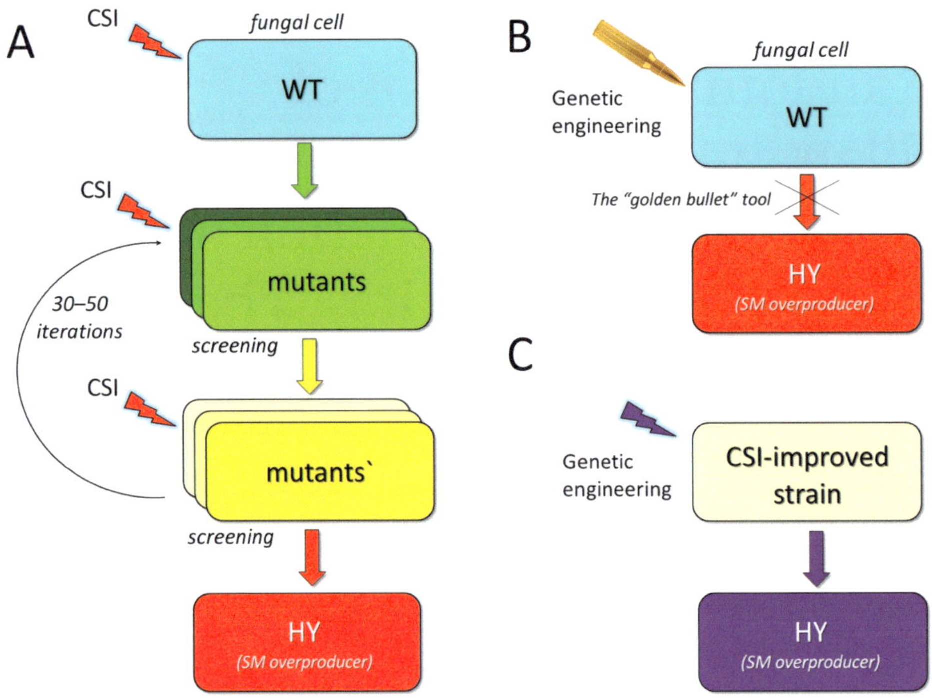

Figure 1.
The improving of filamentous fungi strains for SM production. (A) CSI programs for fungal strain improvement. (B) The WT strain improvement by the "golden bullet" tool from genetic engineering. (C) The combination of SCI and genetic engineering approaches for the developing of novel HY strain. SM: secondary metabolite, CSI: classical strain improvement, WT: wild type, and HY: high yielding.

mutagens and screening [23, 24], and (4) genetic engineering [25–27]. These methods can be applied separately or in various combinations [28]. The first three tools are referred to as classical strain improvement (CSI) methods and have been used in strain improvement programs for filamentous fungi for SM production since the 1950s of the twentieth century (**Figure 1A**). The majority of industrial producers of secondary metabolites in fungi were obtained precisely with the use of CSI [25]. The powerful genetic engineering approach has been available since the end of the twentieth century for targeting the particular genetic determinant to introduce novel properties into an organism [28]. Since the improvement of filamentous fungi strains for SM production is a complex and multistage program that radically changes numerous processes, there is no "golden bullet," any single unique genetic change to produce high yielding (HY) strain from the wild type (WT) strain [29] (**Figure 1B**). However, introducing of novel targeted features into already improved strains enables to create SM-overproducing strains [30]. For instance, the introduction of the compactin pathway from the *Penicillium citrinum*, as well as CYP105AS1 (from *Amycolatopsis orientalis*, for pravastatin hydroxylation) into the β-lactam-negative *P. chrysogenum* DS50662 strain, yielded more than 6 g/L of pravastatin [25]. This seems to be due to the interaction of different tools that are available to improve strains (**Figure 1C**).

2. CSI for SM production in filamentous fungi

For the majority of industrially important filamentous fungi (except members of genera *Aspergillus*, *Claviceps*, and *Emercicellopsis*), the sexual breeding is not available [28]. From the other side, a number of these organisms produce haploid conidia, which provide the ideal material for mutagenic treatment: in the absence of a complementary set of genes, mutations will be easily detected using suitable screening and the stability of the mutant will generally be good [28]. Filamentous fungi turned out to be surprisingly tolerant to strong mutagenic effects, retaining their strength and productivity even after radical rearrangements of their chromosomes [31, 32]. In this case, the main tool of CSI for SM production in filamentous fungi is random mutagenesis mutagens and screening [33].

2.1 The overproduction of target SM in filamentous fungi

The individual species of filamentous fungi under different external and internal signals are able to produce up to 100–150 or more different SMs [34–36]. This is achieved due to the presence in the genomes of these organisms of 30–80 clusters of genes, responsible for various biosynthetic pathways of SMs, so-called biosynthetic gene clusters (BGCs) [37, 38], and by the fine tuning in the regulation of their expression [39, 40]. Currently, more than 20,000 SMs are known to be produced from more than 1000 characterized gene clusters of filamentous fungi [35, 36]. Normally, gene clusters are "silent," the expression level of BGCs is extremely low, and there is practically no biosynthesis of any SMs (**Figure 2A**). For the biosynthesis of particular SM, the corresponding BGC must be "awakened" by some specific signal. For instance, the environmental signal 1 is resulted in the biosynthesis of SM1 (**Figure 2A**). A number of possible SMs, which can be produced in a particular organism after the "awakening" of corresponding BGCs, constitute its biosynthetic capacity for SMs (**Figure 2A**). In order to become an industrial producer, the fungus strain must increase the production the target SM 100- to 1000-fold or more (**Figure 2B**). It is also necessary that under favorable conditions (usually, these are fermentation conditions), the content of spin-off products would be extremely small (**Figure 2B**).

2.2 The molecular mechanisms of SM overproduction in filamentous fungi

An increase in the production of the target SM by 100- to 1000-fold and the elimination of spin-off products under the fermentation conditions in the improved fungal strains (**Figure 2B**) are associated with two main molecular events, the upregulation of genes from target BGC and the knockout of genes from alternative BGC [27, 33, 41, 42]. Since the expression of BGC genes is controlled by the pathway-specific regulation [27, 43, 44], global regulation [45, 46], and global regulation of SM [47–50], the SCI programs are accompanied by changes in such controls. For instance, during CGI program for penicillin G (PenG) production in HY strain (DS17690) two main events occurred, the shift in global regulation of secondary metabolism by introducing mutations in LaeA and VelA and mutations in key enzymes for spin-off SM [33]. That enabled to escape control from the global regulation of SM and involve more than one gene copy of BGC for PenG.

Usually, an increase in the gene dose (introducing several BGC copies for target SM) does not lead to an increase in gene expression. For instance, in the another PenG-overproducing strain (P2niaD18) the enhanced penicillin titer does not strictly depend on the copy number of the cluster [51]. This phenomenon occurs due to the control from the global regulation of SM, which brings only one cluster to work, the rest are silent [35, 52, 53]. Since there are 8 BGC copies for PenG in DS17690 strain, the escape of global regulation resulted in the significant increase in the yield of the target SM [33]. However, the shift in global regulation of SM could also significantly upregulate the expression from alternative BGC [54, 55]. From this point of view, it becomes clear why the CSI program for DS17690 strain

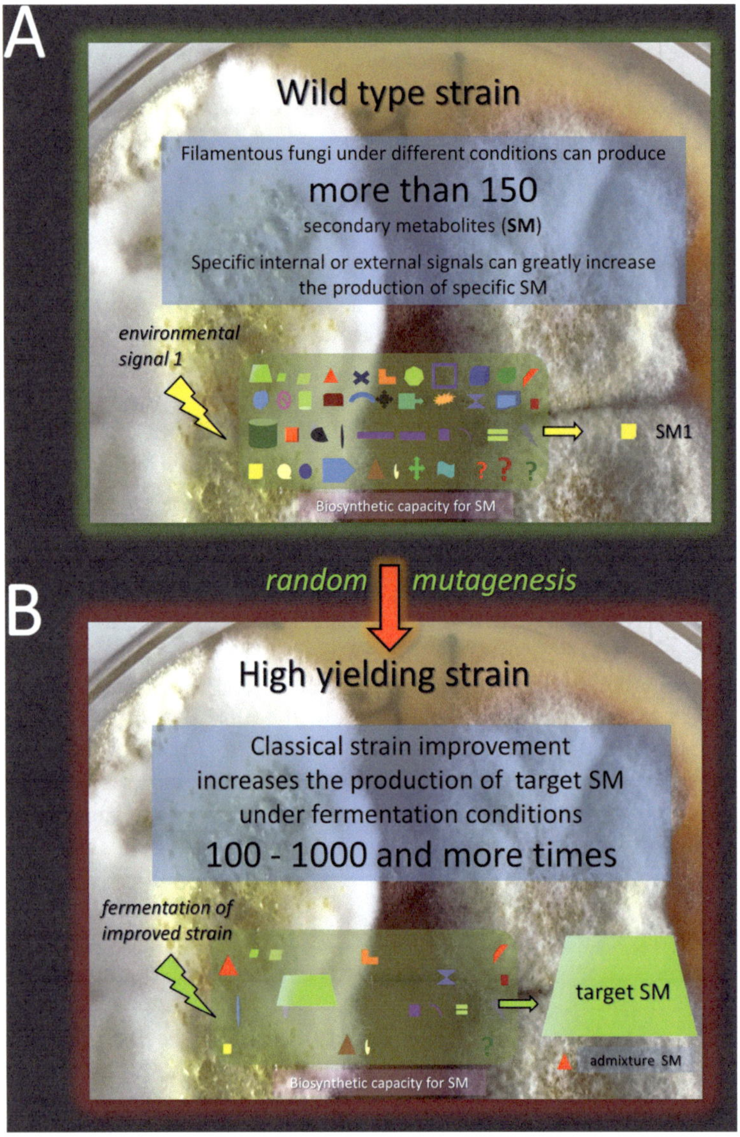

Figure 2.
The shift in biosynthetic capacity for SM production after CSI programs of filamentous fungi. (A) The response of WT strain to the environmental signal 1 and production of SM1. (B) The overproduction of target SM in the HY strain under fermentation conditions. SM: secondary metabolite, CSI: classical strain improvement, WT: wild type, and HY: high yielding.

changes in global regulation of SM also accompanied by mutations in central enzymes for spin-off SM [33]. The shift in global regulation of SM not only took out of control additional BGC copies for PenG, but also – BGC for spin-off SM. Since the screening went against spin-off SM, variants with mutations in central enzymes of alternative BGC were selected [33]. It was demonstrated, that delections in such central enzymes (NRPS or PKS megasynthases) lead by a still unknown mechanism to the silencing of all genes from the corresponding gene cluster [56].

Thus, if the improving of filamentous fungi strains for SM production led to duplication of target BGC, the simultaneous changes both in the system of global regulation of SM and at the level of alternative BGC expression are required [33]. However, in many improved strains, industrial producers of SMs, spin-off products are still formed during fermentation [57, 58]. These impurities are intermediates of the target SM biosynthesis; their amount depends on numerous fermentation conditions [58]. For instance, the cephalosporin C (CPC) yield after fermentation of improved *Acremonium chrysogenum* strains often contaminated with deacetylcephalosporin C (DAC) [57]. DAC is immediate precursor of CPC in the biosynthetic pathway. The conversion from DAC to CPC is catalyzed by deacetylcephalosporin-C acetyltransferase enzyme (CefG; EC 2.3.1.175) by, occurs in the cytoplasm [59] and is utilizes one molecule of cytoplasmic acetyl-CoA per reaction. In HY strains the CPC production increased 200- to 300-fold and the expression from BGC for CPC (*cef* genes) upregulated 20- to 300-fold [41]. In this case the acetyl-CoA content may be depleted in some HY strains [57, 58]. From the other side the screening during CSI programs went the same way against DAC admixture, events that reduce CPC/DAC ratio were selected. In the *A. chrysogenum* HY strain RNCM 408D [60], the CPC/DAC does not exceed 10–15% [61]. Thus, to increase in SM production is accompanied not only by changes in the expression and regulation of BGCs, but by reprogramming the whole organism, starting with changes in the primary metabolism (for the needs of target SM biosynthesis), ending with changes in the transport and assimilation of nutrients, the ability to assimilate oxygen, adaptation to fermentation conditions, and much more [42]. That is why the improvement of the filamentous fungi strain is a multi-step process, involving alterations in many spheres of the strain's vital activity, and there is no "golden bullet," no one cardinal event that converts WT strain to HY (**Figure 1**).

2.3 The technological limit of CSI of filamentous fungi for SM production

Filamentous fungi are a good facility for the improving of SM production by random mutagenesis and screening [2, 28, 62, 63]. Among the most popular mutagens used for fungal strain improvement are DNA alkylating NTG (N′-methyl-N′-nitro-N′-nitrosoguanidine) which typically produces a variety of point mutations and UV irradiation at 254 nm, which causes the formation of pyrimide dimers leading to point mutations and deletions [28]. In general, the CSI program for SM production in filamentous fungi looks as shown in **Figure 3**. The WT strain produce target SM in most cases at a low level, usually it does not exceed 30–50 μg/ml of fermentation medium [27, 41]. On order to convert WT to HY strain a number of independent events, involving BGCs regulation, changes in primary metabolism, strain physiology and so on, must occur. Moreover, all these events do not have to happen simultaneously. There are a number of ways in which the production of target SM gains added benefit. The first round of mutagenesis against WT strain results in a series of mutants, some of them have shift in the production of target SM (**Figure 3**). The majority of alterations lead to decrease or lack of the production change, but some mutants may show the increase in SM production. They are used as origins for the next mutagenesis round, followed by the next stage of screening. For example, on the A′ round of mutagenesis, the production level of SM was increased by A%, on the B′ round of mutagenesis, the production level of SM was increased by B% (**Figure 3**). Thus the CSI gradually leads to the emergence of a whole set of changes leading to an increase in the production. However, along with beneficial changes that increase the production of the target SM, reduce the amount of spin-off products, and others, numerous side changes begin to accumulate in the fungal strain. They can appear in a slow growth on agar and liquid media [27, 64, 65], a decrease in stress resistance [66], reduction in the conidia formation [64] and many other properties, expressed in a decrease in the overall viability of the strain [66, 67]. Finally, the stage comes when the next mutagenic effect no longer leads to further strain improvement. This is the technological limit of CSI method, it comes for each improvement program for a particular strain of filamentous fungus and is usually found at the 10–50th round of mutagenesis [60, 68].

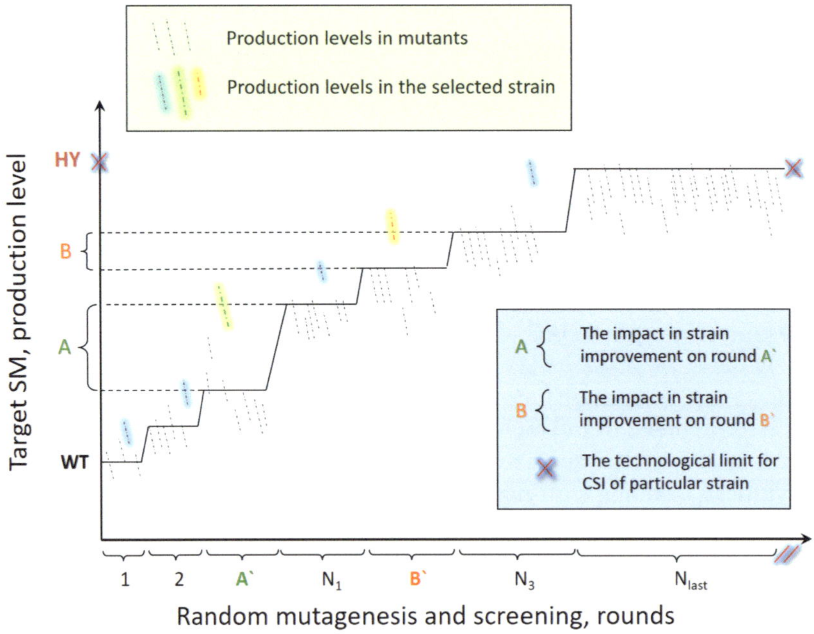

Figure 3.
Random mutagenesis and screening for the improving of filamentous fungi strains for SM production. SM: secondary metabolite, CSI: classical strain improvement, WT: wild type, and HY: high yielding.

3. Role of polyamines in filamentous fungi HY strains (after SCI for SM production)

Aliphatic polyamines (PAs) such as putrescine, spermidine, and spermine are widespread in nature; they are present in all living organisms and are also present in viral particles [69]. Despite the fact that these compounds have long been known as components of biological systems, there is still no clear understanding of their role in various bioprocesses [70]. The most studied functions of PAs are associated with stimulating the growth of microorganisms, increasing membrane stability, interacting with nucleic acids, and regulating the level of heterochromatin in the cell [71–74]. The roles of PAs in fungi cell have also been discussed [71, 75]. The main topics correspond to stress resistance [76], phytopathogenicity [77] and fungal development, including sporulation, growth and other stages of lifecycle [78, 79]. There is tight control of polyamine homeostasis in the cell [80]. For a particular organism, there is a certain content of PAs. For this, there are both biosynthetic and catabolic enzymes of polyamines (**Figure 4**), moreover, the amount of key biosynthetic enzymes, such as ornithine decarboxylase (ODC), or S-adenosylmethionine decarboxylase (AdoMetDC) is regulated at the levels of transcription, translation and turnover rate (half-life) [80, 81].

3.1 Influence of PAs on SM production in improved strains

Recently it was demonstrated, aliphatic PAs, such as 1,3-Diaminopropane (DAP) or spermidine (Spd) may increase the production of target SMs in HY fungi strains [82]. The production level of PenG in *P. chrysogenum* increased by 10–15% [82], the CPC production in *A. chrysogenum* HY strain increased by 10–15% [83] and the production of lovastatin (LOV) by *Aspergillus terreus* HY strain at the particular timepoints of fermentation increased by 20–45% [84]. The addition of 5 mM PAs

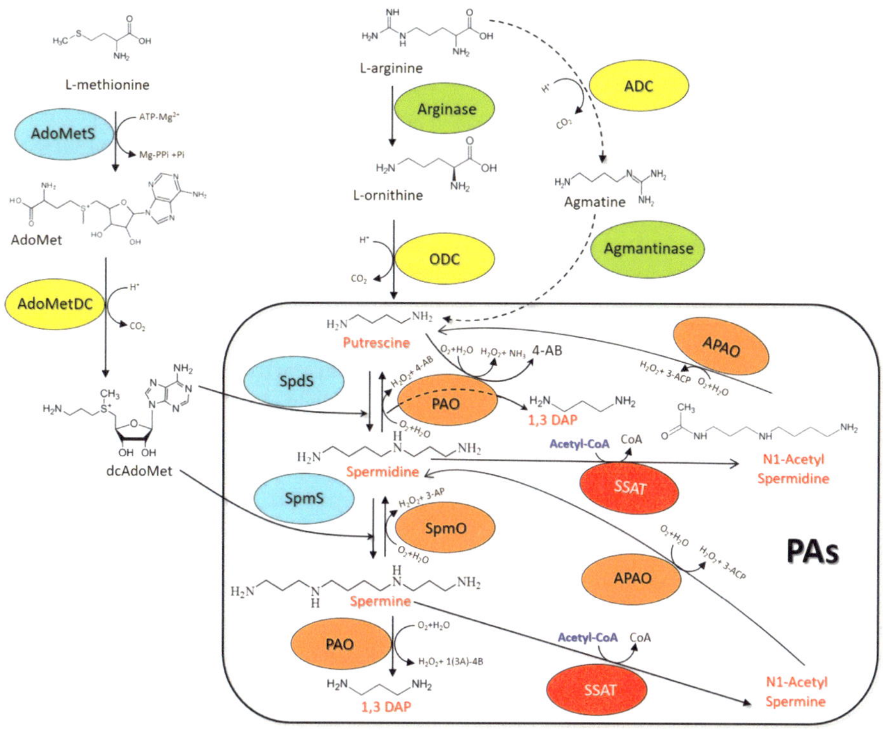

Figure 4.
The metabolism of polyamines in filamentous fungi. PAs: polyamines, ODC: ornithine decarboxylase, ADC: arginine decarboxylase, AdoMetS: S-adenosylmethionine synthetase, AdoMetDC: S-adenosylmethionine decarboxylase, SpdS: spermidine synthase, SpmS: spermine synthase, PAO: polyamine oxidase, SpmO: spermine oxidase, SSAT: spermidine/spermine-N1-acetyltransferase, APAO: N-acetylpolyamine oxidase, DFMO: α-difluoromethylornithine, APA: 1-aminooxy-3-aminopropane, DFMA: α-difluoromethylarginine, and AO-Agm: 1-aminooxy-3-guanidinopropane.

to agar media increased the survival of HY strains, as demonstrated by the drop and dilution assay [83, 84]. The PAs addition during the fermentation of improved strains also led to upregulation of corresponding BGCs (*pen*, *cef* and *lov* genes) [82–84]. This is important because *A. chrysogenum* and *A. terreus* HY strains have reached their technological limit after CSI programs [60, 68] and the possibility of further increasing the production of valuable pharmacologically significant substances as a result of the addition of relatively cheap PAs may be significant in the biotechnology industry.

3.2 Possible mechanisms of influencing of exogenous PAs on SM production

The addition of exogenous PAs also accompanied by the *laeA* upregulation in all studied improved strains [82–84]. LaeA is global regulator of SM in filamentous fungi [50]. It is S-adenosylmethionine (SAMe)-dependent histone methylate, which acts epigenetically, through the chromatin remodeling [85]. Since the biosynthesis of PAs and the work of LaeA require the same substrate, SAMe, the addition of exogenous PAs can lead to a shift in the global regulation of the studied HY strains. It is also known that in all these strains, *P. chrysogenum* Wis 54-1255, *A. chrysogenum* RNCM 408D and *A. terreus* No. 44-62, the only one copy of corresponding BGC is present, one copy of *pen* genes [86], one copy of "early" and "late" *cef* genes [32, 41] and one copy on *lov* genes [84] respectively. In this regard, the CSI programs for these strains could follow a rather different pathway than *P. chrysogenum* DS17690 with eight copies of *pen* genes [30], without significant shifting and removing the global regulation of SM and mutation in LaeA.

In order to confirm this hypothesis we carried out fermentation with PAs for WT, HY and E6 strains of *A. terreus* [44]. The LOV production in *A. terreus* is under the control of two major positive regulators, the LovE pathway-specific regulator and LaeA global regulator of fungi SM [44]. The *A. terreus* E6 strain derived from WT by the genetic engineering introduction the additional copy of *lovE* gene under the control of constitutive promotor [27]. LovE is Zn_2Cys_6 transcription factor for pathway-specific regulation of *lov* genes; in *A. terreus OE::lovE* the LOV production increased 10- to 12-fold [27]. Surprisingly, the addition of PAs during the fermentation of the E6 strain led, on the contrary, to a decrease in LOV production (**Figure 5**). But it is also known that pathway-specific regulators can negatively regulate LaeA [49]. For instance, AflR, a sterigmatocystin pathway-specific transcription factor, negatively regulate the expression of *laeA* [49]. E6 strain has the only one targeted change in the genome of WT, that led to constitutive (which also means LaeA-independent) overexpression of *lovE*. The effects of *laeA* downregulation (due to an increase in the dose of the negative regulator gene) on LOV production in E6 strain are compensated by *lovE* upregulation [49]. However, LovE, unlike LaeA, upregulate only *lov* genes for biosynthesis, not for transport and resistance Therefore, the PAs addition during fermentation of E6 strain causes a toxic effect and the LOV production decreases (**Figure 5**).

3.3 The endogenous polyamines content in *A. chrysogenum* HY strain

Since exogenous PAs are able to influence the production of SM in HY strains, it is important to know if there have been any changes in the metabolism and homeostasis of polyamines into the cells of improved fungi strains. Recently it was demonstrated, that *A. chrysogenum* HY strain shows increased resistance to inhibitors

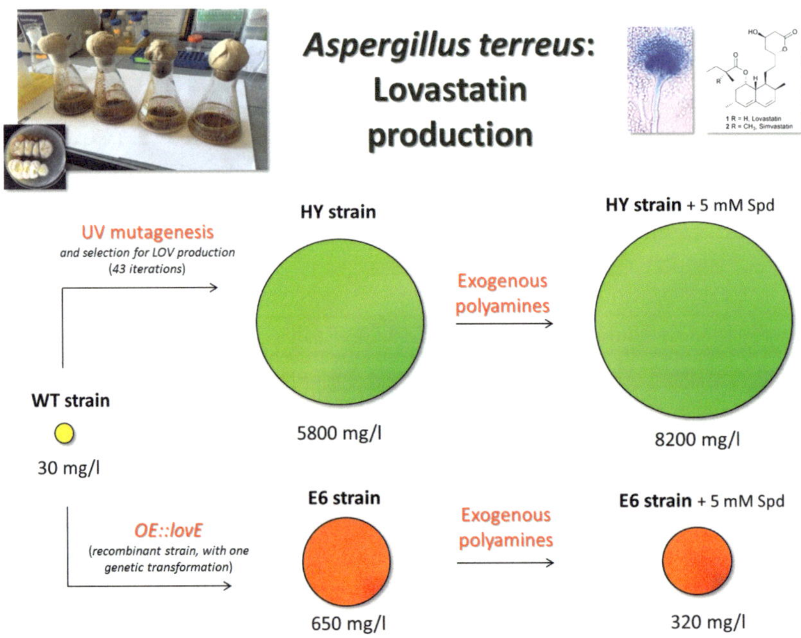

Figure 5.
Effect of exogenous polyamines on lovastatin production in the WT, E6, and HY A. terreus *strains. WT: wild type, E6:* OE::lovE*, HY: high yielding, and Spd: spermidine. Adapted with permission from [44].*

of ODC, the key enzyme of PAs biosynthesis, on minimal agar media [65]. The addition of 5 mM α-difluoromethylornithine (DFMO) or 5 mM of 1-aminooxy-3-aminopropane (APA) completely inhibited the growth of the WT strain, unlike HY strain (**Figure 4**) [65]. Such kind of resistance against inhibiters of key enzyme for PAs production turned out to be rather strange since HY strain is significantly weakened after SCI program [32, 61, 64, 66, 67]. The only previously observed advantage over the WT strain was expressed in CPC overproduction [41]. To explain the phenomenon of the resistance of HY strain to ODC inhibitors, an inhibitory analysis of *A. chrysogenum* WT and HY strains was performed against all pathways of putrescine biosynthesis (**Figure 3**). In filamentous fungi, in addition to the main pathway of putrescine (Put) biosynthesis, via ODC, there is also an additional pathway through arginine decarboxylase (ADC) and biosynthesis of agmatine (**Figure 3**). The inhibitory analysis demonstrated shift from the ADC-dependent to ODC-dependent biosynthesis of Put. During the fermentation for CPC production the total PAs content into HY strain has been increased by about fivefold [65].

The reasons for the increased production of PAs in the HY strain were discussed [65]. One on the reasons may be related to strain improvement techniques. The increasing in PAs content may be spin-o result of mutagenesis and DNA damage. Recently it was demonstrated that PAs can maintain the genome integrity via homology-directed DNA repair, enhancing the DNA strand exchange activity of RAD51 recombinase [87]. PAs also can protect DNA from free-radical damage by reacting direct with the reactive oxygen species [88–90].

4. Conclusions

As a result of CSI programs for filamentous fungi, a number of pharmaceutically significant SMs have been overproduced. One of the side effects of the high yielding strains improvement may be an increase in the content of polyamines (PAs). An increase in the PAs' content could occur as a response to mutagenesis during CSI. The recently discovered increase in the production of targeted SM in some HY strains after the addition of exogenous PAs may occur due to a decrease in endogenous biosynthesis of PAs and the release of additional resources for the biosynthesis of the target SM.

Acknowledgements

This research was funded by the Russian Foundation for Basic Research (grant number 19-04-01173).

Conflict of interest

The author declares no conflict of interest.

Notes/thanks/other declarations

This work is dedicated to the author's teacher and the scientific consultant of doctoral dissertation, Yuri Eduardovich Bartoshevich (passed away in 2014), one of the pioneers in the field of fungi chemical mutagenesis, the author of numerous scientific works, including publications in the Nature journal [90].

Author details

Alexander A. Zhgun
Institute of Bioengineering, Research Center of Biotechnology, Russian Academy of Sciences, Moscow, Russia

*Address all correspondence to: zzhgun@mail.ru

References

[1] Meyer V, Basenko EY, Benz JP, Braus GH, Caddick MX, Csukai M, et al. Growing a circular economy with fungal biotechnology: A white paper. Fungal Biology and Biotechnology. 2020;7:5. DOI: 10.1186/s40694-020-00095-z

[2] Meyer V, Andersen MR, Brakhage AA, Braus GH, Caddick MX, Cairns TC, et al. Current challenges of research on filamentous fungi in relation to human welfare and a sustainable bio-economy: A white paper. Fungal Biology and Biotechnology. 2016;**3**:6. DOI: 10.1186/s40694-016-0024-8

[3] Zhgun A, Avdanina D, Shumikhin K, Simonenko N, Lyubavskaya E, Volkov I, et al. Detection of potential biodeterioration risks for tempera painting in 16th century exhibits from State Tretyakov Gallery. PLoS One. 2020;**15**:e0230591. DOI: 10.1371/journal.pone.0230591

[4] Siegel SM, Galun M, Siegel BZ. Filamentous fungi as metal biosorbents: A review. Water, Air, and Soil Pollution. 1990;**53**:335-344. DOI: 10.1007/BF00170747

[5] Kure CF, Skaar I. The fungal problem in cheese industry. Current Opinion in Food Science. 2019;**29**:14-19. DOI: 10.1016/j.cofs.2019.07.003

[6] Ly S, Kakahi FB, Mith H, Phat C, Fifani B, Kenne T, et al. Engineering synthetic microbial communities through a selective biofilm cultivation device for the production of fermented beverages. Microorganisms. 2019;**7**:206. DOI: 10.3390/microorganisms7070206

[7] Anupma A, Tamang JP. Diversity of filamentous fungi isolated from some amylase and alcohol-producing starters of India. Frontiers in Microbiology. 2020;**11**:905. DOI: 10.3389/fmicb.2020.00905

[8] Geisen R, Färber P. New aspects of fungal starter cultures for fermented foods. Applied Microbiology. 2005:13-29. DOI: 10.1007/0-306-46888-3_1

[9] Sugiharto S. A review of filamentous fungi in broiler production. Annals of Agricultural Science. 2019:1-8. DOI: 10.1016/j.aoas.2019.05.005

[10] Arnau J, Yaver D, Hjort CM. Strategies and challenges for the development of industrial enzymes using fungal cell factories. Grand Challenges in Fungal Biotechnology. 2020:179-210. DOI: 10.1007/978-3-030-29541-7_7

[11] Gudynaite-Savitch L, White TC. Fungal biotechnology for industrial enzyme production: Focus on (hemi) cellulase production strategies, advances and challenges. Fungal Biology. 2016:395-439. DOI: 10.1007/978-3-319-27951-0_19

[12] Hu HL, van den Brink J, Gruben BS, Wösten HAB, Gu JD, de Vries RP. Improved enzyme production by co-cultivation of *Aspergillus niger* and *Aspergillus oryzae* and with other fungi. International Biodeterioration and Biodegradation. 2011;**65**:248-252. DOI: 10.1016/j.ibiod.2010.11.008

[13] Jun H, Kieselbach T, Jönsson LJ. Enzyme production by filamentous fungi: Analysis of the secretome of *Trichoderma reesei* grown on unconventional carbon source. Microbial Cell Factories. 2011;**10**:68. DOI: 10.1186/1475-2859-10-68

[14] Magnuson JK, Lasure LL. Organic acid production by filamentous fungi. Advances in Fungal Biotechnology for Industry, Agriculture, and Medicine. 2004:307-340. DOI: 10.1007/978-1-4419-8859-1_12

[15] Yang L, Lübeck M, Lübeck PS. *Aspergillus* as a versatile cell factory for

organic acid production. Fungal Biology Reviews. 2017;**31**:33-49. DOI: 10.1016/j.fbr.2016.11.001

[16] Calvo AM, Wilson RA, Bok JW, Keller NP. Relationship between secondary metabolism and fungal development. Microbiology and Molecular Biology Reviews. 2002;**66**:447-459. DOI: 10.1128/mmbr.66.3.447-459.2002

[17] Alberti F, Foster GD, Bailey AM. Natural products from filamentous fungi and production by heterologous expression. Applied Microbiology and Biotechnology. 2017;**101**:493-500. DOI: 10.1007/s00253-016-8034-2

[18] Nassiri-Koopaei N, Faramarzi MA. Recent developments in the fungal transformation of steroids. Biocatalysis and Biotransformation. 2015;**33**:1-28. DOI: 10.3109/10242422.2015.1022533

[19] Kristan K, Rižner TL. Steroid-transforming enzymes in fungi. The Journal of Steroid Biochemistry and Molecular Biology. 2012;**129**:79-91. DOI: 10.1016/j.jsbmb.2011.08.012

[20] Kwon-Chung KJ, Sugui JA. Sexual reproduction in *Aspergillus* species of medical or economical importance: Why so fastidious? Trends in Microbiology. 2009;**17**:481-487. DOI: 10.1016/j.tim.2009.08.004

[21] Krijgsheld P, Bleichrodt R, van Veluw GJ, Wang F, Müller WH, Dijksterhuis J, et al. Development in *Aspergillus*. Studies in Mycology. 2013;**74**:1-29. DOI: 10.3114/sim0006

[22] Clutterbuck AJ. Parasexual recombination in fungi. Journal of Genetics. 1996;**75**:281-286. DOI: 10.1007/BF02966308

[23] Guzmán-Chávez F, Zwahlen RD, Bovenberg RAL, Driessen AJM. Engineering of the filamentous fungus *Penicillium chrysogenumas* cell factory for natural products. Frontiers in Microbiology. 2018;**15**:2768. DOI: 10.3389/fmicb.2018.02768

[24] Dikshit R, Tallapragada P. Development and screening of mutants from *Monascus sanguineus* for secondary metabolites production. Beni-Suef University Journal of Basic and Applied Sciences. 2018;**7**:235-240. DOI: 10.1016/j.bjbas.2018.03.001

[25] McLean KJ, Hans M, Meijrink B, van Scheppingen WB, Vollebregt A, Tee KL, et al. Single-step fermentative production of the cholesterol-lowering drug pravastatin via reprogramming of *Penicillium chrysogenum*. Proceedings of the National Academy of Sciences. 2015;**112**:2847-2852. DOI: 10.1073/pnas.1419028112

[26] Anyaogu DC, Mortensen UH. Heterologous production of fungal secondary metabolites in *Aspergilli*. Frontiers in Microbiology. 2015;**6**:77. DOI: 10.3389/fmicb.2015.00077

[27] Zhgun AA, Dumina MV, Voinova TM, Dzhavakhiya VV, Eldarov MA. Role of acetyl-CoA synthetase and LovE regulator protein of polyketide biosynthesis in lovastatin production by wild-type and overproducing *Aspergillus terreus* strains. Applied Biochemistry and Microbiology. 2018;**54**:188-197. DOI: 10.1134/S0003683818020138

[28] Nevalainen KMH. Strain improvement in filamentous fungi - An overview. Applied Mycology and Biotechnology. 2001;**1**:289-304. DOI: 10.1016/S1874-5334(01)80013-7

[29] Nielsen JC, Nielsen J. Development of fungal cell factories for the production of secondary metabolites: Linking genomics and metabolism. Synthetic and Systems Biotechnology. 2017:5-12. DOI: 10.1016/j.synbio.2017.02.002

[30] Skellam E. Strategies for engineering natural product biosynthesis in fungi. Trends in Biotechnology. 2019;**37**:416-427. DOI: 10.1016/j.tibtech.2018.09.003

[31] Zolan ME. Chromosome-length polymorphism in fungi. Microbiological Reviews. 1995;**59**:686-698. DOI: 10.1128/mmbr.59.4.686-698.1995

[32] Dumina MV, Zhgun AA, Domracheva AG, Novak MI, El'darov MA. Chromosomal polymorphism of *Acremonium chrysogenum* strains producing cephalosporin C. Russian Journal of Genetics. 2012;**48**:778-784. DOI: 10.1134/S1022795412050067

[33] Salo OV, Ries M, Medema MH, Lankhorst PP, Vreeken RJ, Bovenberg RAL, et al. Genomic mutational analysis of the impact of the classical strain improvement program on β-lactam producing *Penicillium chrysogenum*. BMC Genomics. 2015;**16**:937. DOI: 10.1186/s12864-015-2154-4

[34] Brakhage AA. Regulation of fungal secondary metabolism. Nature Reviews. Microbiology. 2013;**11**:21-32. DOI: 10.1038/nrmicro2916

[35] Kjærbølling I, Mortensen UH, Vesth T, Andersen MR. Strategies to establish the link between biosynthetic gene clusters and secondary metabolites. Fungal Genetics and Biology. 2019: 107-121. DOI: 10.1016/j.fgb.2019.06.001

[36] Brakhage AA, Schroeckh V. Fungal secondary metabolites - Strategies to activate silent gene clusters. Fungal Genetics and Biology. 2011;**48**:15-22. DOI: 10.1016/j.fgb.2010.04.004

[37] Macheleidt J, Mattern DJ, Fischer J, Netzker T, Weber J, Schroeckh V, et al. Regulation and role of fungal secondary metabolites. Annual Review of Genetics. 2016;**50**:371-392. DOI: 10.1146/annurev-genet-120215-035203

[38] Drott MT, Bastos RW, Rokas A, Ries LNA, Gabaldón T, Goldman GH, et al. Diversity of secondary metabolism in *Aspergillus nidulans* clinical isolates. mSphere. 2020;**5**:e00156-20. DOI: 10.1128/msphere.00156-20

[39] Yu JH, Keller N. Regulation of secondary metabolism in filamentous fungi. Annual Review of Phytopathology. 2005;**43**:437-458. DOI: 10.1146/annurev.phyto.43.040204.140214

[40] Keller NP. Fungal secondary metabolism: Regulation, function and drug discovery. Nature Reviews Microbiology. 2019;**17**:167-180. DOI: 10.1038/s41579-018-0121-1

[41] Dumina MV, Zhgun AA, Novak MI, Domratcheva AG, Petukhov DV, Dzhavakhiya VV, et al. Comparative gene expression profiling reveals key changes in expression levels of cephalosporin C biosynthesis and transport genes between low and high-producing strains of *Acremonium chrysogenum*. World Journal of Microbiology and Biotechnology. 2014;**30**:2933-2941. DOI: 10.1007/s11274-014-1721-1

[42] Terfehr D, Dahlmann TA, Kück U. Transcriptome analysis of the two unrelated fungal β-lactam producers *Acremonium chrysogenum* and *Penicillium chrysogenum*: Velvet-regulated genes are major targets during conventional strain improvement programs. BMC Genomics. 2017;**18**:272. DOI: 10.1186/s12864-017-3663-0

[43] Yin W, Keller NP. Transcriptional regulatory elements in fungal secondary metabolism. Journal of Microbiology. 2011;**49**:329-339. DOI: 10.1007/s12275-011-1009-1

[44] Zhgun AA, Nuraeva GK, Eldarov M. The role of LaeA and LovE regulators in lovastatin biosynthesis with

exogenous polyamines in *Aspergillus terreus*. Applied Biochemistry and Microbiology. 2019;**55**:626-635. DOI: 10.1134/S0003683819060176

[45] Alkan N, Meng X, Friedlander G, Reuveni E, Sukno S, Sherman A, et al. Global aspects of pacC regulation of pathogenicity genes in *Colletotrichum gloeosporioides* as revealed by transcriptome analysis. Molecular Plant-Microbe Interactions. 2013;**26**:1345-1358. DOI: 10.1094/MPMI-03-13-0080-R

[46] Jekosch K, Kück U. Loss of glucose repression in an *Acremonium chrysogenum* beta-lactam producer strain and its restoration by multiple copies of the cre1 gene. Applied Microbiology and Biotechnology. 2000;**54**:556-563. Available from: http://www.ncbi.nlm.nih.gov/pubmed/11092632

[47] Lind AL, Smith TD, Saterlee T, Calvo AM, Rokas A. Regulation of secondary metabolism by the velvet complex is temperature-responsive in *Aspergillus*. G3: Genes, Genomes, Genetics. 2016;**6**:4023-4033. DOI: 10.1534/g3.116.033084

[48] Kosalková K, García-Estrada C, Ullán RV, Godio RP, Feltrer R, Teijeira F, et al. The global regulator LaeA controls penicillin biosynthesis, pigmentation and sporulation, but not roquefortine C synthesis in *Penicillium chrysogenum*. Biochimie. 2009;**91**:214-225. DOI: 10.1016/j.biochi.2008.09.004

[49] Bok JW, Keller NP. LaeA, a regulator of secondary metabolism in *Aspergillus* spp. Eukaryotic Cell. 2004;**3**:527-535. Available from: http://www.pubmedcentral.nih.gov/articlerender.fcgi?artid=387652&tool=pmcentrez&rendertype=abstract

[50] Sarikaya-Bayram Ö, Palmer JM, Keller N, Braus GH, Bayram Ö. One Juliet and four Romeos: VeA and its methyltransferases. Frontiers in Microbiology. 2015;**6**:1. DOI: 10.3389/fmicb.2015.00001

[51] Ziemons S, Koutsantas K, Becker K, Dahlmann T, Kück U. Penicillin production in industrial strain *Penicillium chrysogenum* P2niaD18 is not dependent on the copy number of biosynthesis genes. BMC Biotechnology. 2017;**17**:16. DOI: 10.1186/s12896-017-0335-8

[52] Gacek A, Strauss J. The chromatin code of fungal secondary metabolite gene clusters. Applied Microbiology and Biotechnology. 2012;**95**:1389-1404. DOI: 10.1007/s00253-012-4208-8

[53] Strauss J, Reyes-Dominguez Y. Regulation of secondary metabolism by chromatin structure and epigenetic codes. Fungal Genetics and Biology. 2011;**48**:62-69. DOI: 10.1016/j.fgb.2010.07.009

[54] Collemare J, Seidl MF. Chromatin-dependent regulation of secondary metabolite biosynthesis in fungi: Is the picture complete? FEMS Microbiology Reviews. 2019;**43**:591-607. DOI: 10.1093/femsre/fuz018

[55] Wang B, Lv Y, Li X, Lin Y, Deng H, Pan L. Profiling of secondary metabolite gene clusters regulated by LaeA in *Aspergillus niger* FGSC A1279 based on genome sequencing and transcriptome analysis. Research in Microbiology. 2017;**169**:67-77. DOI: 10.1016/j.resmic.2017.10.002

[56] Chen G, Chu J. Characterization of two polyketide synthases involved in sorbicillinoid biosynthesis by *Acremonium chrysogenum* using the CRISPR/Cas9 system. Applied Biochemistry and Biotechnology. 2019;**188**:1134-1144. DOI: 10.1007/s12010-019-02960-z

[57] Gutiérrez S, Velasco J, Marcos AT, Fernández FJ, Fierro F, Barredo JL, et al. Expression of the cefG gene is

limiting for cephalosporin biosynthesis in *Acremonium chrysogenum*. Applied Microbiology and Biotechnology. 1997;**48**:606-614. DOI: 10.1007/s002530051103

[58] Fujisawa Y, Shirafuji H, Kida M, Nara K, Yoneda M, Kanzaki T. New findings on cephalosporin C biosynthesis. Nature: New Biology. 1973;**246**:154-155. DOI: 10.1038/newbio246154a0

[59] Martín JF. Transport systems, intracellular traffic of intermediates and secretion of β-lactam antibiotics in fungi. Fungal Biology and Biotechnology. 2020;7:6. DOI: 10.1186/s40694-020-00096-y

[60] Patent RU2426793 C12P35/06, C07D501/02, C12R1/75. Method of cephalosporin C biosynthesis by using new *Acremonium chrysogenum* strain; 2011

[61] Dumina MV, Zhgun AA, Kerpichnikov IV, Domracheva AG, Novak MI, Valiachmetov AY, et al. Functional analysis of MFS protein CefT involved in the transport of beta-lactam antibiotics in *Acremonium chrysogenum* and *Saccharomyces cerevisiae*. Applied Biochemistry and Microbiology. 2013;**49**:368-377. DOI: 10.1134/S0003683813040042

[62] Kramer A, Paun L, Imhoff JF, Kempken F, Labes A. Development and validation of a fast and optimized screening method for enhanced production of secondary metabolites using the marine *Scopulariopsis brevicaulis* strain LF580 producing anti-cancer active scopularide A and B. PLoS One. 2014;**9**:e103320. DOI: 10.1371/journal.pone.0103320

[63] Domratcheva AG, Zhgun AA, Novak NV, Dzhavakhiya VV. The influence of chemical mutagenesis on the properties of the cyclosporine a high-producer strain *Tolypocladium inflatum* VKM F-3630D. Applied Biochemistry and Microbiology. 2018;**54**:53-57. DOI: 10.1134/S0003683818010027

[64] Zhgun AA, Ivanova MA, Domracheva AG, Novak MI, Elidarov MA, Skryabin KG, et al. Genetic transformation of the mycelium fungi *Acremonium chrysogenum*. Applied Biochemistry and Microbiology. 2008;**44**:600-607. DOI: 10.1134/S0003683808060070

[65] Hyvönen MT, Keinänen TA, Nuraeva GK, Yanvarev DV, Khomutov M, Khurs EN, et al. Hydroxylamine analogue of agmatine: Magic bullet for arginine decarboxylase. Biomolecules. 2020;**10**:1-16. DOI: 10.3390/biom10030406

[66] Kalebina TS, Selyakh IO, Gorkovskii AA, Bezsonov EE, El'darov MA, Novak MI, et al. Structure peculiarities of cell walls of *Acremonium chrysogenum*-an autotroph of cephalosporin C. Applied Biochemistry and Microbiology. 2010;**46**:614-619. DOI: 10.1134/S0003683810060098

[67] Valiakhmetov AI, Trilisenko LV, Vagabov VM, Bartoshevich IE, Kulaev IS, Novak MI, et al. The concentration dynamics of inorganic polyphosphates during the cephalosporin C synthesis by *Acremonium chrysogenum*. Prikladnaia Biokhimiia i Mikrobiologiia. 2010;**46**:198-204. Available from: http://www.ncbi.nlm.nih.gov/pubmed/20391764

[68] Patent RU2261901 C12N1/14, C12P17/06, C07D309/30. Fungal strain *Aspergillus terreus* No. 44-62 - Producer of lovastatin, industrial method of isolation of lovastatin and method of lactonization of statins; 2005

[69] Cohen SS. A Guide to the Polyamines. 1st ed. NY: Oxford University Press; 1998

[70] Miller-Fleming L, Olin-Sandoval V, Campbell K, Ralser M. Remaining

mysteries of molecular biology: The role of polyamines in the cell. Journal of Molecular Biology. 2015;**427**:3389-3406. DOI: 10.1016/j.jmb.2015.06.020

[71] Rocha RO, Wilson RA. Essential, deadly, enigmatic: Polyamine metabolism and roles in fungal cells. Fungal Biology Reviews. 2019;**33**:47-57. DOI: 10.1016/j.fbr.2018.07.003

[72] Chen D, Shao Q, Yin L, Younis A, Zheng B. Polyamine function in plants: Metabolism, regulation on development, and roles in abiotic stress responses. Frontiers in Plant Science. 2019;**9**:1945. DOI: 10.3389/fpls.2018.01945

[73] Pegg AE. Mammalian polyamine metabolism and function. IUBMB Life. 2009;**61**:880-894. DOI: 10.1002/iub.230

[74] Mounce BC, Olsen ME, Vignuzzi M, Connor JH. Polyamines and their role in virus infection. Microbiology and Molecular Biology Reviews. 2017;**81**:e00029-17. DOI: 10.1128/mmbr.00029-17

[75] Valdés-Santiago L, Ruiz-Herrera J. Polyamines in Fungi: Their Distribution, Metabolism, and Role in Cell Differentiation and Morphogenesis. (Mycology Book 30) 1st Ed. CRC Press; 19 December 2019. p. 186. ISBN: 9780367377106

[76] Valdés-Santiago L, Ruiz-Herrera J. Stress and polyamine metabolism in fungi. Frontiers in Chemistry. 2013;**1**:42. DOI: 10.3389/fchem.2013.00042

[77] Valdés-Santiago L, Cervantes-Chávez JA, León-Ramírez CG, Ruiz-Herrera J. Polyamine metabolism in fungi with emphasis on phytopathogenic species. Journal of Amino Acids. 2012;**2012**:1-13. DOI: 10.1155/2012/837932

[78] Crespo-Sempere A, Estiarte N, Marín S, Sanchis V, Ramos AJ. Targeting *Fusarium graminearum* control via polyamine enzyme inhibitors and polyamine analogs. Food Microbiology. 2015;**49**:95-103. DOI: 10.1016/j.fm.2015.01.020

[79] Guevara-Olvera L, Calvo-Mendez C, Ruiz-Herrera J. The role of polyamine metabolism in dimorphism of *Yarrowia lipolytica*. Journal of General Microbiology. 1993;**139**:485-493. DOI: 10.1099/00221287-139-3-485

[80] Minois N, Carmona-Gutierrez D, Madeo F. Polyamines in aging and disease. Aging (Albany NY). 2011;**3**: 716-732. DOI: 10.18632/aging.100361

[81] Iwami K, Wang JY, Jain R, McCormack S, Johnson LR. Intestinal ornithine decarboxylase: Half-life and regulation by putrescine. American Journal of Physiology. Gastrointestinal and Liver Physiology. 1990;**258**:G309. DOI: 10.1152/ajpgi.1990.258.2.g308

[82] Martín J, García-Estrada C, Kosalková K, Ullán RV, Albillos SM, Martín J-F. The inducers 1,3-diaminopropane and spermidine produce a drastic increase in the expression of the penicillin biosynthetic genes for prolonged time, mediated by the laeA regulator. Fungal Genetics and Biology. 2012;**49**:1004-1013. DOI: 10.1016/j.fgb.2012.10.001

[83] Zhgun AA, Kalinin SG, Novak MI, Domratcheva AG, Petukhov DV, Dzhavakhiya VV, et al. The influence of polyamines on cephalosporine C biosynthesis in *Acremonium chrysogenum* strains. Izvestiya Vuzov. Prikladnaya Khimiya i Biotekhnologiya. 2015;**14**:47-54

[84] Zhgun AA, Nuraeva GK, Dumina MV, Voinova TM, Dzhavakhiya VV, Eldarov MA. 1,3-Diaminopropane and spermidine upregulate lovastatin production and expression of lovastatin biosynthetic genes in *Aspergillus terreus* via LaeA

regulation. Applied Biochemistry and Microbiology. 2019;**55**:244-255. DOI: 10.1134/S0003683819020170

[85] Martín JF. Key role of LaeA and velvet complex proteins on expression of β-lactam and PR-toxin genes in *Penicillium chrysogenum*: Cross-talk regulation of secondary metabolite pathways. Journal of Industrial Microbiology & Biotechnology. 2016;**44**:525-535. DOI: 10.1007/s10295-016-1830-y

[86] Peng Q, Yuan Y, Gao M, Chen X, Liu B, Liu P, et al. Genomic characteristics and comparative genomics analysis of *Penicillium chrysogenum* KF-25. BMC Genomics. 2014;**15**:144. DOI: 10.1186/1471-2164-15-144

[87] Lee C-Y, Su G-C, Huang W-Y, Ko M-Y, Yeh H-Y, Chang G-D, et al. Promotion of homology-directed DNA repair by polyamines. Nature Communications. 2019;**10**:65. DOI: 10.1038/s41467-018-08011-1

[88] Murray Stewart T, Dunston TT, Woster PM, Casero RA. Polyamine catabolism and oxidative damage. The Journal of Biological Chemistry. 2018;**293**:18736-18745. DOI: 10.1074/jbc.TM118.003337

[89] Ha HC, Sirisoma NS, Kuppusamy P, Zweier JL, Woster PM, Casero RA. The natural polyamine spermine functions directly as a free radical scavenger. Proceedings of the National Academy of Sciences of the United States of America. 1998;**95**:11140-11145. DOI: 10.1073/pnas.95.19.11140

[90] Tikchonenko TI, Velikodvorskaya GA, Bobkova AF, Bartoshevich YE, Lebed EP, Chaplygina NM, et al. New fungal viruses capable of reproducing in bacteria. Nature. 1974;**249**:454-456. DOI: 10.1038/249454a0

Chapter 3

Generation, Evaluation, and Prospects of Further Use of Mutations Based on New Homozygous Self-Pollinated Sunflower Lines

Victoria Mykhailenko, Viktor Kyrychenko, Alexander Bragin and Dmitry Chuiko

Abstract

A majority of sunflower lines and hybrids were based on starting material obtained by traditional methods; so the issues of developing new trends in extending the genetic diversity of this crop require constant attention of scientists. At present, induced mutagenesis along with hybridization has become a leading method for generating new forms of crops. Their success depends largely on availability and assortment of starting material. Induction of mutations is a way to create it. The main value of induced mutagenesis for breeding is determined by opportunities to solve problems that are impossible or difficult to solve by traditional methods. The choice of an effective concentration (dose) of a mutagen is very important, since the frequency and range of mutations depend not only on the mutagen itself but also on its dose and exposure. In addition, it is relevant to search for new mutagens with reduced harmful effects at the same level of mutability. Cytological analysis of chromosomal aberrations is an important method of evaluation and identification of mutagenic effects. In this section, studies into chemical and physical mutagenesis in breeding, exemplified by new modern homozygous self-pollinated sunflower lines, are summarized; methodical recommendations on the use of induced mutagenesis in sunflower breeding are presented; and methods of generation, investigation, and further use of mutations are rationalized.

Keywords: gamma rays, dimethyl sulfate, mutagenesis, meiosis, mutation, self-pollinated line, breeding, sunflower

1. Introduction

In comparison with other oil crops, sunflower produces the highest oil yield per unit area (on average 750 kg/ha in Ukraine), which makes this crop a major oil crop. The oil content in seeds of released hybrids is 50–52%, and in breeding hybrids—up to 60%.

The nutritional value of sunflower oil is determined by high content of polyunsaturated fatty linoleic acid (55–60%), which has a significant biological activity and accelerates the metabolism of cholesterol esters in the body, which has a positive effect on health. Sunflower oil also contains ingredients that are very valuable to the human body, such as phosphatides, sterols, and vitamins (A, D, E, K). The nutritional value of sunflower seeds per 100 g is as follows: energy, 2445 kJ; proteins, 20.8 g; fats, 51.5 g (of which saturated fats account for 4.5 g; monounsaturated ones, 18.5 g; and polyunsaturated ones, 23.1 g); and carbohydrates, 20 g. This makes sunflower a valuable food product.

Induced mutagenesis allows developing new starting material with various morphological and physiological features and biochemical parameters, increasing the frequency and expanding the assortment of original mutations within a short time.

Mutations are a source of expansion of the genetic diversity of sunflower, which in its turn is a starting material for the breeding of this crop. Radiation and chemical mutagens are used to produce artificial mutations in sunflower [1].

The strongest chemical mutagens (supermutagens), which cause a several hundred-fold increase in the frequency of mutations, include ethyleneamine, diethyl sulfate, dimethyl sulfate, nitrosoethylurea, nitrosomethylurea, hydrogen peroxide, etc. [2].

Since Wetterer's first attempts to gamma-irradiate sunflower seeds in 1911, Shull and Mitchell's experiments in 1933 [3], Soldatov's achievements [4], reports of contemporary scientists Kalaydzhan [5], Lacombe [6], Soroka [7], Cvejic [8, 9], Lyakh [10], Vasin [11, 12], Kyrychenko [13], Škorić [14], and many others, a considerable progress have been achieved in enriching the sunflower gene pool by induced mutagenesis. However, despite considerable advances, due to continuous refreshment of starting material, induced mutagenesis has been and remains an important method for developing new and improving existent starting material in breeding.

Our purpose was to obtain self-pollinated sunflower lines with genetic mutations induced by chemical and physical mutagens that can be used to improve features of the sunflower crop and to develop methodological approaches for studying mutant generations.

2. Means and mechanisms of experimental mutation induction

When researchers obtain and control new hereditary changes in plants during their experiments, some completely new possibilities to create breeding initial material appear.

Since Watson and Crick decoded the structure of DNA, characterized the mechanism of its replication and discovered the system of recording genetic information, highlighting the genetic nature of mutations, it became evident that the primary cause of any mutation is the primary disorders in the DNA structure, which are in the process of cell metabolism can be realized in true mutations or repaired and restored to their original state.

Primary abnormalities induced in hereditary structures of an organism under the influence of natural or artificial factors can cause the appearance of two types of mutations—point ones, caused by disorders in the original structures of the DNA molecule, and chromosomal ones, caused by qualitative or quantitative changes in the chromosomal systems of cells.

Primary disorders in DNA structures are not repaired to their original state; they initiate the processes of gene (point) mutation formation. Such disorders include replacement of nitrogen base pairs (transversions); the inclusion of additional complementary pairs of nucleotides (duplication); loss of nucleotide pairs in the structure of a DNA molecule (deletions); 1800 rotation of nucleotide pairs (inversions), etc.

Initial DNA integrity disorders may result in chromosome rupture. In this case open sections of chromosomal filaments can be combined reaching their original state or form new combinations. Thus, there are chromosomal mutations that are characterized by a wide diversity.

Mutations can attach a molecule of sugar (deoxyribose), phosphate, or a nitrogenous base to the nucleotides. For example, despite the fact that deoxyribose is the only sugar group in DNA, it is not desirable to exclude the possibility of accidental incorporation of individual ribose molecules into DNA. In such cases, the phosphate and nitrogenous bases of the ribonucleotide may be like those of the dezoxyribonucleotides. Phosphoric acid, as a component of DNA and RNA, may contain radioactive P32 atom instead of a normal phosphorus one.

Disorders induced by irradiation in DNA molecules can affect phosphodiester, sugar-phosphate, glycosyl, and other chemical bonds. As a result, single or double-thread breaks occur, as well as the destruction of nitrogenous bases. For example, when dry seeds are irradiated, the nitrogenous bases included in the DNA structure may be converted in to thymine, guanine radicals, etc., which are sufficiently stable in the dry state and sufficiently reactive when wetted.

The alkylating compounds including DMS are a source to introduce the methyl radicals (CH_3), ethyl (C_2H_5), etc. into the molecules, thereby providing an alkylation reaction. They are characterized by a wide range of mutagenic effects, inducing simple and complex substitutions as well as breaks in DNA molecules. All nitrogenous bases, phosphoric acid residue, and even deoxyribose residue are alkylated. As a result of alkylation reactions, the purine bases are most likely to fall out DNA strand, causing the formation of voids at the corresponding points in the molecule. It is obvious that the mechanism of mutagenesis in the alkylation of DNA bases is associated with a violation in the accuracy of the auto-reproduction of DNA molecules.

All these events eventually result in changes within DNA molecules that manifest themselves as mutations, most of which are lethal. However, many mutations are viable. They are involved in the process of gene recombination, and as a result they are integrated in their functions with other genes of the genotype where they originated.

3. Research methodology: selection of starting material

The plant genotype has a significant effect on the specificity and level of mutations. Therefore, selection of starting material plays a significant role in obtaining valuable mutants. Generally, the best area-specific forms are recommended to use as sources, which need refining in terms of individual characteristics and features. Constant self-pollinated forms are the best for mutational breeding, as their mutations can be easily and reliably identified. Therefore, working with mutagenesis, one should apply different methods of isolation of nurseries and mutant plants in order to prevent biological contamination and occurrence, along with mutations, of possible recombinations.

Twelve new homozygous, self-pollinated sunflower lines from a genetic collection of the Plant Production Institute named after V.Ya. Yuriev, which are of breeding value and differ in several morphological and biochemical features, were taken as study objects.

Chemical supermutagen dimethyl sulfate (DMS) and gamma rays were used to induce genetic variability. Two hundred fifty seeds were used in each variant of treatment.

As to chemical mutagenesis, seeds in capron partly loosened sacs were soaked in 0.01 and 0.05% DMS solutions (prepared on distilled water, as some mutagens tend to degrade rapidly in tap water). We prepared these solutions under a hood, wearing rubber gloves: crushed an ampoule with mutagen in water. Depending on the object, the treatment time ranges 2–24 h. With sunflower seeds, the exposure was 18 hours, with periodic stirring. The mutagen/treated seeds ratio (volume/weight) was 10:1. In addition, to accelerate the process of solution penetration through the seed coat, it is recommended to ultrasound seeds for a short time (1–7 min) [15]. After treatment of seeds, in order to reduce the damaging effect, we washed them out for 1 h in running tap water and then sowed in soil on the same day.

Dimethyl sulfate (DMS) is a chemical supermutagen, an alkylating compound, which breaks chromosomes, leading to a large number of chromosomal inversions.

Studying physical mutagenesis on new sunflower lines, we used gamma rays from the radioactive isotope Co60, which has a relatively high irradiation uniformity. Dry seeds were once irradiated on a "Theratron Elit 80" Ionizing Radiation Source Cobalt 60 at Kharkiv Regional Oncology Hospital.

In a research on induced mutagenesis, a great attention is paid to concentrations (doses) of mutagens, which affect the number and quality of mutations; therefore, we used the most effective for agricultural crops DMS concentrations (0.01 and 0.05%) and doses of gamma rays (120 and 150 Gy).

Seeds of corresponding sunflower lines soaked in distilled water were used as controls.

When working with mutagens, which are poisonous and sometimes volatile, one should strictly follow the safety regulations and have appropriate equipment and rooms [16, 17].

4. Generation, evaluation, and further use of mutations: M_1 generation

Mutagen-treated seeds were sown in mutant nurseries: M_1 nursery (area = 20 m^2; single-row plots comprising 250 plants each), M_2 nursery (area = 40 m^2; single-row plots comprising 25 plants each), and M_3 nursery (area = 50 m^2; single-row plots comprising 25 plants each). The sowing scheme was 70 × 25 cm. Seeds were sown with manual planters within the optimal timeframe (2nd–3rd 10 days of May). Winter wheat was the forecrop. Mutant plants in the experimental plots were harvested by cutting and manually threshed.

We observed the expected decrease in the field germinability in the M_1 generation, and the higher concentration or dose of the mutagenic factor was, the more drastically the germinability is reduced. Our data indicate that the phenotypic effect of gamma rays is stronger than the DMS effect.

The highest frequency of phenotypic changes was noticed with 150 Gy gamma irradiation (42.9%); the frequency of phenotypic changes after DMS treatment was only 27–28%. The plant development was delayed and was followed by death. Among the DMS-treated plants, there were no such phenomena; therefore the used concentrations of this chemical are not lethal (**Table 1**).

Mutagenic factors affect biochemical processes in seeds, impairing metabolism and causing unnatural changes, which in its turn influences vital processes in seeds and plants emerging from them. Therefore, studies of microspore formation (meiosis) are a reliable way to investigate the genetic variability of organisms at the cellular level and to the evaluate effects of mutagenic factors on chromosomes of pollen mother cells (PMC) of sunflower lines.

Mutagen	Concentration (%)/dose (Gy)	Number of treated seeds	Number of plants from treated seeds	Number of phenotypically unchanged plants	Number of phenotypically changed plants	Phenotypic effect (%)
Control	No treatment	250	220	220	0	0.0
DMS	0.01	250	218	157	61	28.0
	0.05	250	208	152	56	27.0
Gamma rays	120	250	38	22	16	42.1
	150	250	28	16	12	42.9

Table 1.
Phenotype effect in the M_1 generation of sunflower (average across lines).

Microspores in anthers of flowering plants are the final result of meiosis, which can be traced on temporary and permanent microslides made from immature anthers.

The genotypes of the new self-pollinated lines—sterility fixers (Kh1002B and Kh1008B) and lines— pollen fertility restorers (Kh06134V and Kh201V) pre-treated with chemical mutagen DMS at concentrations of 0.01 and 0.05% or gamma-irradiated at doses of 120 and 150 Gy were studied.

The steps of microslide preparation to investigate chromosomes in sunflower meiosis were as follows:

1. Collection of specimens in the field—calathidium segments (d = 2–3 cm) with anthers. Green star phase.

2. Fixation of the specimens in Clark's solution (absolute alcohol/glacial acetic acid 3:1) for 24 h.

3. Washing out the specimens in 70% ethanol until the odor of acetic acid disappears.

4. Storage of the specimens in 70% ethanol.

5. Staining the specimens in 2% aceto-orcein for 12–24 h. Aceto-orcein solution was prepared as follows: dissolve 1 g of dye in 45 ml of glacial acetic acid and 55 ml of distilled water. Dissolution is carried out in a reflux flask in a water bath for 30–60 min. After cooling, the solution of aceto-orcein is filtered and placed in a glass stoppered bottle. As a part of the study, we demonstrated that aceto-orcein was more effective for staining sunflower chromosomes than acetocarmine.

6. The stained specimen is placed on a mount in a drop of 45% acetic acid or in a drop of 0.5% aceto-orcein, covered with a cover slip and heated above an alcohol burner until boiling.

7. The slide is carefully crushed with a match to get a cell monolayer under the glass and examined under a microscope.

Meiosis was examined under a Micromed XS-5520 microscope at magnification of 40× and 100×. Oil immersion (special immersion oil, cedar oil, or glycerol) was used to study slides at magnification of 100×. To document and illustrate the results, microphotographs were taken with a Nikon D 3200 kit VR camera equipped with a special Asian Microscope Adapter.

Cells with meiosis disorders were counted by metaphase-anaphase method: the percentage of cells with abnormalities was calculated related to the total number of cells under examination.

Analysis of meiosis in archisporial cells showed considerable effects of DMS and gamma rays on chromosomes in the M_1, which manifested themselves as occurrence of significant chromosomal aberrations compared to the control ($P < 0.99$). The effect level depended on the mutagen exposure.

For example, after DMS treatment, the percentage of cells with abnormalities ranged within 7–14% (0.01%) and 12–20% (0.05%), significantly exceeding the control. After gamma irradiation, the percentage of cells with abnormalities ranged within 16–19% (120 Gy) and 20–25% (150 Gy), significantly exceeding the control.

Comparison of the results showed that the effect of gamma rays on meiosis of the lines under investigation significantly differed ($P < 0.99$) from that of DMS. Gamma rays resulted in the occurrence of more abnormal tetrads in the M_1 compared to DMS treatment. After irradiation, the percentage of abnormal tetrads ranged from 16.00% in line Kh1008B (120 Gy) to 27.10% in line Kh201V (150 Gy), whereas in DMS - treated lines, the percentage of abnormal tetrads ranged from 1.55% in line Kh201V (0.01%) to 21.65% in line Kh1008B (0.05%).

We observed normalization of meiosis and elimination of cells with abnormalities in subsequent mutant generations of sunflower compared to the M_1.

In line Kh06134V, the percentage of cells with abnormalities in different phases of meiosis in the M_2 varied within 8.09–8.69% (0.01 and 0.05% DMS) and within 5.96–8.16% (120 and 150 Gy gamma irradiation). In the M_3, the percentage of aberrations varied within 3.36–4.09% after 0.01 and 0.05% DMS treatment and within 4.29–5.34% after 120 and 150 Gy gamma irradiation.

In line Kh201V, the percentage of cells with abnormalities in the M_2 varied within 4.53–8.45% after DMS treatment and within 7.79–9.48% after gamma irradiation. In the M_3, these values were 2.54–4.96 and 2.15–3.48%, respectively.

In line Kh1002B, the percentage of cells with abnormalities in the M_2 varied within 6.06–4.89% after DMS treatment and within 6.91–7.44% after gamma irradiation. In the M_3, these values were 3.35–4.66 and 3.60–4.83%, respectively.

In line Kh1008B, we noted 4.92–6.95% of cells with abnormalities in the M_2 after DMS treatment and 6.42–10.77% after gamma irradiation. In the M_3, these values were 2.15–3.57 and 3.09–5.26%, respectively (**Figure 1**).

The identified meiotic abnormalities in mutants were manifested as a chromosome lag during the formation of metaphase plate, impaired chromosome distribution in metaphase II, distorted metaphase plates, a chromosome lag in anaphase, asynchronous division during the second stage of meiosis, formation of pentads, triads, dyads, etc. (**Figure 2**).

Note. 1, outsider chromosomes in anaphase I; 2, asynchronous division during the second stage of meiosis; 3, chromosomes outside the metaphase plate in metaphase I; 4, abnormal tetrads.

All the specimens had phenotypic alterations (bent stem, dwarfism, absence of generative organs, chlorophyll deficit, deformation of generative organs, etc.) during subsequent development (**Figure 3**).

To prevent cross-pollination between different sunflower lines, individual inflorescences had been isolated the day before semiflorets opened, the offspring of which were to be examined the next year as the M_2 families. Concurrently, controls, non-treated with mutagens lines, were isolated.

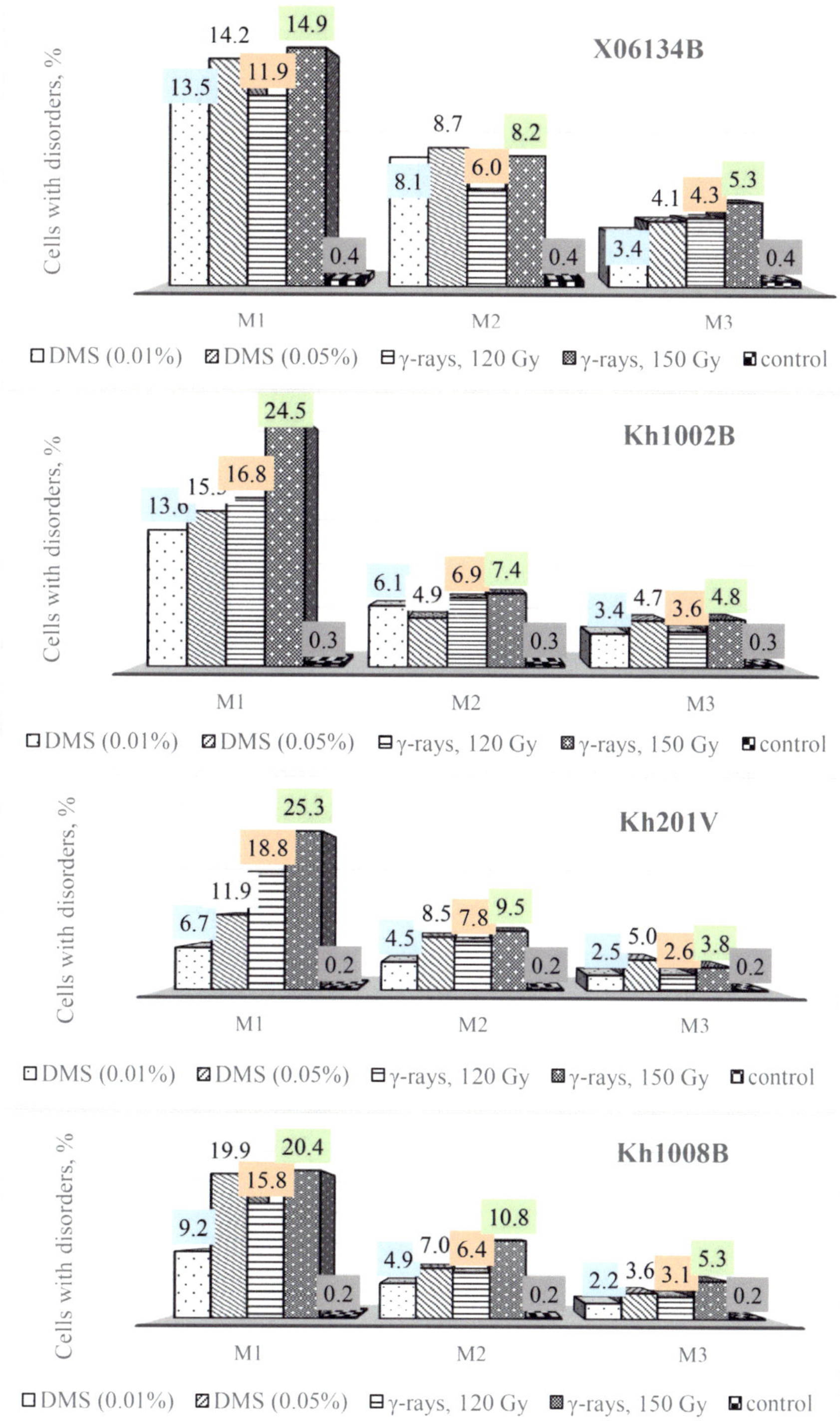

Figure 1.
Normalization of meiosis and gradual attenuation of the mutagenic effects of DMS and gamma rays in the M_1–M_3 sunflower (%).

During the vegetation period, phenological observations of the growth and development of mutant plants were conducted; the field germinability was determined; cytological analysis was performed; and biometric measurements were

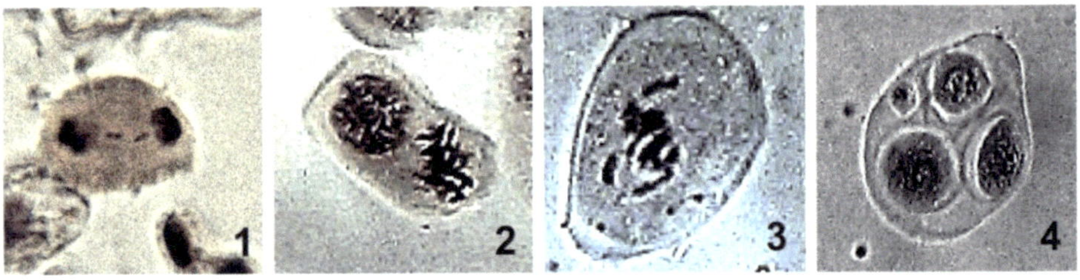

Figure 2.
Microphotographs of meiotic abnormalities in mutant generations of self-pollinated sunflower lines.

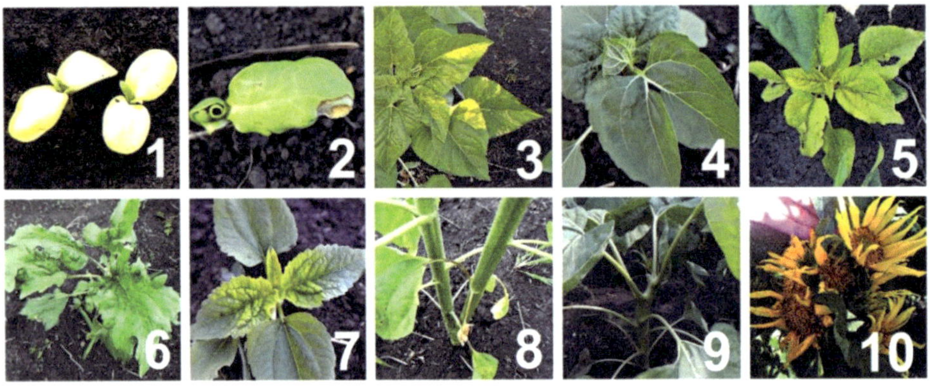

Figure 3.
Phenotypic effects of chemical and physical mutagens in the M_1 sunflower. 1, chlorophyll-deficient shoots from gamma-irradiated seeds (150 Gy); 2, 4, 6, morphoses induced by DMS (0.05%) in the early stages of plant development; 3, 5, 7, chlorophyll morphoses induced by DMS (0.05%); 10, deformation of generative organs induced by DMS (0.01%); 8, stem fasciation induced by DMS (0.05%); 9, absence of generative organs induced by gamma irradiation (120 Gy).

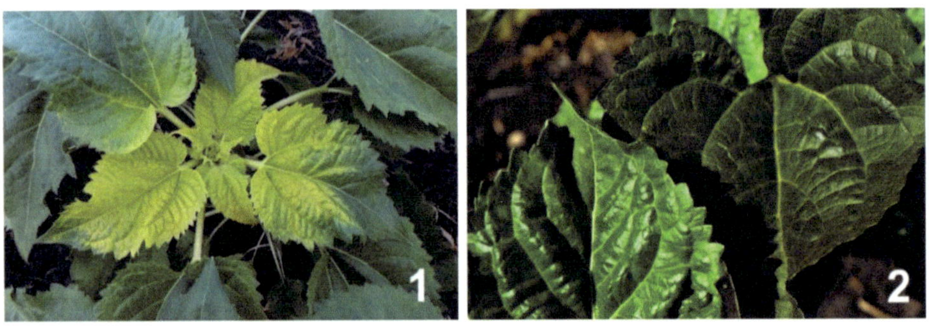

Figure 4.
Morphological changes observed in the M_1 of self-pollinated line Kh06134V: 1, xantha chlorophyll mutation 'golden tip' (0.05% DMS), and 2, "purple tint of leaves" mutation (0.01% DMS).

made (plant height measured 20 days after anthesis, calathidium diameter, and number of leaves per plant). Mutant plants were evaluated for the following parameters: oil content (%), 1000-seed weight, and fatty acid composition of oil.

In the M_1, there were a lot of plants with different phenotypic developmental defects compared to the controls. However, one should keep in mind that most of them were so-called morphoses and consequences of phenotypic variability; such changes are not inherited and disappear in M_2.

It is impossible to detect recessive mutations in M_1 plants, since of 2 alleles of a gene, as a rule, one allele only mutates, and the altered recessive allele is always paired with the unchanged dominant allele (AA–Aa); therefore, selection of mutations is started with M_2.

Only dominant mutations found by some researchers in some crops (usually in wheat) after exposure to chemical supermutagens can be detected in M_1. Thus, examining the M_1 of self-pollinated line Kh06134V, we distinguished some morphological changes: a chlorophyll-deficient mutation (xantha) called "golden top" (0.01% DMS) and a mutation of a purple tint of leaves (0.05% DMS), which is stably expressed in subsequent mutant generations (**Figure 4**).

5. M_2 and M_3 generations, investigation, and use of mutations

M_2 is sown by families and single plants or by continuous sowing according to variants of mutagenic treatment, with optimal convenient density.

Plants were selected in the second mutant generation by visible morphological and physiological alterations to obtain macromutants as well as well-developed plants without visible alterations to find biochemical mutations and micromutations of quantitative traits. In addition, seeds from families without changes in the M_2 were sampled to reveal them in the M_3.

Analysis of the mutant frequency in the M_2 showed that gamma rays (120 and 150 Gy) produced more plants with alterations than DMS (0.01 and 0.05%). The percentage of plants with alterations after gamma irradiation ranged 36.0–36.4%, while the percentage of plants with alterations after DMS treatment was within 9.6–9.8%. We noted the individual genotypic responses of the lines to the increase in the concentration and dose of mutagens. The rise in the number of plants with alterations in the M_2 depended on the increase in the concentration of DMS and the dose of gamma rays (**Table 2**).

In particular, in line Kh1002B, the total frequency of alterations was 3.2% with 0.01% DMS and 3.5% with 0.05% DMS, whereas plants with alterations were much more numerous with gamma rays (120 Gy–22.6%, 150 Gy–27.8%) (**Table 2**).

0.01% DMS-treated line Kh06134V gave the total frequency of plants with alterations of 14.7%, and the total frequency of plants with alterations after 0.05% DMS treatment was 10.0%. Gamma irradiation produced significantly more plants with alterations: 120 Gy produced 36.6% of plants with alterations, and 150 Gy–47.5% (**Table 2**).

In line Kh1334V, the total frequency of plants with alterations was 3.4 and 3.3% with 0.01 and 0.05% DMS, respectively (**Table 2**).

0.01 and 0.05% DMS produced 8.9 and 13.1% of plants with alterations, respectively, in line Kh201V. However, the effect of gamma rays was more conspicuous, and the total frequency of plants with alterations was 32.1 and 37.5% after 120 and 150 Gy exposure, respectively (**Table 2**).

Most of the alterations observed in the M_2 of the gamma-irradiated lines were nonheritable modifications found in early stages of the plant development, which disappeared during growth, whereas most of the DMS-induced alterations detected in different stages of the plant development were stable. The mutation nature of the changes in the M_2 was finally established by inheritance in the M_3 families.

We studied inheritance of mutant traits in the M_3 and subsequent generations. We also assessed the new mutant lines for breeding value and tested them for economically valuable traits, intending to involve constant valuable forms in hybridization and heterosis breeding in order to obtain new sunflower hybrids.

Having evaluated the alterations, we identified mutants noticeable for oil content in seeds, fatty acid composition of oil, 1000-seed weight, and resistance to the pathogen of sunflower downy mildew.

Original line	Mutagen concentration/ dose	The total frequency of mutations (%)	Frequency of chlorophyll mutations (%)	Frequency of morphological mutations (%)	Frequency of economically valuable mutations (%)
Kh1002B	0.01% DMS	3.2	0.6	1.5	1.13
	0.05% DMS	3.5	0.9	2.1	0.6
	120 Gy γ-rays	22.6	10.7*	7.1*	4.8
	150 Gy γ-rays	27.8*	2.8	13.9	11.1*
	LSD 05	1.5	0.8	1.0	0.8
Kh06134V	0.01% DMS	10.0	1.9	3.3	4.7
	0.05% DMS	14.7*	3.5	5.9	5.3
	120 Gy γ-rays	36.6	3.3	20.0	13.3*
	150 Gy γ-rays	47.5*	16.4*	21.3	9.8
	LSD 05	4.6	2.6	3.3	3.0
Kh1334V	0.01% DMS	3.4	0.6	1.5	1.3
	0.05% DMS	3.3	1.7*	0.7	0.9
	LSD 05	1.4	0.8	0.8	0.8
Kh201V	0.01% DMS	8.9	2.0	4.1	2.9
	0.05% DMS	13.1*	4.4*	5.0	3.7
	120 Gy γ-rays	32.1	5.2	18.7	8.2
	150 Gy γ-rays	37.5*	8.6*	18.4	10.5*
	LSD 05	4.1	2.2	3.1	1.6
Average across 12 lines					
DMS	0.01%	9.6	3.1	3.7	2.8
	0.05%	9.8	3.2	3.8	2.8
γ-rays	120 Gy	36.0	11.3	16.3	8.3
	150 Gy	36.4	8.2	18.9	9.3

* *Difference significant at LSD 05.*

Table 2.
Relative frequencies of major mutations induced by DMS and gamma rays in the M_2 sunflower, % (exemplified by 4 lines).

The traits of 1000-seed weight and oil content in seeds followed different patterns, depending on the genotypes of the self-pollinated lines. Thus, in the M_3 there were genotypes, in which DMS treatment and gamma irradiation increased the content of oil in seeds (Od973B, Kh1002B, Mkh845B, X0816B, Kh06135V, Kh1334V, and Kh201V) and 1000-seed weight (Kh808B, Kh1002B, Mkh845B, Kh0816V, Kh785V, Kh1334V, and Kh201V). On the whole, 1000-seed weight insignificantly varied in the M_3 (2–10%).

The mutants with increased content of oil in seeds are listed below: Kh1002B No 224 (0.05% DMS), 50%, and No 876 (150 Gy gamma rays), 48% (46% in the control); Kh0816V No. 422 (0.01% DMS), 50% (53% in the control); Kh1334V No. 609 (0.01% DMS), 48%, and No. 658 (0.05% DMS), 46% (43% in the control); and Kh201V No 685 (0.01% DMS), 54%, and No 1143 (150 Gy gamma rays), 52% (48% in the control) (**Figure 5**).

The mutants with increased 1000-seed weight are listed below: Mkh845B No. 385 (0.05% DMS), 64 g; No. 996 (150 Gy gamma rays), 67 g (48 g in the control);

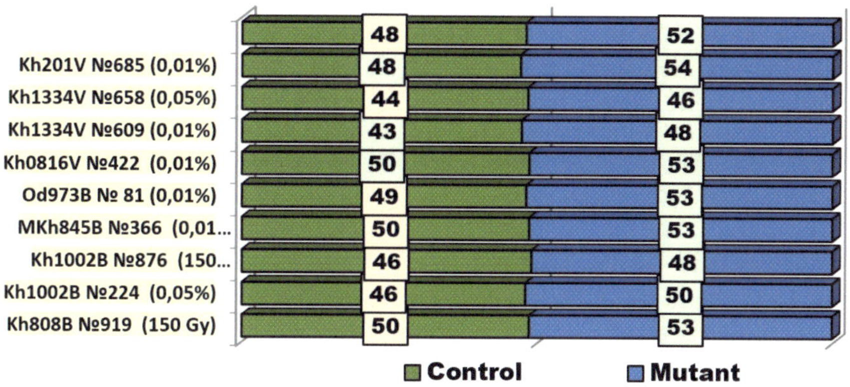

Figure 5.
Oil content in seeds of the mutant families (%).

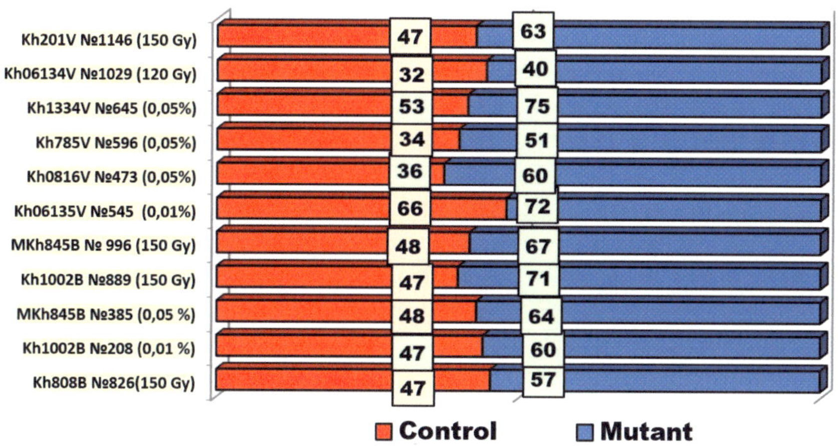

Figure 6.
1000-seed weight in the mutant families (g).

Kh06134V No. 1029 (120 Gy gamma rays), 40 g (32 g in the control); Kh785V No. 596 (0.05% DMS), 51 g (34 g in the control); Kh1334V No. 645 (0.05% DMS), 75 g (53 g in the control); and Kh201V No 1146 (150 Gy gamma rays), 63 g (47.1 g in the control) (**Figure 6**).

Biochemical analysis of oil from mutant sunflower seeds highlighted plants with increased content of linoleic acid of up to 70% (63% in the control) from line Kh201V. Among the mutants obtained from line Kh1334V, there were DMS-induced variants with increased contents of oleic and behenic acids (0.85% vs. 0.64% in the control), and such a combination is valuable for breeding (**Table 3**).

6. Conclusions

As exemplified by the M_1–M_3 mutant generations of sunflower, an important scientific challenge of determining peculiarities of the variability of quantitative and qualitative traits under the influence of DMS (0.01 and 0.05%) and gamma rays (120 and 150 Gy) was theoretically described, and a new solution to it was suggested. The frequency and range of mutational variability in the M_2 were summarized, and the inheritance of the mutant traits in subsequent generations was established. Chromosomal abnormalities in meiosis were characterized, and the

Original line	Mutant	Mutagen, (concentration/dose)	Palmitic	Palmitoleic	Stearic	Oleic	Linoleic	Linolenic	Behenic
			C16:0	C16:1	C18:0	C18:1	C18:2	C18:3	C22:0
Kh201V		Control	6.67	0.47	3.87	25.34	62.75	0.28	0.24
	№742	DMS, 0.05%	6.40	0.41	4.95	16.72	70.79	0.15	0.37
	№694	DMS, 0.01%	6.71	0.56	4.00	25.34	62.85	0.13	0.21
	№1133	γ-rays, 120 Gy	7.25	0.80	3.47	17.55	70.54	0.12	0.11
Kh1334V		Control	3.43	0.11	3.78	87.28	3.51	0.35	0.64
	№659	DMS, 0.05%	3.29	0.11	3.54	89.10	2.00	0.30	0.85
	№642	DMS, 0.05%	3.71	0.12	3.52	88.48	2.15	0.30	0.85
	№628	DMS, 0.01%	3.83	0.17	3.85	87.25	2.75	0.47	0.84
	№609	DMS, 0.01%	3.54	0.15	3.40	86.90	3.92	0.35	0.83

Table 3.
Fatty acid composition of oil from the M_3 sunflower seeds.

breeding-genetic values of induced mutations as well as possibilities of their use in breeding were evaluated. Methodological peculiarities of the mutational breeding of sunflower as a cross-pollinated crop were defined, and new mutants with changed features were detected. In addition, this study allowed us to conclude that DMS was more effective than gamma rays for the induction of valuable for breeding mutations in new homozygous self-pollinated sunflower lines.

Thus, induced mutagenesis is a major component of the complex breeding process of creation of new parental lines and hybrids of sunflower with economically valuable characteristics.

Author details

Victoria Mykhailenko[1]*, Viktor Kyrychenko[2], Alexander Bragin[1] and Dmitry Chuiko[1]

1 Department of Genetics, Selection and Seed Production, Faculty of Agronomy, Kharkiv National Agrarian University Named after V.V. Dokuchayev, Kharkiv, Ukraine

2 Plant Production Institute Named after V.Ya. Yuryev of NAAS of Ukraine, Kharkiv, Ukraine

*Address all correspondence to: toryvasko@gmail.com

References

[1] Olsen O, Wang X, Von Wettstein D. Sodium azide mutagenesis: Preferential generation of A.T--> G.C transitions in the barley antl8 gene. Proceedings of the National Academy of Sciences of the United States of America. 1993;**90**(17):8043-8047

[2] Maliuta SS. Mutagenesis. In: Ecological Encyclopedia: 3 volumes. K.: TOV "Tsentr Ekolohichnoi Osvity ta Informatsii"; 2007. p. 321. (in Ukrainian)

[3] Berezina NM. Pre-sowing irradiation of seeds of agricultural plants. In: Corresponding Member of AS USSR A.M. Kuzin. Moscow: Agropromizdat; 1964. pp. 188-189. (in Russian)

[4] Soldatov KI. Chemical mutagenesis in sunflower breeding. In: Proceeding 7th Internat. Sunflower Conf. 1976. pp. 352-357

[5] Kalaydzhan AA. Chemical mutagenesis in sunflower breeding: Author's abstract of the thesis for a Candidate Degree in Agricultural Sciences: Specialty 06.01.05 "Breeding and Seed Production"; Krasnodar. 1998. 48 p. (in Russian)

[6] Lacombe S. A dominant mutation for high oleic acid content in sunflower (*Helianthus annuus* L.) seed is genetically linked to a single oleate-desaturase RFLP locus. Molecular Breeding. 2001;**8**(2):129-137. DOI: 10.1023/A:1013358711651

[7] Soroka AI. Mutational variability in sunflower after exposure of immature corcules to mutagen. Nauk.-Tekhn. Biul. Instytutu Oliinykh Kultur. 2013;**18**:19-24. (in Russian)

[8] Cvejic S. Radio sensitivity of sunflower restorer lines to different mutagenic treatments. In: Proceed. 5th Confer. of Young Scientists and Specialists; Krasnodar. 2009. pp. 255-259

[9] Cvejić S. Mutation breeding for changed quality in sunflower. In: Cvejić S, Miladinović D, Jocić S, editors. Mutagenesis: Exploring Genetic Diversity of Crops. Wageningen, Netherlands: Wageningen Academic Publishers; 2014. pp. 3379-3388

[10] Lyakh V. Influence of mature and immature sunflower seed treatment with ethylmethanesulphonate on mutation spectrum and frequency. Helia. 2005;**28**(43):87-98

[11] Vasin VA. Genetic variability in sunflower after exposure of mature and immature seeds to ethylmethane sulfonate: Author's abstract of the thesis for a Candidate Degree in Agricultural Sciences: Specialty: 03.00.15; Kyiv. 2008. 48 p. (in Ukrainian)

[12] Vasin VA. Effect of ethylmethane sulfonate exposure of mature and immature seeds of sunflower on the frequency and assortment of mutations in the M_2. Fiziologiya i Biokhimiya Kulturnykh Rasteniy. 2006;**38**(1):34-44. (in Russian)

[13] Kyrychenko VV. Chemical mutagens and improvement of sunflower lines. Selekthiia i Nasinnytstvo.1988;**80**:19-22. (in Ukrainian)

[14] Škorić D et al. Sunflower genetics and breeding: International monography. Novi Sad: Serbian Academy of Sciences and Arts, Branch. 2012;XV:520s

[15] Lysikov VN. Results of using chemical mutagens for breeding and genetic studies on maize in Moldaviya. In: Mutational Breeding. M.: Nauka; 1968. pp. 58-62. (in Russian)

[16] Zoz NN. Methods of using chemical mutagens in agricultural crop breeding.

In: Mutational Breeding. M.: Nauka; 1968. pp. 23-27. (in Russian)

[17] Artemchuk IP. Effects of mutagen exposure on the mutation frequency in winter wheat. Fiziologiya i Biokhimiya Kulturnykh Rasteniy. 2003;**3**:222-228. (in Ukrainian)

Chapter 4

Nefarious, but in a Different Way: Comparing the Ecotoxicity, Gene Toxicity and Mutagenicity of Lead (Pb) and Cadmium (Cd) in the Context of Small Mammal Ecotoxicology

Peter Vladislavov Ostoich, Michaela Beltcheva and Roumiana Metcheva

Abstract

Lead and cadmium are long established toxic and carcinogenic metals. Still, the mechanisms of their interaction with eukaryotic DNA are not unequivocally understood. New data provide evidence on the influence of both metals on DNA repair, particularly non-homologous end joining (NHEJ) and mismatch repair (MMR). This may help explain the weak direct mutagenicity of both Pb^{2+} and Cd^{2+} ions in the Ames test, as opposed to the proven carcinogenicity of both metals; it has long been proposed that lead and cadmium may induce an imbalance in mammalian systems of DNA damage repair and promote genomic instability. While new evidence for mechanistic interactions of metals with DNA repair emerges, some of the old questions involving dose distribution, pathways of exposure and bioaccumulation/detoxification kinetics still remain valid. To help place the current state of the art in the genetic toxicology of lead and cadmium within the context of ecotoxicology, the current authors propose an integrative approach and offer a review of other authors' work as well as some of their own data on systemic and organ-specific toxicities in laboratory mice. The current chapter is a comparative analysis of the state of the art in the specific toxicity and genotoxicity of Pb and Cd, presenting some new and little-known information.

Keywords: lead (Pb), cadmium (Cd), genotoxicity, ecotoxicology, physiological reactions, DNA damage and repair, cell signaling, laboratory mice

1. Introduction

The last several decades have seen an increase in scientific and public interest in the problem of environmental contamination as a consequence of human activities. A wide variety of chemicals is released into the environment from different sources, either intentionally or as a result of accidents, prompting widespread concern about the effects of anthropogenic contamination on the biota. While many organic pollutants such as pesticides and petroleum refining products are subject to environmental degradation by physical, chemical, or biological pathways, heavy metals and their compounds typically retain their toxicity over long periods of time. Recently, important advances have been made in the understanding of the gene toxicity and mutagenicity of heavy metals in the environment [1–6]. For instance, it has been established that the gene toxicity of lead (Pb^{2+}) and cadmium (Cd^{2+}) ions is not due to direct DNA-metal interactions [2, 3]. It has been demonstrated that Cd^{2+} affects DNA repair pathways, particularly the non-homologous end joining (NHEJ) of DNA double-strand breaks (DSBs) at very low concentrations (<30 μmol) in several *in vitro* test systems [4, 5]. Nevertheless, some questions regarding the gene toxicity and mutagenicity of lead and cadmium remain open. For instance, several authors have noted that *in vivo* test systems are much more sensitive than *in vitro* systems (i.e., cell cultures) with respect to lead-induced endpoints for genotoxicity assessment (chromosomal aberrations, micronuclei, sister chromatid exchanges, comet assay endpoints) [7, 8]. In practice this means that animal models, especially rodents, are much more suitable for analysis of the genotoxicity of Pb^{2+} than cell cultures. When considering cadmium, useful mechanistic data on mutagenicity and co-mutagenicity has been obtained with *in vitro* test systems [4, 5]. Still, the question of the importance of Cd^{2+} as genotoxic agent in living mammalian organisms remains open. One study has reported lead-induced genomic instability in the progeny of mice exposed to Pb^{2+} *in utero* [9]. It is still unclear if this phenomenon has been observed by other authors and how common heavy metal-induced genomic instability is. If parental exposure to toxic metals can influence the stability of the genome in subsequent generations, this is potentially very alarming and could influence the current standards and permissible limits for occupational and environmental exposure. Last but not least, toxic metals seldom occur alone in contaminated sites. For instance, non-ferrous metal smelters typically emit a cocktail of toxic chemical elements in the atmosphere. This means that an accurate environmental risk assessment should be performed on a case-by-case basis, and that both ecotoxicological biomonitoring, and more general attempts to resolve the problem of heavy metal genotoxicity and mutagenicity, should be concerned not with a single toxicant but rather a plurality of different toxic agents present in a given locality. A number of studies have been performed with wild rodents exposed environmentally to complex contamination including Pb^{2+} and Cd^{2+} [10–23]. While these studies include endpoints for scoring genetic damage (chromosomal aberrations, micronuclei, comet tail length and tail moment) relatively little is understood about the molecular mechanisms underpinning the genotoxicity of complex mixtures of toxic metals.

In summary, from the perspective of ecotoxicology, it is well-established that Cd^{2+} and Pb^{2+} are genotoxic metal ions, especially in complex organisms. At the same time, knowledge about the mechanisms for heavy metal genotoxicity is scarce, with anecdotal evidence for interactions with DNA repair systems in complex vertebrate organisms, and relatively little knowledge of how the gene toxicity of Pb^{2+} and Cd^{2+} fits into the bigger picture of the specific physiological reactions of terrestrial vertebrates to toxic metals. For the purposes of the current study, the main questions regarding lead and cadmium gene toxicity are the following:

1. What are the specific molecular mechanisms, responsible for the gene toxicity of Pb^{2+} and Cd^{2+}? How does intoxication with heavy metals lead to detectable chromosomal damage and mutagenesis? What are the similarities and differences when considering the gene toxicity of lead and cadmium?

2. Can we draw conclusions about the comprehensive biological effects of heavy metals? For instance, it has long been established that terrestrial vertebrates respond to Pb^{2+} and Cd^{2+} by increased expression of detoxifying proteins (metallothioneins) and increased biosynthesis of glutathione. While there is evidence for adaptive responses, how does this apply to genetic damage induced by heavy metals?

3. What are the effects of complex environmental pollution? How do complex mixtures of metallic toxicants affect organisms?

4. Last but not least, what are the prospects, challenges, and potential answers from future studies dealing with the gene toxicity of Pb^{2+} and Cd^{2+}?

In order to provide, in part, answers to these four questions, the current study aims to analyze the state-of-the-art in what is known about the genotoxicity of lead and cadmium within the context of ecotoxicology. The current authors have employed a wide scope of sources in order to synthesize what is currently known and understood about the gene toxicity of Pb^{2+} and Cd^{2+}, and conduct a comparative analysis of the two metals. In addition, insight and information is provided from a personal set of sources and experience, which are not widely publicized. Finally, the current article discusses several potential directions for future studies in the gene toxicity of heavy metals and proposes an integrated, trans-disciplinary approach to solving the problems, associated with the ecotoxicity and gene toxicity of Pb^{2+} and Cd^{2+}.

2. Lead (Pb)

2.1 Ecotoxicity, bioaccumulation patterns, and specific organ toxicities

Lead (Pb) is present in the Earth's crust at comparatively low concentrations (0.121 ppb) and has four stable isotopes (^{204}Pb, ^{206}Pb, ^{107}Pb, and ^{208}Pb) [24]. Although a comparatively rare metal, it has been historically one of the first industrially mined chemical elements. Contemporary sources estimate annual primary production of lead to be 4.6 million metric tons [25]. While Pb has been released in the atmosphere during manufacturing processes and combustion of fossil fuels, leading to global trace contamination, the main concern has been strong local contamination in the vicinity of mining, refining and smelting processes, as well as localized accidental releases. The toxicity of lead has been suspected since ancient times, with authors arguing mass poisoning from the metal in Ancient Rome due to its use for water pipes, glassmaking, and in winemaking processes [26]. Contemporary ecotoxicological research is concerned mainly with local contamination with Pb, with several important impact sites identified in Europe: Bukowno in Poland, Nitra, Slovakia, Asenovgrad, Bulgaria, and the Coto Doñana area in Spain [12, 15, 16, 18, 19, 22, 27–29]. The studies in these areas have dealt mainly with biomonitor species of wild rodents, and have investigated bioaccumulation of lead and other toxic metals, as well as endpoints for the determination of gene toxicity. Regardless of the zoomonitor used (typically, the wood mouse, *Apodemus sylvaticus*, yellow-necked mouse, *Apodemus flavicollis*, bank vole, *Myodes glareolus*, common vole, *Microtus arvalis*, Algerian mouse, *Mus spretus*), similar tendencies for bioaccumulation of Pb in the organisms of small mammals have been detected, and often correlated with the induction of genetic damage (chromosome aberrations, micronuclei). These studies have demonstrated significant effects of heavy metal contamination on the biota, and have proven the importance of continuing monitoring studies in contaminated ecosystems.

The biokinetics and specific organ and tissue toxicities of Pb have been actively investigated in animal models since the late 1950s, initially employing radioactive tracer isotopes such as ^{203}Pb and ^{210}Pb [30, 31]. This has led to the development of several biokinetic models for the metal in mammalian organisms [31–33]. The Harley-Kneip six-compartent model, developed with the use of primates, is considered to be one of the first informative biokinetic models for lead absorption, distribution and elimination (**Figure 1**).

As evident from the model, a significant percentage of ingested lead (~80%) is excreted without being absorbed by the gut. At the same time, the coefficient for absorption from the bloodstream into bone λ_{12} = 0.34–0.11 is significantly higher than the coefficient for release of Pb from the bones into the bloodstream (λ_{21} = 1.73 x 10^{-3}). In practice, this means that once a significant amount of lead is absorbed into the bones, it is practically impossible to eliminate it. The Harley-Kneip model also emphasizes the differences between juvenile and adult organisms, with juvenile animals much more susceptible to lead bioaccumulation [32]. To a varying level, Pb is also absorbed in the liver, kidneys, and the nervous system. It has been established that, in mammalian organisms, if the metal reaches sustained blood levels above 80 μg/dL, practically every organ and system is affected [24].

The primary targets for lead intoxication are the hematopoietic system, the nervous system and the liver. At sustained blood levels above 50 μg/dL, Pb inhibits

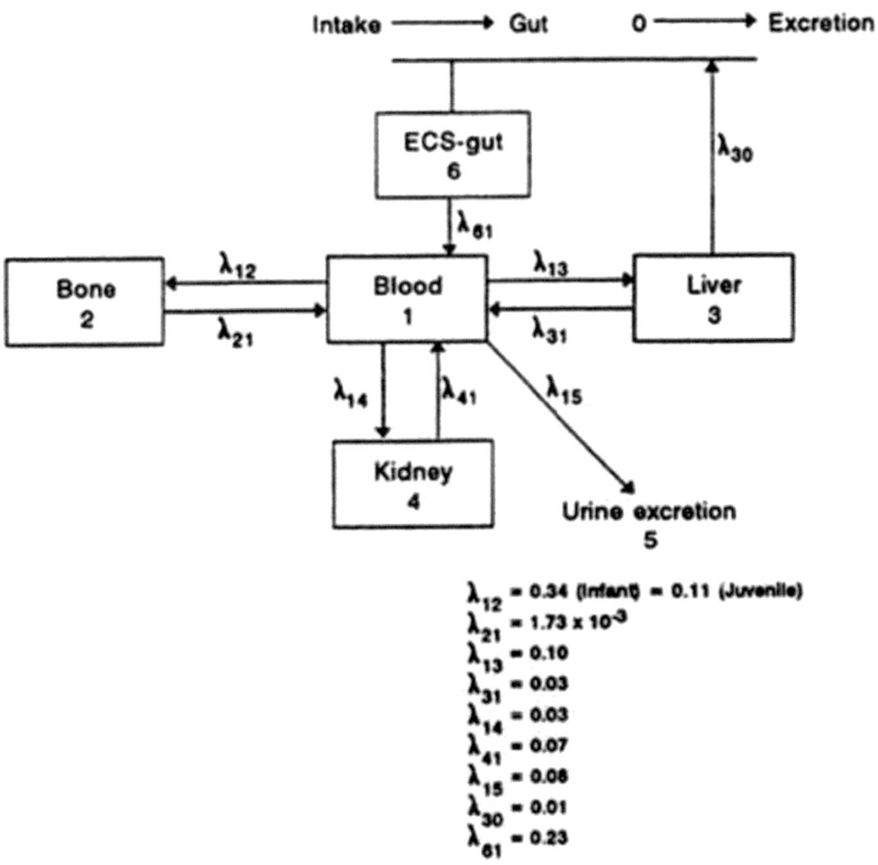

Figure 1.
Biokinetic model for the metabolism of lead in mammalian organisms [32].

the enzymes delta-aminolevulinic acid dehydratase (ALAD) and ferrochelatase, leading to impaired erythrocyte biogenesis, disturbances in erythrocyte kinetics, and anemia [34]. Several authors report an inhibition of the immune system at blood levels above 50 μg/dL, as well as histopathological lesions in the bone marrow at levels exceeding 100 μg/dL [23, 35, 36]. Death from anemia occurs at blood levels above 150 μg/dL. The nervous system is particularly sensitive in young individuals, and it has been established that Pb levels in blood exceeding 18 μg/dL lead to cognitive disturbances; it has been reported that very low doses cause neuronal apoptosis in rats [37]. In cases of chronic and sub-chronic lead intoxication, there is significant liver damage. Macroscopically, the liver increases in size; steatosis, hyperplasia and disruption of the liver microvasculature, as well as focal necrosis, have been observed at doses above 40 μg/dL, with marked changes in the activity of alanine and aspartate transaminase (ALT, and AST) and kidney damage [8].

2.2 Gene toxicity and mutagenicity

Due to low direct mutagenicity levels in the Ames test, lead (Pb) was initially thought not to be directly mutagenic [38]. Nevertheless, evidence soon accumulated that the metal was responsible for producing chromosomal aberrations in occupationally exposed workers and environmentally exposed human populations [31, 35]. Since the 1970s different *in vitro* and *in vivo* studies have been conducted regarding the potential of lead compounds to damage genomic DNA in mammals. The table below presents several informative studies conducted on the gene toxicity of lead using different *in vitro* test systems and endpoints, arranged chronologically (**Table 1**).

The studies cited provide evidence that lead is mutagenic and clastogenic under certain circumstances. While older studies show relatively weak clastogenicity of Pb when considering chromosomal aberrations [39, 40], newer publications report genotoxicity by using more sensitive endpoints, such as the induction of sister chromatid exchanges (SCE), tail length in the comet assay, and induction of γH2AX foci, indicating DNA double-strand breaks [6, 43, 44]. It should be noted that the study indicating the highest toxicity of Pb, uses lead chromate ($PbCrO_4$), which means its effects could be due to the inherent gene toxicity of hexavalent chromium [44].

Several authors have noted the greater sensitivity of *in vivo* test systems when studying the gene toxicity of lead [7, 9]. For the purposes of the current study, several sources dealing with *in vivo* models have been selected (**Table 2**).

It should be noted that, in contrast to *in vitro* test systems not almost all tests with Pb administration to living animals show evidence for genotoxic effects. Not only that, some authors have noted a very close dose dependence of effects on Pb concentrations in living organisms, as well as trans-generational accumulation of chromosomal aberrations after exposure of mice *in utero* [9]. From the viewpoint of ecotoxicology, this means that the risks from environmental exposure to lead compounds are often underestimated when using *in vitro* test systems and only *in vivo* models can provide an accurate assessment of genetic risk to the biota.

Much discussion has taken place concerning the molecular mechanisms of Pb-induced genetic damage. For instance, in the last two decades it has been accepted that lead interferes with the mechanisms for DNA repair, which is evident with studies analyzing Pb as a co-mutagen with other agents such as UV light, X-rays and methylnitronitrosoguanidine (MNNG) [50]. While it is accepter that the metal can inhibit DNA repair, the mechanisms of DNA damage induction *per se* are not well understood. For instance, it has been conclusively demonstrated that Pb and Cd do not interact with DNA directly under physiological conditions [3]. On the other hand, other authors have noted that Pb and other toxic metals can

Authors	Substance tested	Test system	Dose	Exposure	Endpoint	Effect
Bauchinger and Schmid [39]	Lead acetate	CHO cells	10^{-6} to 10^{-3} M	16 h	CA	No effect, except for increase of gaps
Gasiorek and Bauchinger [40]	Lead acetate	lymphocytes	10^{-3} to 10^{-5} M	3 h	CA	No effect
Hartwig et al. [41]	Lead acetate	CH V79 cells	0.5–10 μM	44 h	HPRT mutation	Co-mutagenicity with UV light
					SCE	Increase in SCE
Cai and Arenaz [42]	Lead nitrate	CHO AA8 cells	10^{-6} to 10^{-8} M	48–60 h	CA	No effect
					SCE	Increase in SCE
Wozniak and Blasiak [43]	Lead acetate	lymphocytes	1–100 μM	1 h	Comet assay	Increase in tail length and % tail DNA
Xie et al. [44]	Lead chromate	lung fibroblasts	0.1–5 μM	24–48 h	CA	Increase of % metaphases with damage
					Comet assay	Increased % tail DNA
					γH2AX foci	Dose-dependent increase of γH2AX foci
Pottier et al. [6]	Lead nitrate	EJ30 carcinoma	30–1000 μM	24 h	γH2AX foci	Dose-dependent increase of γH2AX foci
					Telomere score	Telomere instability

Table 1.
Exemplary studies on the genotoxicity of lead compounds in vitro.

induce a pro-oxidative state in living organisms at comparatively low concentrations (<30–50 μmol) [50, 51]. In summary, it can be said that the genotoxicity of lead works at the following levels:

1. Induction of reactive oxygen species (ROS) by Fenton-like reactions; inhibition of key enzymes like glutathione-S-transferase (GST); disruption of lysosomal membranes and induction of apoptosis [51].

2. Induction of genomic DNA damage; inhibition of key DNA repair systems such as base excision repair (BER) and disruption of telomere maintenance [6].

3. Mutagenesis, clastogenesis, tumor initiation and promotion, increase in the levels of apoptosis in some tissues, reproductive toxicity, organ and system toxicities [37].

While the basics of lead genotoxicity have been confirmed, and the metal has been confirmed as reproductively toxic and carcinogenic in mammalian species,

Authors	Substance tested	Test system	Dose	Exposure	Endpoint	Effect
Muro and Goyer [45]	Lead acetate	a/SW mice	1% Pb in food	2 weeks	CA	Increase in CA
Deknudt et al. [46]	Lead acetate	*Macaca fascicularis*	1–15 mg/kg Pb in food	3–16 months	CA	Increase in CA
Sharma et al. [47]	Lead acetate	ICR mice	50–200 mg/kg PB intraperitoneally	Injection	SCE	Increase in SCE
Robbiano et al. [48]	Lead acetate	Sprague-Dawley rats	117 mg/kg in food	3 days	MN test	Increase in MN frequency
Valverde et al. [49]	Lead acetate	CD-1 mice	0.01–1 μM	Inhalation, 3 days	Comet assay	Increase in tail length
Yuan and Tang [9]	Lead acetate	Kunming mice	1 mg/l in drinking water	90 days	Comet assay	Increase in tail length
Tapisso et al. [21]	Lead acetate	*Mus spretus*	21.5 mg/kg Pb in food	17 days	MN test	Increase in MN frequency
					SCE	Increase in SCE

Table 2.
Exemplary studies on the genotoxicity of lead compounds in vivo.

much remains to be investigated regarding the molecular mechanisms of the interactions of Pb^{2+} with mammalian DNA repair systems.

3. Cadmium (Cd)

3.1 Ecotoxicity, bioaccumulation patterns, and specific organ toxicities

Cadmium (Cd) is a malleable, silvery-white metal present in the Earth's crust in concentrations of 01–0.5 ppm, having five stable isotopes (^{108}Cd, ^{110}Cd, ^{111}Cd, ^{112}Cd, and ^{114}Cd) [24]. Discovered as a separate element within zinc ores in 1817, it is a toxicant, associated primarily with the late industrial age. Mined at a large scale since the 1920s, the metal is currently produced at a level of 23,000–24,000 metric tons per year [25]. Similarly to lead, the main concern regarding Cd-associated contamination is local pollution of terrestrial and riverine ecosystems. The toxicity of cadmium was discovered after the start of its extraction from polymetallic ores, with one example being the "itai-itai" disease in the Toyama prefecture of Japan, attributed after 1950 to Cd poisoning [52]. In Europe sites, severely polluted with cadmium are comparatively rare. One exception is the area of Bukowno in Poland, where there is significant local contamination [16, 53, 54]. Several studies deal with the ecotoxicity of Cd with the use of zoomonitors (mainly yellow-necked mice, *Ap. flavicollis* and bank voles, *M. glareolus*, but also the common magpie, *Pica pica*) [53, 54]. While in Europe the element is mostly present as a trace contaminant in cases of polymetallic pollution, the main concern for cadmium contamination are the countries where most of it is mined and produced, namely China, South Korea, Japan, Mexico, Canada and Kazakhstan.

The toxicity of cadmium was discovered after animal studies in the period 1955–1970 [52, 55, 56]. In mammalian organisms, the metal affects primarily the kidneys, liver, pancreas, and, at higher levels, the nervous system [55]. As an established IARC Group 1 carcinogen, Cd increases the risk of lung cancer at low doses, and causes pneumonitis and lung edema at higher doses [52]. Nevertheless, the main target organ for chronic Cd intoxication are the kidneys, where the metal is accumulated, causing proteinuria, hypophosphatemia, histopathological changes in the kidney tissue, and loss of kidney function [57]. High chronic and sub-chronic dose burdens cause histopathological changes in the liver [58, 59]. Due to its antagonistic and antimetabolic activity against necessary elements such as Zn, Cu, and Ca, as well as its interference with a variety of DNA-binding enzymes, cadmium is considered toxic at high levels to all organs and systems [24, 57]. Unlike Pb, which has a strong tendency for bioaccumulation in the animal organism, Cd has higher rates of clearance from mammalian organisms due to the action of metallothionein (MT) proteins—low molecular-weight, highly conserved molecules, which bind non-specifically to dietary elements such as Zn, Se, Cu, as well as toxic elements like Cd, Hg, Ag, As, and, to a much lesser extent, Pb [54, 60]. Metallothioneins bind Cd^{2+} ions in mammals, form Cd-MT complexes, which are excreted through the kidneys, thereby detoxifying, to some extent, low levels of cadmium. Nevertheless, although this system is inducible and upregulated by the presence of toxic metals in the body, it gets saturated at high doses, being unable to compensate high dose burdens of toxic metals [54]. Due to the inefficiency of existing biological detoxication systems, as well as the tendency of the metal for bioaccumulation in plants and animals, Cd is considered very dangerous even at low doses where no physical symptoms are present. It is, therefore, not surprising that a variety of biomonitoring studies for Cd have been conducted [22, 61].

3.2 Gene toxicity and mutagenicity

The debate regarding the genotoxicity of cadmium continued for decades until recently [52]. This was due primarily to the fact that initially, using the Ames test, Cd was demonstrated to have very low mutagenicity. This, on the other hand, contradicted data demonstrating that the metal was a powerful carcinogen in mammals [24, 62]. At the same time, cadmium-induced inhibition of DNA repair systems and, consequently, co-genotoxicity, has been reported consistently since the late 1980s [56, 63]. Due to these relatively early observations on DNA repair inhibition, most *in vitro* studies have focused on the role of Cd as a co-genotoxin when combined with other genotoxic agents, for instance, ionizing and UV radiation, DNA intercalators and DNA alkylating agents [5, 63]. Data on cadmium-induced genotoxicity from several investigations with *in vitro* test models are presented in **Table 3**.

All the studies cited typically provide evidence for co-mutagenicity of Cd with known mutagens such as UV light, DNA alkylating agents such as methylnitronitrosoguanidine (MNNG), and ionizing radiation. Comparably to *in vitro* studies with Pb, older experimental work with cadmium provides evidence for co-mutagenicity (although not direct mutagenicity) of the metal, while newer work, utilizing more sensitive endpoints, provides evidence for specific mechanisms such as DNA repair inhibition [4, 5].

While *in vitro* studies highlight Cd as a powerful co-mutagen due to DNA repair inhibition, several *in vivo* studies have shown that cadmium can be genotoxic (particularly clastogenic) at low doses. The results of several such investigations are presented in **Table 4**.

The *in vivo* studies above demonstrate cadmium genotoxicity at acute sublethal doses. It should be noted that in these studies, no separate co-mutagen is required, unlike in the *in vitro* models. Even though they prove conclusively that cadmium is genotoxic to mammals, they have a major shortcoming from an ecotoxicological point of view. Namely, the dose administration is either by injection or by oral gavage, which means that the observed effects of cadmium are due to acute exposure, as opposed to chronic and sub-chronic intoxication, which can be achieved by dosing the animal with food, water, or by inhalation means. One of the studies deals with minisatellite DNA instability, demonstrating that Cd intoxication can lead to instability in the non-coding segments of mammalian genomic DNA [69]. Nevertheless, this methodology is still very controversial.

To some extent, the molecular mechanisms of DNA damage induction by Cd^{2+} ions are better understood than those of Pb^{2+}-induced gene toxicity. It has been demonstrated that, at doses above 30 μM, cadmium down-regulates a key system for DNA DSB repair, namely non-homologous end-joining [4, 5]. Evidence suggests that the kinetics and formation of γH2AX foci are impaired at doses greater than 30 μM, with DNA-PKcs catalytic activity falling off at cadmium concentrations at doses of 200 μM [4, 5]. It has been established, as well, that at these doses the metal initially over-activates the system of homologous recombination repair, which may promote genomic instability [4]. Nevertheless, the induction of DNA damage in *in vivo* models by cadmium alone does not show a clear dose-response curve [52]. El-Ghor et al. have demonstrated a significant increase in microsatellite instability in rats exposed to cadmium [69]. Nevertheless, this methodology is controversial, both due to the unknown relationship of microsatellite DNA stability to the overall

Authors	Substance tested	Test system	Dose	Exposure	Endpoint	Effect
Takahashi et al. [64]	Cadmium chloride	*E. coli* CHS26	10^{-8} to 10^{-4} M	4 h	Mutagenicity	β-Gal gene inactivation
Nocentini [56]	Cadmium chloride	Human fibroblasts	10^{-7} to 10^{-2} M	24 h	DNA repair	Inhibition of DNA DSB repair
					DNA synthesis	Inhibition of DNA synthesis
Snyder et al. [65]	Cadmium chloride	HeLa cells	10^{-8} to 10^{-3} M	24 h	UV damage	Co-mutagenicity with UV light
					X-ray damage	Inhibition of DNA DSB repair
Viau et al. [4]	Cadmium chloride, cadmium acetate	HMEC-1 endothelial cells	1–100 μM	24 h	NHEJ activity	Inhibition of DNA DSB repair by NHEJ
					HR activity	Upregulation of homologous recombination
Pereira et al. [5]	Cadmium chloride	ZF-4 zebrafish cells	1–100 μM	24 h	γH2AX foci	Disruption of γH2AX foci kinetics
					Micronuclei	Dose-dependent increase of micronuclei
					DNA repair	Inhibition at doses above 30 μM

Table 3.
Exemplary studies on the genotoxicity of cadmium compounds in vitro.

Authors	Substance tested	Test system	Dose	Exposure	Endpoint	Effect
Mukherjee et al. [66]	Cadmium chloride	Swiss albino mice	0.4–6.75 mg/kg body weight	Injection	SCE	Increase in SCE
					CA	Increase in CA
					MN test	Increase in MN frequency
Privezentsev et al. [67]	Cadmium chloride	ICR mice	1 mg/kg body weight	Injection	MN test	Increase in MN frequency
					CA	Increase in CA
Fahmy and Aly [68]	Cadmium chloride	Swiss albino mice	1–7.6 mg/kg body weight	Injection	SCE	Increase in SCE
					CA	Increase in CA
El-Ghor et al. [69]	Cadmium chloride	Wistar rats	2.93 mg/kg body weight	Oral gavage	Minisatellite DNA	Minisatellite instability
Wada et al. [70]	Cadmium chloride	Sprague-Dawley rats	40–80 mg/kg body weight	Oral gavage	Comet assay	Increase in tail length

Table 4.
Exemplary studies on the genotoxicity of cadmium compounds in vivo.

stability of coding genomic DNA, and the method of Cd intoxication used (oral gavage versus the more common method of administering via food or water). The available literature leads the current authors to believe that cadmium acts as a *tumor promoter*, with initiating events being diverse other factors (ionizing radiation background, metabolic reactive oxygen species, or other genotoxic factors). With respect to reproductive toxicity and cadmium-induced genomic instability, there is reason to believe that cadmium is reproductively toxic at high doses and can cause transmissible genetic damage in the progeny of exposed individuals. Still, much more research (both mechanistic studies and eco-toxicological experimentation) is needed to demonstrate conclusively the potential of the metal to change the genetic structure of exposed populations.

4. Comparing lead and cadmium as genotoxic agents

4.1 Induction of DNA damage

It has been demonstrated that both Pb and Cd do not bind DNA directly, nor induce DNA damage due to DNA-metal interactions [3, 41]. At the same time, it is well-established that the metals promote the generation of reactive oxygen species and interact with redox signaling, disrupting cell homeostasis in organs and tissues and promoting a pro-oxidative state [41, 71]. In addition, specific target enzymes for Cd^{2+} have been identified—these include specifically several zinc-finger proteins like p53, XPA, PARP-1 and NF-κB. This would indicate increased potential of cadmium ions to act as tumor promoters even at low concentrations [41, 71].

On the other hand, it has been observed that Cd alone, at physiological concentrations, is a more significant causal agent of chromosomal aberrations in *in vivo* models, thereby acting more strongly as a mutagen and clastogen [3]. This is probably due to stronger induction of ROS and disruption of cellular redox signaling [72].

4.2 Interactions with DNA repair systems

Little is understood about the interactions of lead with DNA repair systems. While several studies show disruption of γH2AX foci kinetics and, therefore, disruption of DNA DSB repair, and one study highlights a disruption of telomere maintenance, no mechanistic data exists to suggest how exactly Pb^{2+} ions interfere with DNA repair and the DNA damage response [6, 44].

Much more is known about the influence of Cd^{2+} ions with DNA repair. For instance, the tendency of this metal ion to displace zinc from zinc-finger DNA-binding enzymes leads to a disruption in the nucleotide-excision repair system (NER), which can explain the co-mutagenicity of cadmium with agents such as UV light and DNA alkylating chemicals [56, 63]. There have been a few studies analyzing the effects of cadmium on key DNA DSB repair systems [4, 5]. What these authors have established that, in selected *in vitro* models, even at concentrations lower than 30 μM, cadmium chloride inhibits non-homologous end-joining (NHEJ), over-activates the MRE-11-dependent homologous recombination (HR) and telomere maintenance, and leads to a general disturbance in γH2AX foci kinetics (a very sensitive indicator for DNA damage and repair), as well as a sharp decrease in DNA-PKcs catalytic activity, indicating inability to repair double-strand breaks.

While cadmium has undoubtedly been better studied as a genotoxic and co-genotoxic agent, lead (Pb) is also a significant genotoxin, albeit at significantly higher concentrations (>10-fold or more). Pointing out the exact mechanisms of the interaction of Pb with mammalian DNA repair system remains a valid topical area for future research.

5. Gene toxicity of lead and cadmium in the context of ecotoxicology

Mechanistic studies, both *in vivo* and *in vitro*, are informative when trying to understand the basic principles of heavy metal genotoxicity. Nevertheless, what is the significance of environmental exposure to Pb and Cd? Typically environmental exposure occurs chronically or sub-chronically through food, drinking water and inhalation, and happens at comparatively low doses. In addition, exposure patterns are complex. For instance, pollution is often polymetallic, with an added variety of other organic and inorganic chemicals. Studies have been conducted in localities where pollution from lead-zinc smelters and mines is present, such as Asenovgrad in Bulgaria and Bukowno in Poland [10, 12, 14, 16, 18, 22, 27] as well as in areas, polluted by ecological accidents [15, 19].

The answers that these studies give us is that each studied locality has its own pollution pattern, leading to its own "fingerprint" of systemic toxicity and gene toxicity. For instance, it has been demonstrated that for BALB/c laboratory mice, exposed to 1% polymetallic industrial dust through food, the contents of the heavy metals Pb and Cd increase steadily in a 90-day experiment, while at the same time the incidence of chromosome aberrations peaks at the 45-day midpoint, indicating the possibility of an adaptive response [18]. Similar results have been obtained with wild rodents from the same locality in different time frames [20]. Another area of research, which is currently active and productive, is heavy metal detoxification, particularly with the use of zeolite sorbents [29]. From the viewpoint of ecotoxicology, it is already known how chronic and sub-chronic doses of Pb and Cd affect the organism separately, but more research (including mechanistic studies) is needed in order to understand the effects of complex pollution patterns on living organisms.

The available data on the gene toxicity and eco-toxicity of Pb and Cd leads the current authors to believe that more significant research needs to be done in two main areas:

1. Mechanistic studies dealing with the specific effects of the two metals on DNA repair systems. This is especially true for Pb, since lead-induced chromosomal aberrations in mammalian cells at low doses are a well-established fact, but no concrete mechanistic studies on the effects of Pb on DNA repair systems have been conducted.

2. Ecotoxicological studies highlighting the effects of different cocktails of pollutants in a given locality on a standardized test system. Suitable *in vitro* systems, which have been proposed include metabolically competent human and rat hepatoma cell lines, which have been used for the study of metabolically activated genotoxins for over two decades [73].

Finally, connections should be made to existing occupational safety and environmental legislation regarding the use of Pb and Cd worldwide. Some of the safety concerns regarding the two elements stem from the fact that heavy metals and their compounds are highly persistent in the environment. Additionally, gene toxicity, especially in the case of cadmium, have caused EU authorities to propose banning the use, mining and refining of Cd within the EU entirely. Since effects of Pb and Cd on genomic instability in the progeny of mammalian species have been observed [9, 69], but are not well understood, it is advisable that safety approaches to Cd and Pb have a "conservative approach," meaning that exposure tolerance limits and environmental releases should be as low as possible in order to mitigate risk to humans and the biosphere.

6. Conclusion

The current work has analyzed the state-of-the art in what is known about the gene toxicity of lead and cadmium in an ecotoxicological context. Cd has been demonstrated as a powerful co-mutagen in *in vitro* test systems and as a direct mutagen *in vivo*. While Pb is generally a less potent inductor of chromosome aberrations, it has still been demonstrated to be genotoxic, particularly *in vivo*. While many studies have been conducted on the environmental exposure to Pb and Cd and their compounds, the interactions of the two metals as genotoxic agents are not yet fully understood. Two main challenges remain for future research in ecotoxicology and toxicogenetics: the combination of mechanistic *in vivo* and *in vitro* studies with ecotoxicological research, in order to understand better the specific pathways of heavy metal-induced gene toxicity, and future research on the detoxication of Pb and Cd and the mitigation of their gene toxicity.

Acknowledgements

This work is supported by the National Science Fund of the Republic of Bulgaria, Project DN 04/1, 13.12.2016: "Study of the combined effect of the natural radioactivity background, the UV radiation, the climate changes and the cosmic rays on model groups of plant and animal organisms in mountain ecosystems".

Author details

Peter Vladislavov Ostoich*, Michaela Beltcheva and Roumiana Metcheva
Institute of Biodiversity and Ecosystem Research, Bulgarian Academy of Sciences, Sofia, Bulgaria

*Address all correspondence to: p.ostoich@gmail.com

References

[1] Ferraro M, Fenocchio A, Mantovani M, Ribeiro C, Cestari M. Mutagenic effects of tributyltin and inorganic lead (Pb II) on the fish *H. Malabaricus* as evaluated using the comet assay and the piscine micronucleus and chromosome aberration tests. Genetics and Molecular Biology. 2004;**27**(1):27-33

[2] Valverde M, Fortoul T, Diaz-Barriga F, Mejia J, Rojas E. Induction of genotoxicity by cadmium chloride inhalation in several organs of CD-1 mice. Mutagenesis. 2000;**15**:109-114

[3] Valverde M, Trejo C, Rojas E. Is the capacity of lead acetate and cadmium chloride to induce genotoxic damage due to direct DNA–metal interaction? Mutagenesis. 2001;**16**(3):265-270

[4] Viau M, Gastaldo J, Bencokova Z, Joubert A, Foray N. Cadmium inhibits non-homologous end-joining and over-activates the MRE-11-dependent repair pathway. Mutation Research. 2008;**654**:13-21

[5] Pereira S, Cavalie I, Camilleri V, Gilbin R, Adam-Guillermin C. Comparative genotoxicity of aluminium and cadmium in embryonic zebrafish cells. Mutation Research. 2013;**750**:19-26

[6] Pottier G, Viau M, Ricoul M, Shim G, Bellamy M, Cuceu C, et al. Lead exposure induces telomere instability in human cells. PLoS One. 2013;**8**(6):1-8

[7] Garcia-Leston J, Mendez J, Pasaro E, Laffon B. Genotoxic effects of lead: An updated review. Environment International. 2010;**36**(1):623-636

[8] Wang L, Li J, Li J, Liu Z. Effects of lead and/or cadmium on the oxidative damage of rat kidney cortex mitochondria. Biological Trace Element Research. 2010;**137**:69-78

[9] Yuan X, Tang C. The accumulation effect of lead on DNA damage in mice blood cells of three generations and the protection of selenium. Journal of Environmental Science and Health. 2001;**36**(1):501-508

[10] Wlostowski T. Heavy metals in the liver of *Clethrionomys glareolus* (Schreber, 1780) and *Apodemus sylvaticus* (Pallas, 1771) from forests contaminated with coal-industry fumes. Ekologia Polska. 1987;**35**:115-129

[11] Ma W, Denneman W, Faber J. Hazardous exposure of ground-living small mammals to cadmium and lead in contaminated terrestrial ecosystems. Archives of Environmental Contamination and Toxicology. 1991;**20**:266-270

[12] Topashka-Ancheva M, Metcheva R. Bioaccumulation of heavy metals and chromosome aberrations in small mammals from industrially polluted region in Bulgaria. In: Contributions to the Zoogeography and Ecology of the Eastern Mediterranean Region. Vol. 1. 1999. pp. 69-74

[13] Gdula-Argasinska J, Sawicka-Kapusta K. Effect of heavy metals pollution on rodents from six forest sites of Malopolska district. In: 11th Annual Meeting of SETAC Europe, Madrid, Spain. 2001. pp. 1-5

[14] Ieradi L, Zima J, Allegra F, Kotlanova E, Campanella L, Grossi R, et al. Evaluation of genotoxic damage in wild rodents from a polluted area in the Czech Republic. Folia Zoologica. 2003;**52**(1):57-66

[15] Tanzarella C, Degrassi F, Cristaldi M, Moreno S, Lascialfari A, Chiuchiarelli G, et al. Genotoxic damage in free-living Algerian mouse (*Mus spretus*) after the Coto Doñana ecological

disaster. Environmental Pollution. 2001;**115**(1):43-48

[16] Damek-Poprawa M, Sawicka-Kapusta K. Damage to the liver, kidney and testis with reference to burden of heavy metals in yellow-necked mice from areas around steelworks and zinc smelters in Poland. Toxicology. 2003;**186**:1-10

[17] Sánchez-Chardi A, Penarroja-Matutano C, Oliveira Ribeiro CA, Nadal J. Bioaccumulation of metals and effects of a landfill in small mammals. Part II. The wood mouse, *Apodemus sylvaticus*. Chemosphere. 2007;**70**:101-110

[18] Metcheva R, Topashka-Ancheva M, Teodorova S. Influence of lead and cadmium on some genetic and physiological parameters of laboratory mice. In: Cato M, editor. Environmental Research Trends. 2007. pp. 205-230

[19] Udroiu I, Ieradi L, Tanzarella C, Moreno S. Biomonitoring of Doñana National Park using the Algerian mouse (*Mus spretus*) as a sentinel species. Fresenius Environmental Bulletin. 2008;**17**(9):1519-1525

[20] Topashka-Ancheva M, Metcheva R, Teodorova S. A comparative analysis of the heavy metals loading of small mammals in different Bulgarian regions. II. Chromosomal aberrations and blood pathology. Ecotoxicology and Environmental Safety. 2003;**54**(2):188-193

[21] Tapisso J, Marques C, da Luz Mathias M, Ramalhinho M. Induction of micronuclei and sister chromatid exchange in bone-marrow cells and abnormalities in sperm of Algerian mice (*Mus spretus*) exposed to cadmium, lead and zinc. Mutation Research/Fundamental and Molecular Mechanisms of Mutagenesis. 2009;**678**(1):59-64

[22] Martiniakova M, Omelka R, Stawarz R, Formicki G. Accumulation of lead, cadmium, nickel, iron, copper and zinc in bones of small mammals from polluted areas in Slovakia. Polish Journal of Environmental Studies. 2012;**21**(1):153-158

[23] Tete N, Durfort M, Reiffel D, Scheifler A, Sanchez-Chardi M. Histopathology related to cadmium and lead bioaccumulation in chronically exposed wood mice, *Apodemus sylvaticus*, around a former smelter. Science of the Total Environment. 2014;**481**(1):167-177

[24] Luckey T, Venugopal B. Metal Toxicity in Mammals: Physiologic and Chemical Basis for Metal Toxicity. New York: Plenum Press; 1977. 238p

[25] Graedel T. Metal stocks in society: Scientific synthesis. International Resources Workshop Proceedings. 2010;**1**(1):59-90

[26] Nriagu J. Saturnine gout among Roman aristocrats: Did lead poisoning contribute to the fall of the empire? New England Journal of Medicine. 1983;**308**(1):660-663

[27] Metcheva R, Teodorova S, Topashka-Ancheva M. A comparative analysis of the heavy metals and toxic elements loading indicated by small mammals in different Bulgarian regions. Acta Zoologica Bulgarica. 2001;**53**:61-80

[28] Festa F, Cristaldi M, Ieradi L, Moreno S, Cozzi R. The comet assay for the detection of DNA damage in *Mus spretus* from Doñana National Park. Environmental Research. 2003;**91**:54-61

[29] Beltcheva M, Metcheva R, Topashka-Ancheva M, Popov N, Teodorova S, Heredia-Rojas J, et al. Zeolites versus lead toxicity. Journal of Bioequivalence & Bioavailability. 2015;7(1):12-29

[30] Catellino N, Aloj S. Determination of the elimination constants of Pb-210 from various rat tissues. Folia Medica. 1964;**47**(1):238-248

[31] Rabinowitz M. Historical perspective on lead biokinetic models. Environmental Health Perspectives. 1998;**106**(6):1461-1465

[32] Kneip T, Mallon R, Harley N. Biokinetic modeling for mammalian metabolism. Neurotoxicology. 1983;**4**:189-192

[33] O'Flaherty E. Physiologically based models for bone seeking elements. V: Lead absorption and disposition in childhood. Toxicology and Applied Pharmacology. 1995;**131**:297-308

[34] Goyer R, Rhine B. Pathological effects of lead. International Review of Experimental Pathology. 1973;**12**(1):23-37

[35] ZelikoffJ,ThomasP.Immunotoxicology of Environmental and Occupational Metals. London: Taylor and Francis; 2005. 382p

[36] Tham C, Chakravarthy S, Haleagrahara N, De Alvis R. Morphological study of bone marrow to assess the effects of lead acetate on haemopoiesis and aplasia and the ameliorating role of *Carica papaya* extract. Experimental and Therapeutic Medicine. 2013;**5**(2):648-654

[37] Ahmed M, Ahmed M, Meki A, Abd-Raboh N. Neurotoxic effects of lead on rats: Relationship to apoptosis. International Journal of Health Sciences. 2013;**7**(2):192-199

[38] Winder C, Bonin T. The genotoxicity of lead. Mutation Research. 1993;**285**(1):117-124

[39] Bauchinger M, Schmid E. Chromosome analysis of cultures of Chinese hamster cells after treatment with lead acetate. Mutation Research. 1972;**14**:95-100

[40] Gasiorek K, Bauchinger M. Chromosome changes in human lymphocytes after separate and combined treatment with divalent salts of lead, cadmium, and zinc. Environmental Mutagenesis. 1981;**3**:513-518

[41] Hartwig A, Schlepegrell R, Beyersmann D. Indirect mechanism of lead-induced genotoxicity in cultured mammalian cells. Mutation Research. 1990;**241**:75-82

[42] Cai M, Arenaz P. Antimutagenic effect of crown ethers on heavy metal-induced sister chromatid exchanges. Mutagenesis. 1998;**13**(1):27-32

[43] Wozniak K, Blasiak J. In vitro genotoxicity of lead acetate: Induction of single and double DNA strand breaks and DNA-protein cross-links. Mutation Research. 2003;**535**:127-139

[44] Xie H, Wise S, Holmes A, Xu B, Wakeman T, Pelsue S. Carcinogenic lead chromate induces DNA double-strand breaks in human lung cells. Mutation Research. 2005;**586**:160-172

[45] Muro L, Goyer R. Chromosome damage in experimental lead poisoning. Archives of Pathology. 1969;**87**:660-663

[46] Deknudt G, Colle A, Gerber G. Chromosomalabnormalitiesinlymphocytes from monkeys poisoned with lead. Mutation Research. 1977;**45**:77-83

[47] Sharma R, Jacobson-Kram D, Lemmon M, Bakke J, Galperin I, Blazak W. Sister chromatid exchange and cell replication kinetics in fetal and maternal cells after treatment with chemical teratogens. Mutation Research. 1985;**158**:217-231

[48] Robbiano L, Carrozzino R, Porta Puglia C, Corbu C, Brambilla G.

Correlation between induction of DNA fragmentation and micronuclei formation in kidney cells from rats and humans, and tissue-specific carcinogenic activity. Toxicology and Applied Pharmacology. 1999;**161**:153-159

[49] Valverde M, Fortoul T, Diaz-Barriga F, Mejia J, del Castillo E. Genotoxicity induced in CD-1 mice by inhaled lead: Differential organ response. Mutagenesis. 2002;**17**:55-61

[50] Hartwig A. Role of DNA repair inhibition of lead and cadmium-induced genotoxicity: A review. Environmental Health Perspectives. 1994;**102**(3):45-50

[51] Van den Bussche J, Soarez E. Lead induces oxidative stress and phenotypic markers of apoptosis in *Saccharomyces cerevisae*. Applied Microbiology and Biotechnology. 2011;**90**(2):679-687

[52] Waalkes M. Cadmium carcinogenesis in review. Journal of Inorganic Biochemistry. 2000;**79**:241-244

[53] Wlostowski T, Krasowska A, Bonda E. Photoperiod affects hepatic and renal cadmium accumulation, metallothionein induction, and cadmium toxicity in the wild bank vole (*Clethrionomys glareolus*). Ecotoxicology and Environmental Safety. 2004;**58**:29-36

[54] Wlostowski T, Dmowski K, Bonda-Ostaszewska E. Cadmium accumulation, metallothionein and glutathione levels, and histopathological changes in the kidneys and liver of magpie (*Pica pica*) from a zinc smelter area. Ecotoxicology. 2010;**19**:1066-1073

[55] Friberg L, Piscator M, Nordberg G, Kjellstrom T. Cadmium in the Environment. 2nd ed. Cleveland, Ohio: Chemical Rubber Co.; 1974. 176p

[56] Nocentini S. Inhibition of DNA replication and repair by cadmium in mammalian cells. Protective interaction of zinc. Nucleic Acids Research. 1987;**15**:4211-4225

[57] Nordberg G. Historical perspectives on cadmium toxicology. Toxicology and Applied Pharmacology. 2009;**238**:192-200

[58] Rikans L, Yamano T. Mechanisms of cadmium-mediated acute hepatotoxicity. Journal of Biochemical and Molecular Toxicology. 1999;**14**(2):110-117

[59] Salinska A, Wlostowski T, Zambrzyczka E. Effect of dietary cadmium and/or lead on histopathological changes in the kidneys and liver of bank voles *Myodes glareolus* kept in different group densities. Ecotoxicology. 2012;**21**(8):2235-2243

[60] Bremner I. Mammalian absorption, transport and excretion of cadmium. In: Webb M, editor. The Chemistry, Biochemistry and Biology of Cadmium. Amsterdam: Elsevier Holland; 1979. pp. 175-193

[61] Shore R, Douben P. The ecotoxicological significance of cadmium intake and residues in terrestrial small mammals. Ecotoxicology and Environmental Safety. 1994;**29**:101-112

[62] Rossmann T, Roy N, Lin W. Is cadmium genotoxic? IARC Publications. 1992;**118**:367-375

[63] Hartwig A, Asmuss A, Ehleben I, Herzer U, Kostelac D, Pelzer A, et al. Interference of toxic metal ions with DNA repair processes and cell cycle control: Molecular mechanisms. Environmental Health Perspectives. 2002;**110**(5):797-799

[64] Takahashi K, Imaeda T, Kawazoe Y. Effect of metal ions on the adaptive

response induced by N-methyl-N-nitrosourea in *Escherichia coli*. Biochemical and Biophysical Research Communications. 1988;**157**:1124-1130

[65] Snyder RD, Davis GF, Lachmann PJ. Inhibition by metals of X-ray and ultraviolet-induced DNA repair in human cells. Biological Trace Element Research. 1989;**21**:389-398

[66] Mukherjee A, Giri A, Sharma A, Talukder G. Relative efficacy of short-term tests in detecting genotoxic effects of cadmium chloride in mice *in vivo*. Mutation Research. 1988;**206**(2):285-295

[67] Privezentsev K, Sirota N, Gaziev A. The genotoxic effects of cadmium studied *in vivo*. Tsitologiya i genetika. 1996;**30**(3):45-51

[68] Fahmy A, Aly F. *In vivo* and *in vitro* studies on the genotoxicity of cadmium chloride in mice. Journal of Applied Toxicology. 2000;**20**:231-238

[69] El-Ghor A, Noshy M, El Ashmaoui H, Eid J, Hassanane M. Microsatellite instability at three microsatellite loci (D6mit3, D9mit2 and D15Mgh1) located in different common fragile sites of rats exposed to cadmium. Mutation Research. 2010;**696**(2):160-166

[70] Wada K, Fukuyama T, Nakashima N, Matsumoto K. Assessment of the *in vivo* genotoxicity of cadmium chloride, chloroform, and D,L-menthol as coded test chemicals using the alkaline comet assay. Mutation Research. 2015;**786**:114-119

[71] Xu J, Wise J, Wang L, Schumann K, Zhang Z, Shi X. Dual roles of oxidative stress in metal carcinogenesis. Journal of Environmental Pathology, Toxicology and Oncology. 2017;**36**(4):345-376

[72] Hartwig A. Metal interaction with redox regulation: An integrating concept in metal carcinogenesis? Free Radical Biology and Medicine. 2013;**55**:63-72

[73] Knasmüller S, Parzefall W, Sanyal R, Ecker S, Schwab C, Uhl M, et al. Use of metabolically competent human hepatoma cells for the detection of mutagens and antimutagens. Mutation Research. 1998;**402**:185-202

Chapter 5

DCLK1 and DNA Damage Response

Janani Panneerselvam, Dongfeng Qu, Courtney Houchen, Michael Bronze and Parthasarathy Chandrakesan

Abstract

Genome integrity is constantly monitored by sophisticated cellular networks, collectively termed as the DNA damage response (DDR). The DDR is a signaling network that includes cell cycle checkpoints and DNA repair and damage tolerance pathways. Failure of the DDR or associated events causes various diseases, including cancer. DDR is primarily mediated by phosphatidylinositol-3-kinase-like protein kinase (PIKKs) family members ataxia-telangiectasia mutated (ATM) and ataxia telangiectasia and Rad3-related protein (ATR). However, one of the many unanswered questions regarding these signal-transduction pathways is: how does the cell turn the DDR signals on? There was no conclusive demonstration of the involvement of a specific sensory kinase in DDR signals until our recent research on the DCLK1 role in regulating ATM after genotoxic injury. Currently, various studies are demonstrating the importance of DCLK1 in DNA damage response. Here, we discuss the novel insights into the role of DCLK1 in DNA damage response.

Keywords: DNA damage, DDR, ATM, ATR, DCLK1

1. Introduction

DNA damage exists in all cellular organisms, and DNA, the genetic material in each living cell is the fundamental unit of life and its integrity and stability are essential to life [1]. However, DNA is not passive; rather, it is a chemical unit subject to be attacked from a range of endogenous and environmental damaging agents. The endogenous damages are the damage caused by reactive oxygen species or metabolic byproducts, and DNA metabolization; exogenous damages are caused by external agents, like radiations, toxins, chemicals, and microorganisms [2]. In response to the DNA damage, cells rapidly recruit a sophisticated network which is called DNA damage-response (DDR) systems. DDR systems include DNA repair mechanisms, damage tolerance processes, and cell-cycle checkpoint pathways [3]. Failure of DDR causes genomic instability which results in various diseases including immune deficiency, neurological degeneration, premature aging, and severe cancer susceptibility [2, 4]. Indeed, great progress has been made towards understanding the mechanisms of DDR in homeostasis, carcinogenesis and cancer advancement but much remains to delineate how the DDR network systems are regulated. Furthermore, how the DDR network is formed and how it is fine-tuned by upstream and downstream mediators or signaling pathways that support the homeostasis or disease progression required to understand. While the rapid activation of DDR against the

DNA damage is expected, it is unclear how and who activates or gives the instruction to DDR network systems? Gaining knowledge about DDR and its regulators will not only enhance our understanding of DDR functions but will undoubtedly giving us opportunities to better manage human diseases. Although, very few studies reported that protein kinases and DNA adaptor molecules or DNA regulators may influence or send signals to DDR after DNA gets damaged [5, 6]. DCLK1 is a member of the protein kinase superfamily and the doublecortin family, that belongs to the group of microtubule-associated proteins [7]. Our novel findings that DCLK1 regulate DNA damage response and cell survival following genotoxic injury opens many windows of how DDR is regulated [8]. In this chapter we will highlight the functional role of DCLK1 in injury, DDR and cell survival, which will lead us to a better understanding of DCLK1 expression in helping genomic stability in normal and neoplastic cells.

2. DNA damage, DNA damage response, and DNA repair

DNA is the source of genetic information in all living cells, its integrity and fidelity are essential to life. Because DNA is not passive, it is a chemical entity subject to be assaulted from various reactive agents, causing DNA damage [9]. DNA damage can be subdivided into two types: (1) endogenous damage caused by reactive oxygen species (ROS) that are derived from metabolic byproducts and (2) exogenous damage caused by radiation (UV, X-ray, gamma), hydrolysis, plant toxins, and viruses, chemical toxins [9, 10]. Most of the DNA damage can be repaired by the host systems called the DNA damage response (DDR) and DNA repair systems. Such systems also face failure and not 100% efficient, which resulted in either cell death or cell survival with un-repaired DNA causing mutation and eventually cancer [11]. In some cases, the un-repaired DNA damage accumulates in non-replicating cells, such as neurons or myocytes of adult mammals, and can cause aging [12]. The DDR is a sophisticated cellular network, which constantly monitors the integrity of the genome, in response to DNA damage [13]. Once the DDR gets activated it rapidly recruit downstream protein sensors and adaptors establishing the sensing, activating repair, tolerating damage and apoptosis (**Figure 1**). DDR is primarily mediated by phosphatidylinositol-3-kinase-like protein kinase (PIKKs) family members, ataxia-telangiectasia mutated (ATM) and ataxia telangiectasia and Rad3-related protein (ATR) and DNA-dependent protein kinase catalytic subunit (DNA-PKcs) [13, 14]. The ATM pathway for homologous recombination (HR) repair is activated after a double-stranded break. The ATR pathway for nonhomologous end-joining (NHEJ) is associated with single-stranded DNA and stalled DNA replication forks. ATM pathway is a higher-fidelity repair pathway than the ATR. For lesions repaired by the HR, double-strand breaks (DSBs) are detected and processed by the MRE11–RAD50–NBS1 (MRN) complex [15, 16]. For lesions repaired by the NHEJ, DNA breaks are detected and the process by the ATR interacting protein (ATRIP) complex. ATM and ATR transduce the most upstream DDR signal by phosphorylating the checkpoint kinases CHK1/CHK2 and the tumor suppressor protein p53, which resulted in cell cycle arrest to allow time for DNA repair. The main function of DNA-PK activated under the ATM/ATR pathway is to induce cell cycle arrest and DNA repair [17]. DNA repair is a vital cellular process required for the maintenance of genomic integrity and fidelity [18]. Living cells employ several DNA repair pathways for distinct types of DNA damage. There are five major DNA repair pathways: (1) mismatch repair (MMR), (2) nucleotide excision repair (NER), (3) base excision repair (BER), (4) homologous recombinational repair (HR), and (5) non-homologous end joining (NHEJ) [19, 20]. MMR's primary

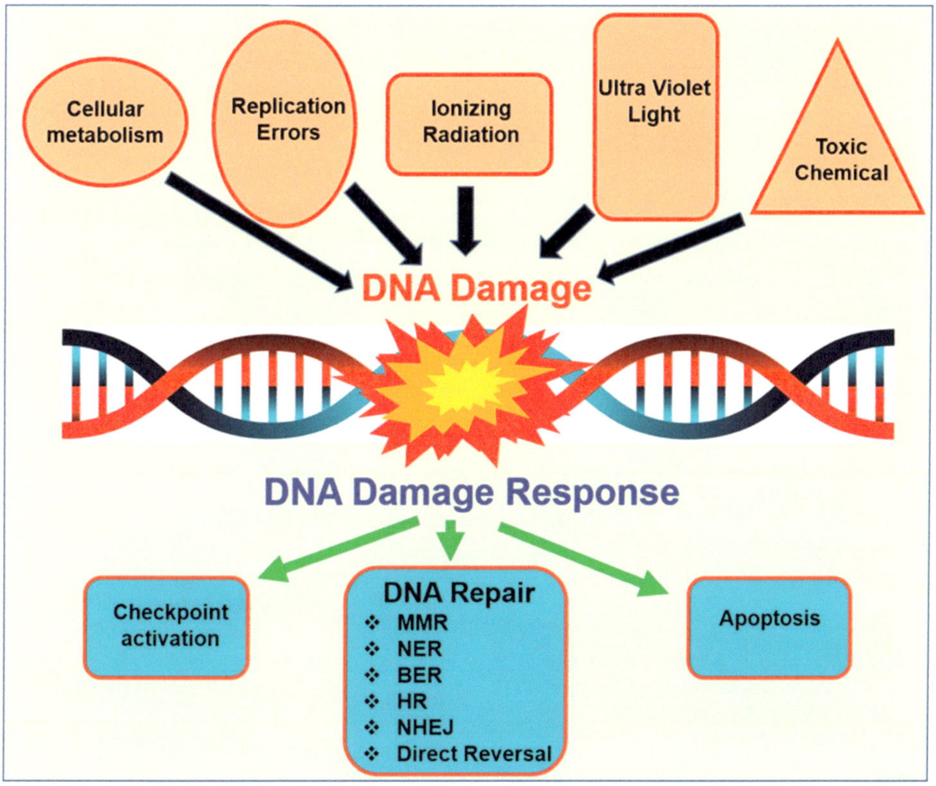

Figure 1.
DNA damage, DNA damage response, and repair. Graphical illustration demonstrating the DNA damage caused by different sources and the cellular response to DNA damage.

function is to remove base mismatches and small insertion and deletion loops which is introduced during replication. The NER pathway is a multistep process that serves to repair a variety of DNA damage, including DNA lesions caused by UV radiation, toxic chemicals, or chemotherapeutic drugs that form huge DNA adducts. BER primarily repairs non-bulky lesions produced by alkylation, oxidation or deamination of bases. The BER pathway deals with base damage, the most common insult to cellular DNA. DSBs can be repaired by either HR or NHEJ. HR uses a homologous DNA template and is highly accurate, whereas NHEJ rejoins the broken ends without using a template and is often accompanied by loss of some nucleotides. Direct reversal of DNA damage is one repair mechanism used to restore damaged DNA without using excision, resynthesis, and ligation [21, 22].

3. DCLK1

The human doublecortin (DCX) gene family comprises members that share the tubulin-binding domain and known to have limited functions in microtubule-associated regulation and neuronal-regulation [23]. One of the best known and most interesting members of this DCX family is doublecortin-like kinase 1 (DCLK1 also known as DCAMKL1), a gene encoding for a protein that is 70% identical to doublecortin in the microtubule-binding N-terminal domain. However, unlike doublecortin, the DCKL1 gene also encodes for a serine–threonine kinase C-terminal domain that is similar to Ca^{2+}/calmodulin-dependent protein kinase II but lacks a canonical calmodulin-binding site [24, 25]. DCLK1 gene also encodes

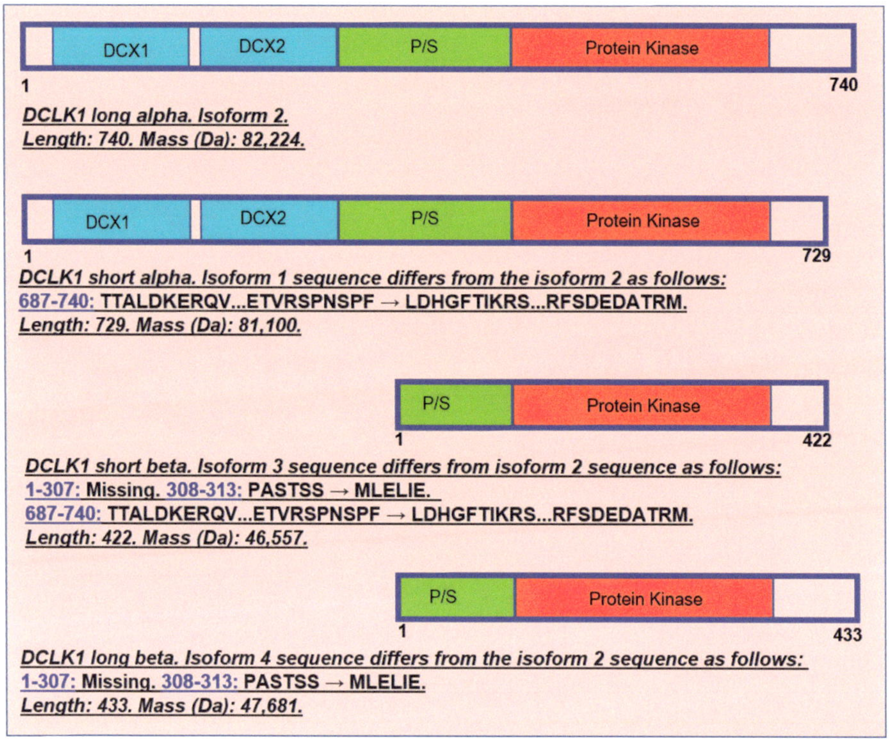

Figure 2.
Human DCLK1-isoforms. Graphical illustration demonstrating the length of each isoform and shared protein kinase domain between DCLK1 isoforms referenced in UniProt; www.uniprot.org/uniprot/O15075. DCX1 = Doublecortin1; DCX2 = Doublecortin2; and P/S = pro/Ser rich domain and a protein kinase domain.

for a serine/proline-rich domain in between the doublecortin and the protein kinase domains, which mediates multiple protein–protein interactions. In humans, DCLK1 consists of four primary isoforms with a shared kinase domain-driven from two promoter regions termed α and β (**Figure 2**) [26–28]. The α-promoter drives the expression of isoforms termed α-long (isoform 2) and α-short (isoform 1) which contain an N-terminal microtubule-binding region with high homology to DCX. Importantly, the α-promoter isoforms are specifically expressed in the DCLK1+ tuft cells that eventually give rise to tumor stem cells following relevant mutagenesis in the colon and pancreatic cancer [29–31]. The β-promoter drives the expression of two isoforms termed β-long (isoform 4) and β-short (isoform 3) that can be used to predict survival in colon cancer [32]. Although these isoforms likely play a significant role in tumorigenesis through their kinase activity, there is no evidence that they are functionally involved in the regulation of DDR, until our first report to demonstrate its direct interaction with ATM.

4. DCLK1 and DDR following injury and inflammation

Cell survival after severe injury requires highly coordinated complex interplay between the diverse molecular signaling responses to repair the injury [15, 33]. We discussed three fundamental standards about the critical role of DCLK1 in intestinal epithelial cell survival after severe genotoxic injury: (1) how intestinal epithelial cells respond to severe DNA damage because intestinal epithelial cells are the most affected cells after bone marrow during radiotherapy or accidental or incidental radiation exposure [34] and (2) how DCLK1 a kinase protein expression play key role in injury response, because DCLK1 expressing cells survive high dose radiation and DSS-induced inflammation [29]. It is reported that the deletion of DCLK1 ($Villin^{Cre}$;$DCLK1^{f/f}$ mice) in the intestinal epithelial cells does not confer a significant deleterious phenotype in adult mice, compared with their wild-type littermates [35]. However, after 24 h of 12 Gy total body irradiation (TBI), none of the intestinal epithelial-specific DCLK1 knockout mice survived longer than 5 days [35]. The best-known primary defense mechanism against the genotoxic injury-induced DNA damage is the DDR, which repairs the damaged DNA and increased the survival of intestinal epithelial cells [36]. Indeed studies demonstrated that deficient DDR has been suggested to increase intestinal epithelial death and loss of survival [37]. During the early event of DNA damage, the ATM-H2AX axis gets activated, generating gamma-H2AX and other adaptors, providing a stage for efficient homologous recombinant repair [38]. Recently, ATM knockout or loss of Rad50 and Mre11 was reported to increase intestinal injury and lethality [39, 40]. But how these DDR signaling pathways were regulated following radiation injury is not well known. Chandrakesan et al. reported that the absence of DCLK1 expression in the intestinal epithelial cells abrogated the activation and expression of ATM, gamma-H2AX, and downstream adopter proteins BRCA1, Rad50, and MRE11 in the intestinal epithelial cells 24 h post-TBI [8]. Furthermore, it is reported that this reduction persisted up to 3.5 days post-TBI. It is suggested that there is a profound defect in intestinal DDR in DCLK1 knock-out mice, which

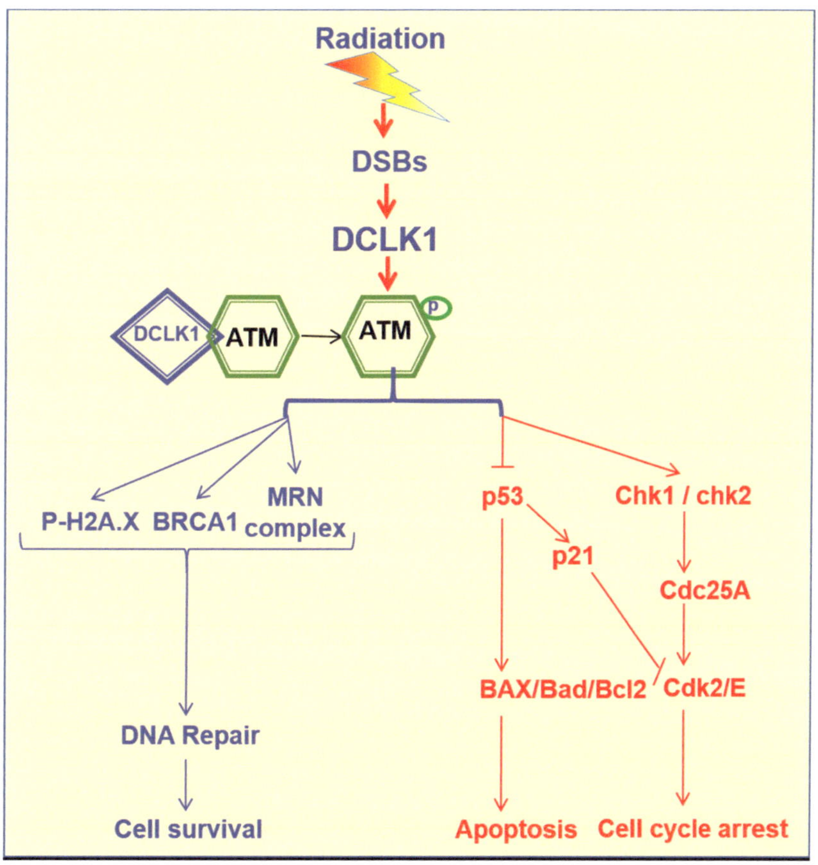

Figure 3.
DCLK1 and DDR. Graphical illustration demonstrating the regulatory role of DCLK1 in DDR following radiation injury.

might contribute to defective epithelial survival and overall survival. Interestingly they established that phosphorylation of ATM which is critical for its activation is reduced in the intestinal epithelial cells of DCLK1 knock-out mice, under physiological conditions, and discovered that DCLK1 can directly interact with ATM for its activation. ATM activation during and or after radiation injury directly depends on the ratio of DCLK1-ATM interaction [8]. Furthermore, DCLK1 knockdown and overexpression experiments with the YAMC cell line in vitro established that DCLK1 interaction is important for ATM activation. It is the first study to establish a direct link between DCLK1 and ATM mediated DDR, for the survival of cell in response to severe genotoxic injury (**Figure 3**).

5. DCLK1 in the regulation of DDR in cancers

A faulty DDR system can initiate cancer development [41]. Cancer cells with a DDR deficiency are profoundly dependent on remaining DDR [42, 43], for example in the case of ATM deficiency cancer cell relies on the ATR pathway. Therefore, DDR inhibition in cancers exploits these defects by inhibiting the remaining DDR system, and which in turn causes cancer cell death. Indeed the healthy cells are not vulnerable to DDR targeted therapies because normal cells can have higher expression of DDR only if they exposed to injury [44, 45]. Most cancer cells depend on their enhanced DDR activation for their survival, mainly activation of ATM and ATR pathways, and associated, CHK2, histone H2AX, and p53 [46, 47].

The present conventional radiotherapy and chemotherapies including platinum-based therapies are used to kill cancer cells by inducing DNA damage. A huge problem that arises when using conventional therapies is the development of resistance by these cancer cells whose DDR repair the genomic instability, which causes conventional therapies to fail [48, 49]. Cancer cells as a short-term solution can bypass the DNA damage caused by chemotherapeutic agents by a mechanism known as translesion synthesis [50, 51]. Cancer cells with high DNA damage tolerance allow DNA replication to proceed in the presence of DNA damage include the convergence of adjacent replicons, re-priming of DNA synthesis downstream of lesions on the leading strand and discontinuous synthesis of Okazaki fragments on the lagging DNA strand [52, 53]. Given the fundamental role of DDR in the gain of chemo-resistance, the novel strategies of combination therapies including DDR targeted therapies will be effective [41]. Recent regulatory approval of olaparib (Lynparza), a poly (ADP ribose) polymerase (PARP) inhibitor, which inhibits PARP enzyme activity and forms severe DSBs [54]. In cancers, PARP inhibitor increases genomic instability that results in tumor cell death [55, 56]. Although, the pharmacological inhibitors of PARP have shown promising results in preclinical studies and in clinical trials, the gain of resistance in cancer cells to PARP inhibitors, is inevitable [57]. However, the combination of PARP inhibitors with other DDR agents including ATR inhibitors, CHK1 inhibitors, ATM inhibitors, and DNA-PKs inhibitors, or with chemotherapeutic agents are novel strategies currently investigated to overcome resistance to PARP inhibitors [57] (**Table 1**—[58]). However, while the DDR targeted therapies are expected to cause DNA damage in tumor cells, it is unclear how these DDR networks are regulated in cancer cells? DDR regulators in cancers are reported recently, (1) MORC2 (MORC Family CW-Type Zinc Finger 2) is required for DNA damage-induced PAR production and PAR-dependent DNA repair signaling cascades and stimulates chromatin remodeling [59, 60]. Inhibition of MORC2 in breast cancer cells impaired DDR and sensitize cancer cells to PARP inhibitors. (2) MYB is an oncogene that plays an important role in regulating DDR in ER+ breast cancers and inhibition of MYB induces DNA

ClinicalTrials.gov identifier	Title	Phase	Drug target
NCT02797964	A Phase 1 Trial of SRA737 in Subjects with Advanced Cancer	I	CHK1 inhibitor
NCT02797977	A Phase 1 Trial of SRA737 in Combination with Gemcitabine Plus Cisplatin or Gemcitabine Alone in Subjects with Advanced Cancer	I	CHK1 inhibitor Chemotherapy
NCT03057145	Combination Study of Prexasertib and Olaparib in Patients with Advanced Solid Tumors	I	CHK1 inhibitor PARP inhibitor
NCT02516813	Phase 1 Trial of MSC2490484A, an Inhibitor of a DNA-dependent Protein Kinase, in Combination with Radiotherapy	I	DNA-PK inhibitor Radiotherapy
NCT03308942	Phase 2, Multi-Arm Study of Niraparib Administered Alone and in Combination with PD-1 Inhibitor in Patients with Non-Small Cell Lung Cancer	II	PARP Inhibitor PD-1 Inhibitor
NCT02660034	The Safety, Pharmacokinetics and Antitumor Activity of BGB-A317 in Combination with BGB-290 in Subjects with Advanced Solid Tumors	I	PARP Inhibitor PD-1 Inhibitor
NCT02264678	Ascending Doses of AZD6738 in Combination with Chemotherapy and/or Novel Anti Cancer Agents	I	ATR Inhibitor Chemotherapy PDL-1 Inhibitor
NCT01844986	Olaparib Maintenance Monotherapy in Patients with BRCA Mutated Ovarian Cancer Following First Line Platinum Based Chemotherapy. (SOLO-1)	III	PARP inhibitor
NCT02282020	Olaparib Treatment in Relapsed Germline Breast Cancer Susceptibility Gene (BRCA) Mutated Ovarian Cancer Patients Who Have Progressed at Least 6 Months After Last Platinum Treatment and Have Received at Least 2 Prior Platinum Treatments (SOLO3)	III	PARP inhibitor
NCT02446704	Study of Olaparib and Temozolomide in Patients With Recurrent Small Cell Lung Cancer Following Failure of Prior Chemotherapy	I	PARP inhibitor
NCT02789332	Assessing the Efficacy of Paclitaxel and Olaparib in Comparison to Paclitaxel/Carboplatin Followed by Epirubicin/Cyclophosphamide as Neoadjuvant Chemotherapy in Patients with HER2-negative Early Breast Cancer and Homologous Recombination Deficiency (GeparOla)	II	PARP inhibitor Chemotherapy
NCT02264678	Ascending Doses of AZD6738 in Combination With Chemotherapy and/or Novel Anti Cancer Agents Drug: administration of AZD6738 in combination with carboplatin Drug: administration of AZD6738 Drug: administration of AZD6738 in combination with olaparib Drug: administration of AZD6738 in combination with MEDI4736	I/II	PARP inhibitor Chemotherapy

ClinicalTrials. gov identifier	Title	Phase	Drug target
NCT00535353	AZD2281 and Irinotecan in Treating Patients with Locally Advanced or Metastatic Colorectal Cancer	I	PARP inhibitor Chemotherapy
NCT00678132	AZD2281 and Cisplatin Plus Gemcitabine to Treat Solid Tumor Cancers	I	PARP inhibitor Chemotherapy
NCT00515866	Study to Assess the Safety & Tolerability of a PARP Inhibitor in Combination with Gemcitabine in Pancreatic Cancer	I	PARP inhibitor Chemotherapy
NCT01460888	Radiotherapy & Olaparib in COmbination for Carcinoma of the Oesophagus (ROCOCO)	I	PARP inhibitor Radiotherapy
NCT02308072	Phase I Study of Olaparib Combined with Cisplatin-based Chemoradiotherapy to Treat Locally Advanced Head and Neck Cancer (ORCA-2)	I	PARP inhibitor Chemoradiotherapy

Selected clinical studies involving DDR inhibitors as a single agent or adjuvant therapy in combination with conventional chemotherapy or radiotherapy in cancer patients.

Table 1.
Ongoing DDR inhibitor trials.

damage and tumor cell death [61]. (3) IKKα directly activates ATM via BRAF regulates DNA damage and inhibition of IKKα induces DNA damage associated cell death in colon cancer [62]. Although these signaling molecules are involved in the regulation of DDR in cancers, their mechanism and therapeutic efficiency are yet to develop.

DCLK1, a protein kinase is overexpressed in various tumor cancers [63–65]. DCLK1 plays a critical role in injury response for repair via regulating DDR [8]. However, recently the role of DCLK1 in the regulation of DDR in cancers has established by many investigators [66–68]. In an in vitro mechanistic study, it is reported that DCLK1 caused chromatin instability, and chromatin rearrangement in colon, lung, and breast cancer cell lines, which drives the advancement of cancer cells for progression and this function is independent of its kinase activity [68]. In another study, it is reported that DCLK1 regulates the phosphorylation of CHK1 in pancreatic cancer cells. Inhibition of DCLK1 enhanced the sensitivity to gemcitabine treatment [67]. In a parallel study, it is shown that DCLK1 by regulating the phosphorylation of CHK1 enhances the sensitivity of 5-FU in colon cancer [69]. Taken together these reports suggest that DCLK1 plays a critical role in the regulation of DDR for cancer cell survival and progression. Novel therapies in the combination of targeting DCLK1 along with chemotherapeutic agents or targeting DCLK1 plus targeting an ATM or ATR with chemotherapeutic agents will be beneficial for the most effective treatment against cancers particularly the resistant cancers.

6. DCLK1 and radiation mitigators

Radiation therapy has been used for the treatment of a wide range of malignancies, especially cancers. Radiation not only kills cancer cells, but it also kills/affects normal healthy cells. Exposure of normal tissues to a substantial amount of radiation may cause both acute and chronic damage that can result in adverse effects for intended treatment [70, 71]. For example, radiation enteritis (RE) is an intestinal inflammatory process that occurs in response to radiotherapy [72]. It is a major health concern characterized by abdominal pain, diarrhea, and rectal bleeding [73]. It can be complicated by translocation of gut bacteria into the circulation due to the loss of intestinal epithelial cells, disruption of intraepithelial tight junctions, and loss of regenerative ability resulting in severe impairment of gut function and even death. Relatively little is known about the mechanisms underlying the intestinal epithelial injury repair, cell survival and crypt regeneration in RE. Besides the severe side effects resulted in gastrointestinal mucosal damage, ionizing radiation also impairs the bone marrow-derived hematopoietic cells and immune response, which causes a significant increase in morbidity and mortality [74]. Prevention and amelioration of radiation-induced adverse effects would improve the quality of life for patients and would help cancer curability by allowing more intense therapies [75].

There are three types of chemical/biological agents used to interfere with radiation effects. Agents used before or at the time of radiation treatment are called radioprotectors, whereas agents used post-treatment are called radiation mitigators, agents used to ameliorate established normal tissue toxicity are considered treatment [76]. Currently, Amifostine is the only radioprotector in clinical use, and a few radiation mitigators been used [76]. DCLK1 can be a novel target for radiation mitigators for action, as it is mentioned above, deletion of DCLK1 within intestinal epithelial cells results in the premature death of mice following severe radiation injury, suggesting that DCLK1 is a major mediator of the crypt epithelial survival to severe genotoxic injury via a DDR-ATM mediated mechanism [8]. Recently, single-cell analysis in the intestine has revealed that the DCLK1 expressing epithelial cells in the intestine is the primary source of Cox1 (Ptgs1) and Cox2 (Ptgs2) for PGE2 synthesis [77]. PGE2 increases the survival of murine intestinal stem cells when given before photon radiation [78, 79]. It is reported that the treatment of dimethyl-PGE2 to the intestinal epithelial cells increased the survival of the colonic epithelial cells by enhancing DCLK1 expression and reduced the DNA damage [8]. Qu et al. reported that Notch signaling in the intestinal epithelium prevents the death of epithelial cells expressing DCLK1 following radiation injury [80]. Also, dietary pectin has been demonstrated to increase intestinal crypt stem cell survival following radiation injury via a DCLK1 [81]. Kantara et al. have reported that a novel regenerative peptide TP508 can significantly increase survival and delay mortality by mitigating radiation-induced intestinal and colonic toxicity, and its mechanism of action via upregulating the expression of DCLK1 in the intestinal epithelial cells which are responsible for maintaining and regenerating intestinal crypts [82]. In summary, DCLK1 could be a potential radiation mitigator by regulating DDR to ameliorate radiation-induced adverse effects.

7. Conclusion

It is becoming clear that DCLK1 contributes to DNA damage response and repair via direct and indirect mechanisms that are distinct from its role as a stem cell marker. A long-standing question of how DDR is regulated in response to DNA damage is now getting a new clarity. Furthermore, (i) DCLK1 and ATM direct interaction for ATM activation following DSBs and (ii) radiation mitigators enhance the survival of cells following DSBs via a DCLK1 dependent mechanism, which expects that DCLK1 can be a potential target for radiation mitigators in radiotherapy. Finally, in the expanding field of DDR, it is important to consider how DCLK1 is involved in the repair of DNA in cancer and homeostatic injure conditions. This will allow clinical and non-clinical researchers and practitioners to avoid possible issues with DCLK1 therapeutics, such as enhanced cancer survival and cancer advancement with DCLK1 dependent mitigators during radiotherapy, and, more excitingly, inhibition of DCLK1 along with DDR following chemo-therapy or radiotherapy in cancers will lead the way to develop novel strategies for the effective treatment of cancer.

Acknowledgements

This work was supported by DOD grant # W81XWH-18-1-0457 (PI: Chandrakesan).

Conflict of interest

The authors declare no conflict of interest.

Author details

Janani Panneerselvam, Dongfeng Qu, Courtney Houchen, Michael Bronze and Parthasarathy Chandrakesan*
Department of Medicine, University of Oklahoma Health Sciences Center, Oklahoma City, OK, USA

*Address all correspondence to: parthasarathy-chandrakesan@ouhsc.edu

References

[1] Cimprich KA, Cortez D. ATR: An essential regulator of genome integrity. Nature Reviews. Molecular Cell Biology. 2008;**9**(8):616-627

[2] Jackson SP, Bartek J. The DNA-damage response in human biology and disease. Nature. 2009;**461**(7267):1071-1078

[3] Derks KW, Hoeijmakers JH, Pothof J. The DNA damage response: The omics era and its impact. DNA Repair (Amst). 2014;**19**:214-220

[4] Ribezzo F, Shiloh Y, Schumacher B. Systemic DNA damage responses in aging and diseases. Seminars in Cancer Biology. 2016;**37**-**38**:26-35

[5] Bensimon A, Aebersold R, Shiloh Y. Beyond ATM: The protein kinase landscape of the DNA damage response. FEBS Letters. 2011;**585**(11):1625-1639

[6] Mahajan K, Mahajan NP. Cross talk of tyrosine kinases with the DNA damage signaling pathways. Nucleic Acids Research. 2015;**43**(22):10588-10601

[7] Lin PT, Gleeson JG, Corbo JC, Flanagan L, Walsh CA. DCAMKL1 encodes a protein kinase with homology to doublecortin that regulates microtubule polymerization. The Journal of Neuroscience. 2000;**20**(24):9152-9161

[8] Chandrakesan P, May R, Weygant N, Qu D, Berry WL, Sureban SM, et al. Intestinal tuft cells regulate the ATM mediated DNA damage response via Dclk1 dependent mechanism for crypt restitution following radiation injury. Scientific Reports. 2016;**6**:37667

[9] Chatterjee N, Walker GC. Mechanisms of DNA damage, repair, and mutagenesis. Environmental and Molecular Mutagenesis. 2017;**58**(5):235-263

[10] Gupta D, Lin B, Cowan A, Heinen CD. ATR-Chk1 activation mitigates replication stress caused by mismatch repair-dependent processing of DNA damage. Proceedings of the National Academy of Sciences of the United States of America. 2018;**115**(7):1523-1528

[11] Basu B, Yap TA, Molife LR, de Bono JS. Targeting the DNA damage response in oncology: Past, present and future perspectives. Current Opinion in Oncology. 2012;**24**(3):316-324

[12] Pan MR, Li K, Lin SY, Hung WC. Connecting the dots: From DNA damage and repair to aging. International Journal of Molecular Sciences. 2016;**17**(5):685

[13] Petsalaki E, Zachos G. DNA damage response proteins regulating mitotic cell division: Double agents preserving genome stability. The FEBS Journal. 6 February 2020. DOI: 10.1111/febs.15240

[14] Scully R, Panday A, Elango R, Willis NA. DNA double-strand break repair-pathway choice in somatic mammalian cells. Nature Reviews. Molecular Cell Biology. 2019;**20**(11):698-714

[15] Hoeijmakers JH. DNA damage, aging, and cancer. The New England Journal of Medicine. 2009;**361**(15):1475-1485

[16] Maynard S, Schurman SH, Harboe C, de Souza-Pinto NC, Bohr VA. Base excision repair of oxidative DNA damage and association with cancer and aging. Carcinogenesis. 2009;**30**(1):2-10

[17] Kerzendorfer C, O'Driscoll M. Human DNA damage response and repair deficiency syndromes: Linking genomic instability and cell cycle checkpoint proficiency. DNA Repair (Amst). 2009;**8**(9):1139-1152

[18] Sirbu BM, Cortez D. DNA damage response: Three levels of DNA repair regulation. Cold Spring Harbor Perspectives in Biology. 2013;**5**(8):a012724

[19] Fleck O, Nielsen O. DNA repair. Journal of Cell Science. 2004;**117** (Pt 4):515-517

[20] Marti TM, Fleck O. DNA repair nucleases. Cellular and Molecular Life Sciences. 2004;**61**(3):336-354

[21] Eker AP, Quayle C, Chaves I, van der Horst GT. DNA repair in mammalian cells: Direct DNA damage reversal: Elegant solutions for nasty problems. Cellular and Molecular Life Sciences. 2009;**66**(6):968-980

[22] Mishina Y, Duguid EM, He C. Direct reversal of DNA alkylation damage. Chemical Reviews. 2006;**106**(2):215-232

[23] Matsumoto N, Pilz DT, Ledbetter DH. Genomic structure, chromosomal mapping, and expression pattern of human DCAMKL1 (KIAA0369), a homologue of DCX (XLIS). Genomics. 1999;**56**(2):179-183

[24] Burgess HA, Reiner O. Alternative splice variants of doublecortin-like kinase are differentially expressed and have different kinase activities. The Journal of Biological Chemistry. 2002;**277**(20):17696-17705

[25] Engels BM, Schouten TG, van Dullemen J, Gosens I, Vreugdenhil E. Functional differences between two DCLK splice variants. Brain Research. Molecular Brain Research. 2004;**120**(2):103-114

[26] Sossey-Alaoui K, Srivastava AK. DCAMKL1, a brain-specific transmembrane protein on 13q12.3 that is similar to doublecortin (DCX). Genomics. 1999;**56**(1):121-126

[27] Weygant N, Qu D, Berry WL, May R, Chandrakesan P, Owen DB, et al. Small molecule kinase inhibitor LRRK2-IN-1 demonstrates potent activity against colorectal and pancreatic cancer through inhibition of doublecortin-like kinase 1. Molecular Cancer. 2014;**13**:103

[28] Omori Y, Suzuki M, Ozaki K, Harada Y, Nakamura Y, Takahashi E, et al. Expression and chromosomal localization of KIAA0369, a putative kinase structurally related to Doublecortin. Journal of Human Genetics. 1998;**43**(3):169-177

[29] Westphalen CB, Asfaha S, Hayakawa Y, Takemoto Y, Lukin DJ, Nuber AH, et al. Long-lived intestinal tuft cells serve as colon cancer-initiating cells. The Journal of Clinical Investigation. 2014;**124**(3):1283-1295

[30] Nakanishi Y, Seno H, Fukuoka A, Ueo T, Yamaga Y, Maruno T, et al. Dclk1 distinguishes between tumor and normal stem cells in the intestine. Nature Genetics. 2013;**45**(1):98-103

[31] Westphalen CB, Takemoto Y, Tanaka T, Macchini M, Jiang Z, Renz BW, et al. Dclk1 defines quiescent pancreatic progenitors that promote injury-induced regeneration and tumorigenesis. Cell Stem Cell. 2016;**18**(4):441-455

[32] O'Connell MR, Sarkar S, Luthra GK, Okugawa Y, Toiyama Y, Gajjar AH, et al. Epigenetic changes and alternate promoter usage by human colon cancers for expressing DCLK1-isoforms: Clinical implications. Scientific Reports. 2015;**5**:14983

[33] Hasty P. The impact of DNA damage, genetic mutation and cellular responses on cancer prevention, longevity and aging: Observations in humans and mice. Mechanisms of Ageing and Development. 2005;**126**(1):71-77

[34] DiCarlo AL, Tamarat R, Rios CI, Benderitter M, Czarniecki CW,

Allio TC, et al. Cellular therapies for treatment of radiation injury: Report from a NIH/NIAID and IRSN Workshop. Radiation Research. 2017;**188**(2):e54-e75

[35] May R, Qu D, Weygant N, Chandrakesan P, Ali N, Lightfoot SA, et al. Brief report: Dclk1 deletion in tuft cells results in impaired epithelial repair after radiation injury. Stem Cells. 2014;**32**(3):822-827

[36] Yu J. Intestinal stem cell injury and protection during cancer therapy. Translational Cancer Research. 2013;**2**(5):384-396

[37] Kenyon J, Gerson SL. The role of DNA damage repair in aging of adult stem cells. Nucleic Acids Research. 2007;**35**(22):7557-7565

[38] Lee JH, Paull TT. Activation and regulation of ATM kinase activity in response to DNA double-strand breaks. Oncogene. 2007;**26**(56):7741-7748

[39] Ch'ang HJ, Maj JG, Paris F, Xing HR, Zhang J, Truman JP, et al. ATM regulates target switching to escalating doses of radiation in the intestines. Nature Medicine. 2005;**11**(5):484-490

[40] Rotolo JA, Mesicek J, Maj J, Truman JP, Haimovitz-Friedman A, Kolesnick R, et al. Regulation of ceramide synthase-mediated crypt epithelium apoptosis by DNA damage repair enzymes. Cancer Research. 2010;**70**(3):957-967

[41] Broustas CG, Lieberman HB. DNA damage response genes and the development of cancer metastasis. Radiation Research. 2014;**181**(2):111-130

[42] Sun S, Osterman MD, Li M. Tissue specificity of DNA damage response and tumorigenesis. Cancer Biology & Medicine. 2019;**16**(3):396-414

[43] Biss M, Xiao W. Selective tumor killing based on specific DNA-damage response deficiencies. Cancer Biology & Therapy. 2012;**13**(5):239-246

[44] Bhattacharya S, Asaithamby A. Repurposing DNA repair factors to eradicate tumor cells upon radiotherapy. Translational Cancer Research. 2017;**6**(Suppl 5):S822-SS39

[45] O'Connor MJ. Targeting the DNA damage response in cancer. Molecular Cell. 2015;**60**(4):547-560

[46] Bartek J, Bartkova J, Lukas J. DNA damage signalling guards against activated oncogenes and tumour progression. Oncogene. 2007;**26**(56):7773-7779

[47] Bartkova J, Horejsi Z, Koed K, Kramer A, Tort F, Zieger K, et al. DNA damage response as a candidate anti-cancer barrier in early human tumorigenesis. Nature. 2005;**434**(7035):864-870

[48] Housman G, Byler S, Heerboth S, Lapinska K, Longacre M, Snyder N, et al. Drug resistance in cancer: An overview. Cancers (Basel). 2014;**6**(3):1769-1792

[49] Periti P, Mini E. Drug resistance in cancer: An overview of the clinical aspects. Journal of Chemotherapy. 1989;**1**(1):5-9

[50] Goodman MF, Woodgate R. Translesion DNA polymerases. Cold Spring Harbor Perspectives in Biology. 2013;**5**(10):a010363

[51] Waters LS, Minesinger BK, Wiltrout ME, D'Souza S, Woodruff RV, Walker GC. Eukaryotic translesion polymerases and their roles and regulation in DNA damage tolerance. Microbiology and Molecular Biology Reviews. 2009;**73**(1):134-154

[52] Bianchi J, Rudd SG, Jozwiakowski SK, Bailey LJ, Soura V, Taylor E, et al. PrimPol bypasses UV

photoproducts during eukaryotic chromosomal DNA replication. Molecular Cell. 2013;**52**(4):566-573

[53] Heller RC, Marians KJ. Non-replicative helicases at the replication fork. DNA Repair (Amst). 2007;**6**(7):945-952

[54] Cerrato A, Morra F, Celetti A. Use of poly ADP-ribose polymerase [PARP] inhibitors in cancer cells bearing DDR defects: The rationale for their inclusion in the clinic. Journal of Experimental & Clinical Cancer Research. 2016;**35**(1):179

[55] Ceccaldi R, Liu JC, Amunugama R, Hajdu I, Primack B, Petalcorin MI, et al. Homologous-recombination-deficient tumours are dependent on Poltheta-mediated repair. Nature. 2015;**518**(7538):258-262

[56] Mateos-Gomez PA, Gong F, Nair N, Miller KM, Lazzerini-Denchi E, Sfeir A. Mammalian polymerase theta promotes alternative NHEJ and suppresses recombination. Nature. 2015;**518**(7538):254-257

[57] Francica P, Rottenberg S. Mechanisms of PARP inhibitor resistance in cancer and insights into the DNA damage response. Genome Medicine. 2018;**10**(1):101

[58] Minchom A, Aversa C, Lopez J. Dancing with the DNA damage response: Next-generation anti-cancer therapeutic strategies. Therapeutic Advances in Medical Oncology. 2018;**10**:1758835918786658

[59] Liu J, Zhang Q, Ruan B, Chen W, Zheng J, Xu B, et al. MORC2 regulates C/EBPalpha-mediated cell differentiation via sumoylation. Cell Death and Differentiation. 2019;**26**(10):1905-1917

[60] Li DQ, Nair SS, Ohshiro K, Kumar A, Nair VS, Pakala SB, et al. MORC2 signaling integrates phosphorylation-dependent, ATPase-coupled chromatin remodeling during the DNA damage response. Cell Reports. 2012;**2**(6):1657-1669

[61] Yang RM, Nanayakkara D, Kalimutho M, Mitra P, Khanna KK, Dray E, et al. MYB regulates the DNA damage response and components of the homology-directed repair pathway in human estrogen receptor-positive breast cancer cells. Oncogene. 2019;**38**(26):5239-5249

[62] Colomer C, Margalef P, Villanueva A, Vert A, Pecharroman I, Sole L, et al. IKKalpha kinase regulates the DNA damage response and drives chemo-resistance in cancer. Molecular Cell. 2019;**75**(4):669-682

[63] Chandrakesan P, Panneerselvam J, Qu D, Weygant N, May R, Bronze MS, et al. Regulatory roles of Dclk1 in epithelial mesenchymal transition and cancer stem cells. Journal of Carcinogenesis & Mutagenesis. 2016;**7**(2):257

[64] Chandrakesan P, Weygant N, May R, Qu D, Chinthalapally HR, Sureban SM, et al. DCLK1 facilitates intestinal tumor growth via enhancing pluripotency and epithelial mesenchymal transition. Oncotarget. 2014;**5**(19):9269-9280

[65] Chandrakesan P, Yao J, Qu D, May R, Weygant N, Ge Y, et al. Dclk1, a tumor stem cell marker, regulates pro-survival signaling and self-renewal of intestinal tumor cells. Molecular Cancer. 2017;**16**(1):30

[66] Mohammadi C, Najafi R. DCLK1 as a promising marker for radioresistance in colorectal cancer. Journal of Gastrointestinal Cancer. 17 August 2019. DOI: 10.1007/s12029-019-00292-z

[67] Kawamura D, Takemoto Y, Nishimoto A, Ueno K, Hosoyama T, Shirasawa B, et al. Enhancement of

cytotoxic effects of gemcitabine by Dclk1 inhibition through suppression of Chk1 phosphorylation in human pancreatic cancer cells. Oncology Reports. 2017;**38**(5):3238-3244

[68] Lu Y, Maruyama J, Kuwata K, Fukuda H, Iwasa H, Arimoto-Matsuzaki K, et al. Doublecortin-like kinase 1 compromises DNA repair and induces chromosomal instability. Biochemistry and Biophysics Reports. 2018;**16**:130-137

[69] Suehiro Y, Takemoto Y, Nishimoto A, Ueno K, Shirasawa B, Tanaka T, et al. Dclk1 inhibition cancels 5-FU-induced cell-cycle arrest and decreases cell survival in colorectal cancer. Anticancer Research. 2018;**38**(11):6225-6230

[70] Bray FN, Simmons BJ, Wolfson AH, Nouri K. Acute and chronic cutaneous reactions to ionizing radiation therapy. Dermatology and Therapy. 2016;**6**(2):185-206

[71] Lam SY, Peppelenbosch MP, Fuhler GM. Prediction and treatment of radiation enteropathy: Can intestinal bugs lead the way? Clinical Cancer Research. 2019;**25**(21):6280-6282

[72] Harb AH, Abou Fadel C, Sharara AI. Radiation enteritis. Current Gastroenterology Reports. 2014;**16**(5):383

[73] Huang Y, Guo F, Yao D, Li Y, Li J. Surgery for chronic radiation enteritis: Outcome and risk factors. The Journal of Surgical Research. 2016;**204**(2):335-343

[74] Dainiak N. Hematologic consequences of exposure to ionizing radiation. Experimental Hematology. 2002;**30**(6):513-528

[75] Koukourakis MI. Radiation damage and radioprotectants: New concepts in the era of molecular medicine. The British Journal of Radiology. 2012;**85**(1012):313-330

[76] Citrin D, Cotrim AP, Hyodo F, Baum BJ, Krishna MC, Mitchell JB. Radioprotectors and mitigators of radiation-induced normal tissue injury. The Oncologist. 2010;**15**(4):360-371

[77] Haber AL, Biton M, Rogel N, Herbst RH, Shekhar K, Smillie C, et al. A single-cell survey of the small intestinal epithelium. Nature. 2017;**551**(7680): 333-339

[78] Hanson WR. Radiation protection of murine intestine by WR-2721, 16,16-dimethyl prostaglandin E2, and the combination of both agents. Radiation Research. 1987;**111**(2):361-373

[79] Hanson WR, Grdina DJ. Radiation-induced DNA single-strand breaks in the intestinal mucosal cells of mice treated with the radioprotectors WR-2721 or 16-16 dimethyl prostaglandin E2. International Journal of Radiation Biology and Related Studies in Physics, Chemistry, and Medicine. 1987;**52**(1):67-76

[80] Qu D, May R, Sureban SM, Weygant N, Chandrakesan P, Ali N, et al. Inhibition of notch signaling reduces the number of surviving Dclk1+ reserve crypt epithelial stem cells following radiation injury. American Journal of Physiology. Gastrointestinal and Liver Physiology. 2014;**306**(5):G404-G411

[81] Sureban SM, May R, Qu D, Chandrakesan P, Weygant N, Ali N, et al. Dietary pectin increases intestinal crypt stem cell survival following radiation injury. PLoS One. 2015;**10**(8):e0135561

[82] Kantara C, Moya SM, Houchen CW, Umar S, Ullrich RL, Singh P, et al. Novel regenerative peptide TP508 mitigates radiation-induced gastrointestinal damage by activating stem cells and preserving crypt integrity. Laboratory Investigation. 2015;**95**(11):1222-1233

Chapter 6

Oxidative Stress and Vanadium

Marcela Rojas-Lemus, Patricia Bizarro-Nevares, Nelly López-Valdez, Adriana González-Villalva, Gabriela Guerrero-Palomo, María Eugenia Cervantes-Valencia, Otto Tavera-Cabrera, Norma Rivera-Fernández, Brenda Casarrubias-Tabarez, Martha Ustarroz-Cano, Armando Rodríguez-Zepeda, Francisco Pasos-Nájera and Teresa Fortoul-van der Goes

Abstract

Air pollution is a worldwide health problem, and metals are one of the various air pollutants to which living creatures are exposed. The pollution by metals such as: lead, cadmium, manganese, and vanadium have a common mechanism of action: the production of oxidative stress in the cell. Oxidative stress favors the production of free radicals, which damage biomolecules such as: DNA, proteins, lipids, and carbohydrates; these free radicals produce changes that are observed in different organs and systems. Vanadium is a transition element delivered into the atmosphere by the combustion of fossil fuels as oxides and adhered to the PM enters into the respiratory system, then crosses the alveolar wall and enters into the systemic circulation. In this chapter, we will review the oxidative stress induced by vanadium—as a common mechanism of metal pollutants—; in addition, we will review the protective effect of the antioxidants (carnosine and ascorbate).

Keywords: air pollution, metals, vanadium, oxidative stress damage, ascorbate, carnosine

1. Introduction

Air pollution is a worldwide concern because of the health problems associated with its uncontrolled emissions that affect all the biological systems. Within the wide range of pollutants, the suspended particles or particulate matter (PM) are of particular interest, which became more important since IARC listed them as carcinogens. The toxicity of PM is the consequence of the elements adhered to its surface [1]. An example of this are the particles generated by the combustion of fossil fuels and its derivatives, these particles usually consist of a carbon core on which complex mixtures of compounds are adhered, such as: polyaromatic hydrocarbons, toxins, sulfates, nitrates, and especially transition metals like vanadium, manganese, chromium, among others [2]. Metals are considered to play an important role in the induction of toxic effects reported in the literature [3].

Metals are the largest category of globally distributed pollutants with a tendency to accumulate in some human tissues and with a high toxic potential at relatively low concentrations. Constant exposure to certain metals has been linked to inflammation, cell damage, and cancer [4]. Each metal has its own mechanisms of action [5]. Some of them produce its adverse effects alone, while others interact with various factors resulting in greater damage in different organs and systems [4]. It is known that metals, including vanadium, have different toxic pathways, and oxidative stress is the most frequent mechanism [5].

Oxidative stress is the consequence of an imbalance between the production of free radicals and the antioxidant capacity of an organism [6]. It may result from the increase in exposure to oxidants, due to the decrease in the protection against oxidants, or because both events occur simultaneously [7].

A free radical represents any chemical species of independent existence that has one or more missing electrons spinning in its external atomic orbitals. This electrochemical configuration is unstable and gives them property of being a highly reactive and short-lived chemical species [8]. Most of the free radicals of biological interest are usually extremely reactive and have a very short life span (microsecond fractions). When a radical reacts with a non-radical compound, it results in other free radicals, thus generating chain reactions that produce biological effects [9], coupled with the fact that when they collide with a biomolecule and subtract an electron (oxidizing it), it loses its specific function in the cell [8].

Regardless of the origin, free radicals can interact with the biomolecules found in the cell such as nucleic acids [10], proteins, lipids, and carbohydrates [9], thereby causing potentially serious modifications and consequences in the cell [10].

Vanadium is an element that is find in various oxidation states and participates in reactions that lead to the production of free radicals such as superoxide, peroxovanadyl, and the highly reactive radical hydroxyl [8].

2. Oxidative stress, vanadium, and cellular and systemic damages

The increasing production of free radicals leads the cell to an imbalance in its redox state and thus generating oxidative stress; therefore, the cellular dysfunction will be reflected in the failure of organs and systems.

2.1 Oxidative stress and cellular damage

The cell is the basic functional unit of life and its dysfunction induced by oxidative stress might produce DNA damage and cell death.

2.2 Oxidative stress, vanadium, and DNA damage

The International Agency for Research on Cancer lists vanadium pentoxide (V_2O_5) as "a possible carcinogen for humans" in group 2B. The above was based on evidence of lung cancer generation in mice that was published by the National Toxicology Program [11]. However, evidence on the carcinogenicity of vanadium has been widely questioned by Duffus in 2007 [12] and Starr et al. [13]. Information related to the carcinogenic and genotoxic potential of vanadium pentoxide (V_2O_5) is limited [14]. In both animal and human models, the effects on the DNA caused by vanadium include single strand breaks, micronuclei, chromosomal aberrations (structural and numerical), and oxidation of nitrogenous bases [15, 16]. The spectrum of alterations that DNA might have as a consequence of free radicals interaction, in this case caused by vanadium, are: deoxyribose oxidation, modification of nitrogen bases, chain cross-linking, and ruptures [6]. The double or single chain breaks that are generated by the interaction of free radicals with DNA are produced by the fragmentation of the sugar-phosphate skeleton or indirectly by the cleavage of oxidized bases [17].

The above indicates that vanadium is an element with mutagenic potential, because its genotoxic, aneugenic, and clastogenic effects, although there are not strongly data supporting that vanadium is carcinogenic, this possibility should not be eliminated, because the DNA damage caused by the exposure and therefore genetic instability, processes closely related to the generation of malignancy [18].

2.3 Oxidative stress, vanadium, and cellular death

Cell death is central to physiological homeostasis; the balance between cellular differentiation, proliferation, and death support aspects of biology, including embryogenesis, organ function, tissue remodeling, immune regulation, and carcinogenesis. Cell death was once believed to be the result of one of three different processes: apoptosis, autophagy or necrosis; however, in the last decade about 15 different types have been reported, highlighting that a cell can die via different pathways which depends on the intensity of the stimuli [19]. Reactive oxygen species (ROS) activates cell death and plays different roles in the biological systems which can be either injurious or beneficial. Generation of ROS might be caused by metals such as: arsenic, cadmium, chromium, cobalt, copper, gold, iron, nickel, rhodium titanium or vanadium [8]. Vanadium compounds can interconvert into different species (vanadyl and vanadate) event which is constantly occurring inside the cell in the presence of ROS [20].

Studies *in vivo* and *in vitro* showed that vanadium compounds induce cell death in leukemia [21], lung cancer [22] cervical and breast carcinoma [23], neuroblastoma [24], liver carcinoma [25], osteosarcoma [26], and pancreatic ductal adenocarcinoma [27]. *In vitro* studies demonstrated that the cell lines stimulated with vanadium compounds produce H_2O_2 and O_2 and induce autophagy, necroptosis, and mitotic catastrophe [27]. Apoptosis is the main type of cell death associated with vanadium compounds, reporting the release of cytochrome c from mitochondria [21] and the disruption of the mitochondrial membrane potential [25]. This type of cell death is mediated through the activation of p53 and p21 [27], which modulate the activation or inactivation of phosphorylation of some proteins such as MEK, ERK 1/2, PI3K, p38, JNK, TNF-alpha, and NFkB [28].

2.4 Oxidative stress and vanadium in different systems

The systemic vanadium effects observed *in vivo* and *in vitro* are briefly described below.

2.4.1 Reproductive system

The reprotoxic effects of vanadium in male reproductive system in laboratory animals include interruption of spermatogenesis [29], morphological and biochemical changes in spermatogenic cells [30], abnormalities in the shape and movement of sperm, as well as decrease in the weight of the testis, epididymis, and prostate [31].

One of the mechanisms of vanadium toxicity includes imbalance in the cellular redox state [30]; testicular cells are highly susceptible to free radical actions because its membranes are rich in polyunsaturated fatty acids, which limits the fluidity of the membrane and alters the functioning of integral membrane proteins [32].

In rat's testis, after given sodium metavanadate ($NaVO_3$), an increase in malondialdehyde (MDA) was found, which is a product of lipid peroxidation, as well as a decrease in the activity of superoxide dismutase (SOD) and catalase [33]. Intraperitoneal administration of $NaVO_3$ caused in the testis a decrease in the number of germ cells, the presence of degenerated cells, and necrosis of the seminiferous tubules, associated to the increase in testicular lipid peroxidation and inhibition of the activity of antioxidant enzymes (SOD and catalase) [34]; alteration in spermatogenesis, decrease in serum testosterone, LH and FSH levels, inhibition of steroidogenic enzyme activity, increase in testicular vanadium concentration, inhibition of antioxidant enzymes (SOD, catalase and GPx), increased levels of lipid peroxidation [29], and abnormalities in the form of sperm have also been reported [35].

During female reproductive processes, such as ovarian follicle development, ovarian steroid synthesis, ovulation, fertilization, and implantation, require certain amounts of ROS [36]; however, due to the oxidizing effects of vanadium, the delicate balance between ROS generation and the cellular antioxidant system can be altered.

In the case of the female reproductive system of rats, it has been observed that the administration of vanadium sulfate ($VOSO_3$) causes oxidative stress and biochemical alterations in uterine cells, such as the decrease in the activity of alkaline phosphatase and adenosine triphosphatase; while in the ovary, the damage of the oocyte and ovarian follicles was observed, as well as stromal fibrosis [37]. In an inhalation model of vanadium in non-pregnant females, histological alterations were found in the ovary and uterus and lipid peroxidation, indicated by the increase in the levels of 4-hydroxynonenal (4-HNE) a marker of oxidative stress [30].

Vanadium crosses the placental barrier and exerts its toxic effects on embryos and fetuses; in rats, it has been observed that fetal weight decreases and the number of implants and fetuses, while the number of resorptions, malformations, and dead fetus increases [31]. The fetotoxic and embryotoxic effects of vanadium have also been associated with oxidative stress since both in fetuses and in mothers exposed to vanadyl sulfate ($VOSO_4$), and lipid peroxidation was observed in the liver [37].

2.4.2 Urinary system

Kidney chronic disease (CKD) has increased worldwide. The main risk factors for the development of this disease are diabetes, metabolic syndrome, and hypertension. However, there are a segment of population that has none of these risk factors and there are other factors that are being studied as a possible cause of renal injury. One of them is the environmental pollution, particularly pollution by metals in atmosphere and water. Arsenic, cadmium, mercury, lead, and vanadium have been reported as nephrotoxic metals because of the production of ROS and the induction of oxidative stress. These metals enter the body by oral or inhaled exposure, then they are absorbed, enter into the systemic circulation, and distributed into the organs where they may accumulate. Finally, most of them are eliminated by the kidney, reason why this organ is one of the most affected structures by metals [38]. Also, there are reports that in CKD when there is a problem to eliminate pollutant metals, these can concentrate into kidney cells and the damage worsened when it occurs in humans, both in children and adults [39]. Oxidative stress and inflammation are the principal mechanisms of renal injury; in addition, arsenic, cadmium, mercury, and lead are associated to hyperglycemia that may aggravate the oxidative stress and the renal damage. Vanadium is an exception because it has a hypoglycemic effect, but this does not ameliorate its toxicity [40].

Vanadium is nephrotoxic, as it has been proved mainly in animal models, but also in humans [41]. In a report of human acute poisoning by oral ammonium metavanadate, hypoglycemia, bronchoconstriction, and acute renal insufficiency were the causes of death; in a chronic model of vanadium exposure reported glomerulonephritis, glomerular and tubular necrosis that lead to renal insufficiency and hypertension [42]. The reported findings in other study with ammonium metavanadate *p.o.* at doses of 30, 45, and 60 mg/kg were edema, vacuolization, and degeneration of epithelial tubular cells at 21st day of exposure [43]. Another research group, using different compounds and doses of vanadium (45 and 90 mg/kg) reported thickening of glomerular basement membrane, pyknotic nuclei, cellular vacuolization, and pyelonephritis [44]. In our group, in a subchronic model of vanadium inhalation, we found foci of inflammatory cells, vacuolation, loss of microvilli of epithelial tubular cells, and changes in urine parameters as proteinuria and hematuria associated to the increase, in a time dependent manner, of 4-hidroxynonenal (4-HNE) [45] (**Figure 1A** and **B**). Oxidative stress is also the toxic vanadium mechanism reported by other groups, for example, Marouane et al. [46] found lipid peroxidation, protein denaturation, DNA degradation, and cell membrane disintegration; in addition, Scibior et al. [47] reported elevated malonaldehyde (MDA) as a marker of oxidative stress and enhanced total antioxidant status in a rat model of 12-week oral sodium metavanadate exposure.

2.4.3 Immune system

The immune system is an interactive network of lymphoid organs, cells, humoral factors, and cytokines whose function is to distinguish between self and non-self-antigens in the host system, thus providing mechanisms against infections and tolerance to the components of the host. When an antigen attacks the host, two distinct, yet interrelated, branches of the immune system are activated, the nonspecific/innate and specific/adaptive immune response. Both of these systems

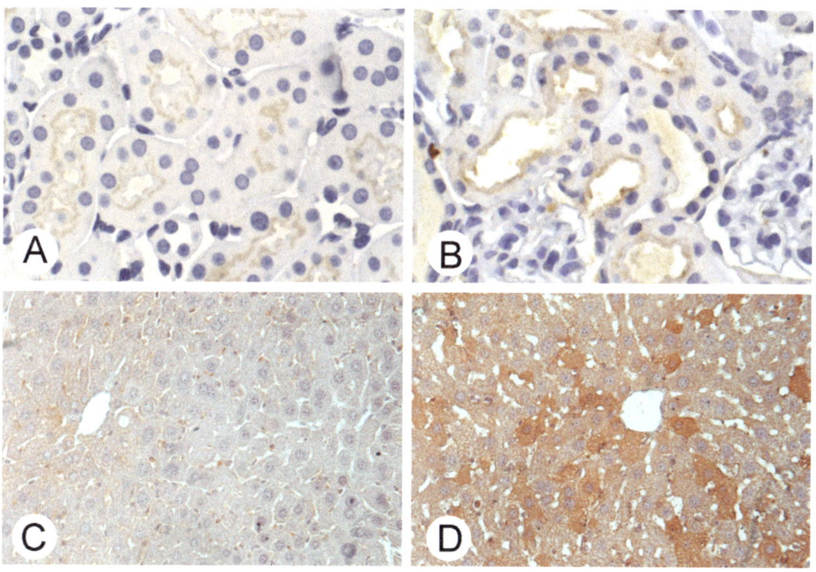

Figure 1.
4-hydrxynonenal (4-HNE) in kidney and liver as a marker of oxidative stress. (A) Kidney tubules in control group with a basal 4-HNE immunoreactivity. (B) In vanadium group, 4-HNE immunoreactivity increased in microvilli of proximal tubules after 8th-week exposure. (C) Liver of control group with a basal 4-HNE immunoreactivity. (D) Liver of vanadium group after 8th-week exposure with increase in 4-HNE immunoreactivity in hepatocytes, some of them with a very intense mark.

have certain physiological mechanisms, which enable the host to recognize foreign materials as foreign materials and to neutralize, eliminate, or metabolize them [48]. The immune system is a target of air pollutants, such as vanadium that might impair its function and induce oxidative stress.

In previous studies, effects from vanadium inhalation on the immune system have been demonstrated. Changes in the spleen morphology and a decrease in humoral immune responses have been reported [49], as well as a decrease in the number of thymic dendritic cells, its expression of CD11c and MHC-II biomarkers, and an increase of thymic medullar epithelial cells [50]. Oxidative stress could be an important mechanism involved in these effects and some mechanisms are described as follows:

Sodium metavanadate ($NaVO_3$) induced oxidative stress through generation of ROS and depletion of the antioxidant defense systems. When the exposure is chronic, the oxidative stress turns out in severe damage [51].

The effect of vanadyl sulfate ($VOSO_4$) in blood glucose and in the spleen, in streptozotocin (STZ)-induced diabetic rats was evaluated. The levels of lipid peroxidation (LPO) and glutathione (GSH) in the spleen were analyzed. After 60 days of treatment, spleen LPO significantly increased, but spleen GSH levels significantly decreased in the diabetic group. On the other hand, treatment with $VOSO_4$ reversed these effects in STZ diabetic animals [52]. These studies show that vanadium induced oxidative stress in the spleen, which might disrupt the immune response.

2.4.4 Digestive system

The liver as the major site for metabolism, biotransformation and detoxification of drugs and foreign compounds, is constantly exposed to ROS resulting in oxidative stress and frequently, permanent and irreversible tissue damage [53]. Studies have shown that liver is one of the most important target tissues for vanadium toxicity with its capacity to form ROS by interacting with mitochondrial redox centers, mainly in mitochondrial respiratory processes I, II, and III [54]. Studies with HepG2 cell line have shown that exposure to vanadium causes damage to nuclear and mitochondrial DNA, as well as decreased cell viability [55]. *In vivo* studies from our group demonstrate that vanadium increases lipid peroxidation in V-exposed animals [56]. **Figure 1C** and **D** show the oxidative marker 4-HNE in liver parenchyma.

As a heavily irrigated, highly connected organ with neural, endocrine, digestive, absorptive, and immune functions, the gut can enter oxidative cycles mostly by two well-defined mechanisms:

1. Ambient-polluting microparticle swallowing: especially in heavily polluted areas (industrial centers, cities, mines, etc.), the air is charged with carbon PM, whose size varies between 10 and 2.5 (or even less) micrometers. Such particles are normally covered by metals (vanadium, for instance), which get trapped via natural defense mechanisms in the nasal and oral mucosa, slowly, descending into the pharynx and into the digestive tract carried on through saliva [30].

2. Direct toxic ingestion: recent research relates ingestion of food ingredients—especially sugar (sucrose or high fructose) present mostly in sugar-sweetened beverages (SSB)—with tissue damage. Although there is no specific data on gut tissue damage, it has been reported in other bodily systems—e.g., kidney [45]. This represents a particularly severe problem in a world where no matter the country, the SSB consumption increases steadily year after year [57].

Research on this matter has still a long path to walk. However, preliminary results from ongoing protocols at our laboratory show a significant rise in 4-HNE levels in the gut epithelium in response to air pollution and SSB consumption mice models, which indicate higher oxidative stress levels vs. control groups.

2.4.5 Cardiovascular system

Air pollution has been associated to thrombosis and cardiovascular risk. Pollutants, including PM and metals may induce oxidative stress and inflammation predisposing to endothelial dysfunction, platelet activation, and procoagulant state [58]. There is epidemiological evidence that elevated concentrations of pollutants, e.g., vanadium, are associated to an increase in ER visits for acute cardiovascular effects or exacerbations of preexisting cardiovascular diseases [59].

Vanadium induces oxidative stress, and there is evidence of their toxic effects on endothelium, platelets, and myocardium. An *in vitro* study using HUVEC (human umbilical vein endothelial cells) exposed to different V_2O_5 concentrations reported an increase in ROS that damaged endothelial cells leading to apoptosis and diminished proliferation. This might be involved in endothelial dysfunction and increased cardiovascular risk associated to metals [60]. An *in vivo* vanadium inhalation mice model, from our group, reported thrombocytosis that is an increase in platelet number, but also the presence of giant platelets that are associated to increase reactivity [61]. Also, we found a megakaryocytosis with an increase in megakaryocytes size and granularity because of the activation of JAK/STAT pathway [40, 62, 63]. Platelet aggregation after subchronic vanadium inhalation diminished, but activation markers of platelets P-selectin or CD-62p were increased after the 4th week of exposure, maybe because of the slow elimination of vanadium, so it is possible that this metal has on platelet aggregation a long-term effects [64]. Another effect of vanadium on cardiovascular system is arrhythmia; in our group, we studied its effect on myocardium N-cadherin and connexin-43, important proteins in the intercalated discs. The reduction of both proteins and its effect on the electric stimuli conduction was proposed to explain the pathophysiology of the arrhythmias induced by vanadium [65]. Vanadium and other metals induce oxidative stress that may damage several cells of cardiovascular system.

2.4.6 Respiratory system

The lung is one of the main targets of air pollution damage because it is the first site in contact with the pollutants suspended in the air. After reaching the alveolar epithelium, the pollutants can cross the alveoli-capillary barrier. There are various reports that demonstrate the damage caused to this organ by exposure to specific contaminants, such as vanadium that is part of the suspended particles.

In vivo, it has been reported that inhaled exposure to vanadium, mainly in the form of pentoxide induces histopathological changes in the lung, such as fibrosis [66], inflammation [30, 66, 67], hyperplasia and epithelial metaplasia [30, 67] and apoptotic cell death [68], among others.

Experimental evidence supports that exposure to V_2O_5 increases the production of ROS in lung cells. Wang et al. [68] reported increase in ROS production in mice bronchoalveolar lavage cells treated with a concentration of 10 μm of sodium metavanadate ($NaVO_3$), in a time-exposure dependent manner (3, 10, 30, and 60 minutes) through a spin trapping essay.

On the other hand, other evidence shows that exposure to V modifies in the lung glutathione concentrations, both in its oxidized (GSSG) and reduced (GSH) forms. It is known that oxidative stress results in the depletion of GSH and the increase in

GSS; so, the determination of their respective concentrations in blood and other tissues is considered a measure of intracellular oxidative stress [69].

Schuler et al. reported that in their inhalation model of V_2O_5 at exposure concentrations of 0.25, 1, and 4 mg/m^3, there was an increase in the levels of oxidized glutathione (GSSG) in lung tissue, with the consequent reduction in the ratio between reduced and oxidized glutathione (GSH/GSSG) concentrations [70]. Kulkarni and colleagues reported the same finding in relation to GSH concentration in lung tissue in a model of exposure to V_2O_5 nanoparticles [66]. In addition to this finding in the same study, the significant increase in MDA levels in plasma was identified. The MDA is a final product of lipid peroxidation.

Another biomarker of oxidative damage that has been identified is the 8-oxo-7,8-dihydro-2-deoxyguanosine (8-oxoGuo) in the DNA. Schuler demonstrated the increase in the formation of 8-oxoGuoin at exposure concentrations of 1 and 4 mg/m^3 of V_2O_5 in lung cells [70].

2.4.7 Nervous system

Neurotoxic metals as vanadium can induce oxidative damage in the brain and develop blood brain barrier disruption, neuropathology, and neuronal damage that can trigger central nervous system alterations as depression, increase in anger, fatigue, and tremors between other clinical features [71]. Also, a decrease in tyrosine hydroxylase and dopamine levels has been reported after vanadium exposure [72]. Chronical exposure to $NaVO_3$ can cause, in mice, metal accumulation in the olfactory bulb, brain stem, and cerebellum, as well as histopathological alterations like nuclear shrinkage in the prefrontal cortex and cell death of the hippocampal pyramidal cells and cerebellum Purkinje cells [71]. The accumulation of vanadium in the brain depends more on the exposure time than on the concentration of the metal. In fact, it is reported that disruption of ependymal cells is observed after long periods of vanadium inhalation [73].

Recently, behavioral alterations due to vanadium occupational exposure have been reported. Vanadium exposed workers exhibited poor performance in the simple reaction time, digit span memory, and Benton visual retention tests [74]. Memory loss in mice exposed to vanadium for 3 months was observed; nevertheless, in these animals, memory was recovered 9 months after vanadium was removal [75]. Increased incidence of Parkinson's disease is related to environmental metal exposure. It has been reported that vanadium pentoxide (V_2O_5) is neurotoxic to dopaminergic neurons via caspase-3-dependent PKCδ cleavage, so maybe vanadium can promote nigral dopaminergic degeneration [76].

2.5 Antioxidative action of carnosine and ascorbate

The cells exposed continuously to oxidative stress are not defenseless against free radicals. All aerobic organisms count with a series of mechanisms protecting them against oxidative damage; among them are antioxidant molecules which represent a first line of defense. If the antioxidant mechanisms fail, the cell uses others such as: transient cell arrest, biomolecular repair systems or apoptosis death processes [7].

An antioxidant is any substance that when is present in low concentrations, compared to the oxidizable substrate, decreases or prevents the substrate oxidation. Oxidizable substrates comprise everything that is found in living tissues including proteins, lipids, carbohydrates, and nucleic acids [77].

Cells use a series of antioxidant compounds that react directly with oxidizing agents, functioning as "sweepers" or chemical shields [7]; these molecules have enzymatic or non-enzymatic actions. Non-enzymatic antioxidants carry out the reduction of free radicals through electron donation, thus avoiding oxidative reactions. Glutathione (GSH), alpha-tocopherol (vitamin E), ascorbic acid (vitamin C), carnosine, bilirubin, and uric acid are the main molecules performing this function.

Ascorbate is an important water-soluble antioxidant in biological fluids, because it eliminates reactive oxygen species and radicals such as: alkoxy, hydroxyl, peroxyl, and hydroperoxyl radicals, singlet oxygen, superoxide anion, and ozone. It also eliminates reactive species and radicals derived from nitrogen and chlorine and even radicals that come from other antioxidants [78].

In general, a large number of studies have been carried out to show the beneficial effects of ascorbate. Evidence indicates that supplementation with this compound protects against lipid oxidation *in vivo*, particularly in individuals exposed to exacerbated conditions of oxidative stress, such as smokers [79].

Epidemiological studies of treatment with this antioxidant have shown consistently favorable effects in patients with cardiovascular disease or coronary risk. In addition, it has been suggested that the increase in ascorbate consumption significantly decreases the incidence and mortality from cardiovascular diseases. Even in pathologies related to free radicals and the inability of the organism defenses against them, as is the case of cancer, epidemiological studies show that increased consumption of ascorbate decreases the incidence and mortality from cancer [79].

Experimental evidence indicates that ascorbic acid works as an antidote against acute vanadium poisoning. In mice, Jones and Basinger [80] examined several compounds and concluded that ascorbate was the most promising for human use.

Domingo et al. [81] administered $NaVO_3$ to mice intraperitoneally and observed, as did Jones and Basinger, that ascorbate proved to be the most effective antidote against vanadium poisoning. In another study, Domingo et al. [82] showed that ascorbate stimulates urinary excretion of vanadium when mice are injected intramuscularly with $VOSO_4$.

Another water-soluble antioxidant is carnosine which is a dipeptide composed of β-alanine and L-histidine; it is found naturally in many mammalian species, mainly in the skeletal muscle. It is estimated that 99% of the carnosine in the organism is found in muscular tissue [83].

It has been reported that carnosine may form complexes with transition metals and has antioxidant activity, which implies mechanisms such as chelation of metals, scavenging of ROS, and peroxyl radicals [83].

The antioxidant efficiency of carnosine in the nervous system, when mice are exposed to vanadium inhalation was successfully tested by our group. It was observed that in those groups with carnosine treatment, a larger size granulose cells with a greater number of dendritic spines, and in general less adverse ultrastructural morphological changes, as well as less lipid peroxidation were observed [84].

3. Conclusions

Air pollution has been continuously mentioned as one of the problems that decrease the quality and life expectancy of all living organisms, included humankind. It is true that not all the sources of pollution are from anthropological origin; however, a great deal of it are generated by humans and can be prevented or controlled by those who generate it.

The use of fossil fuels as the quasi unique source of energy and limited use of other sources of energy will maintain the air pollutant levels high enough to keep its deleterious health effects.

As it is revised in this chapter, metals are one of the air pollutants that enter through the respiratory tract, reaching by the systemic circulation every cell in living organisms. Vanadium is one of the elements adhered to PM which results from the incomplete combustion of fossil fuels. PM generates ROS, mainly those that contains transition metals (e.g., Fe, V, and Mn).

Reported previously in this chapter, one of the main toxic mechanisms of metals is oxidative stress which affects all biomolecules. DNA oxidative damage may conduct the cell to genotoxic and mutagenic changes and further to cell death or cancer.

When proteins are oxidized: cell structure, cell signaling modification, and/or disruption of cellular enzymatic processes could be noticed. The reactive molecules which results from these interactions with proteins and ROS may interplay with specific peptide residues such as: lysines, arginines, histidines, and cysteines. The result of these actions causes the formation of reactive carbonyls and protein carbonylation, and its accumulations have been related with chronic diseases and aging.

If lipids are in contact with ROS, peroxidation occurs producing MDA, a biomarker of oxidative stress that could interact with proteins forming protein adducts and inactivating the protein. Another lipid peroxidation product is 4-HNE with cytotoxic effects and the induction of pro-inflammatory cytokines, which could result in cellular dysfunction and death [85].

If the sources of V or other pollutants are not reduced and the oxidative insults prevail, we can supplement our system with antioxidants such as vitamin C. This water-soluble molecule is not synthesized by humans, and its supplementation is obtained by different dietary sources such as fruits and vegetables or by vitamin C supplements. One of the benefits of vitamin C is its antioxidant action, scavenging ROS and NOS species. In addition, it helps to regenerate alpha-tocopherol and coenzyme Q; also, vitamin C inhibits NAD(P)H oxidase decreasing ROS formation [86]. Another less known endogenous and exogenous antioxidant is carnosine that in our laboratory showed promising antioxidant effects in the nervous system [84].

The systems and organs affected by the oxidative potential of vanadium and the protective effect of antioxidants are summarized in **Figure 2**.

While humankind decide to work together in order to find a common solution for controlling air pollution, scientist should be working in finding more and better

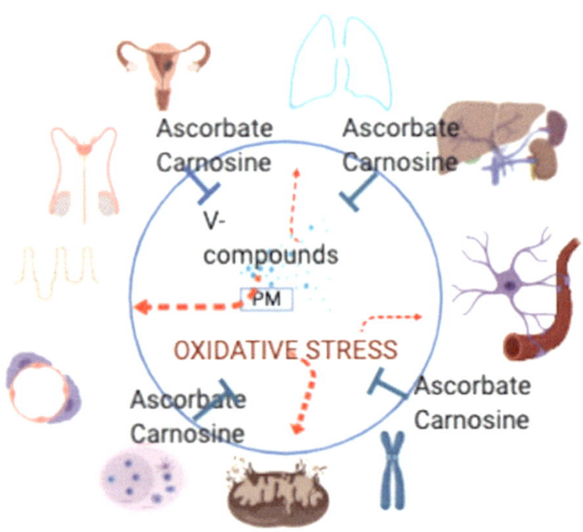

Figure 2.
Oxidative stress by vanadium and antioxidants protective effects (this figure was created by Biorender software in www.biorender.com).

antioxidants to prevent and ameliorate the effects that metals, such as V adhered to PM, have on living organisms, that meanwhile might reduce oxidative stress, its injurious effects and improves the quality of life on the planet.

Acknowledgements

This work was partially supported by project PAPIIT-DGAPA UNAM IN200418.

Author details

Marcela Rojas-Lemus[1], Patricia Bizarro-Nevares[1], Nelly López-Valdez[1,3], Adriana González-Villalva[1], Gabriela Guerrero-Palomo[1], María Eugenia Cervantes-Valencia[1,4], Otto Tavera-Cabrera[1], Norma Rivera-Fernández[2], Brenda Casarrubias-Tabarez[1,3], Martha Ustarroz-Cano[1], Armando Rodríguez-Zepeda[1], Francisco Pasos-Nájera[1] and Teresa Fortoul-van der Goes[1]*

1 Department of Cellular and Tissular Biology, Faculty of Medicine, National Autonomous University of Mexico (UNAM), Mexico City, Mexico

2 Department of Microbiology and Parasitology, Faculty of Medicine, National Autonomous University of Mexico (UNAM), Mexico City, Mexico

3 Doctoral Fellow, Biological Sciences, UNAM

4 Postdoctoral Fellow, Faculty of Medicine, UNAM

*Address all correspondence to: fortoul@unam.mx

References

[1] Fernandez A, Wendt JOL, Wolski N, Hein KRG, Wang S, Witten ML. Inhalation health effects of fine particles from the co-combustion of coal and refuse derived fuel. Chemosphere. 2003;**51**:1129-1137. DOI: 10.1016/S0045-6535(02)00720-8

[2] Sorensen M, Schins RPF, Hertel O, Loft S. Transition metals in personal samples of PM2.5 and oxidative stress in human volunteers. Cancer Epidemiology, Biomarkers and Prevention. 2005;**14**:1340-1343. DOI: 10.1158/1055-9965.EPI-04-0899

[3] Marconi A. Materiale particellare aerodisperso: definizioni, effetti sanitari, misura e sintesi del leindagani ambientali effettuate a Roma. Annali dell'Istituto Superiore di Sanità. 2003;**39**:329-342

[4] Leonard SS, Bower JJ, Shi X. Metal-induced toxicity, carcinogenesis, mechanisms and cellular responses. Molecular and Cellular Biochemistry. 2004a;**255**:3-10. DOI: 10.1023/b:mcbi.0000007255.72746.a6

[5] Leonard SS, Harris GK, Shi X. Metal-induced stress and signal transduction. Free Radical Biology and Medicine. 2004b;**37**:1921-1942. DOI: 10.1016/j.freeradbiomed.2004.09.010

[6] Chihuailaf RH, Contreras PA, Wittwer FG. Patogénesis del estrés oxidativo: consecuencias y evaluación en salud animal. Veterinaria México. 2002;**33**:265-283

[7] Davies KJ. Oxidative stress, antioxidant defenses, and damage removal, repair, and replacement systems. IUBMB Life. 2000;**50**:279-289. DOI: 10.1080/713803728

[8] Valko M, Rhodes CJ, Moncol J, Izakovic M, Mazur M. Free radicals, metals and antioxidants in oxidative stress-induced cancer. Chemico-Biological Interactions. 2006;**160**:1-40. DOI: 10.1016/j.cbi.2005.12.009

[9] Martínez-Cayuela M. Toxicidad de xenobióticos mediada por radicales libres de oxígeno. Ars Pharmaceutica. 1998;**39**:5-18

[10] Cooke MS, Evans MD, Dizdaroglu M, Lunec J. Oxidative DNA damage: Mechanism, mutation and disease. The FASEB Journal. 2003;**17**:1195-1214. DOI: 10.1096/fj.02-0752rev

[11] NTP. Technical Report on the Toxicology and Carcinogenicity Studies of Vanadium Pentoxide (CAS No. 1314-62-1) in F344/N Rats and B6C3F1 Mice (Inhalation Studies). National Toxicology Program, Research Triangle Park NC. NTP TR 507, NIH Publication No. 03-44412002. p. 352

[12] Duffus JH. Carcinogenicity classification of vanadium pentoxide and inorganic vanadium compounds, the NTP study of carcinogenicity of inhaled vanadium pentoxide, and vanadium chemistry. Regulatory Toxicology and Pharmacology. 2007;**47**:110-114. DOI: 10.1016/j.yrtph.2006.08.006

[13] Starr TB, Macgregor JA, Ehman KD, Kikiforov AI. Vanadium pentoxide: Use of relevant historical control data shows no evidence for carcinogenic response in F344/N rats. Regulatory Toxicology and Pharmacology. 2012;**64**:155-160. DOI: 10.1016/j.yrtph.2012.06.017

[14] Rodríguez-Mercado JJ, Mateos-Nava RA, Altamirano-Lozano MA. DNA damage induction in human cells exposed to vanadium oxides in vitro. Toxicology In Vitro. 2011;**25**:1996-2002. DOI: 10.1016/j.tiv.2011.07.009

[15] Altamirano-Lozano M, Valverde M, Alvarez BL, Molina B, Rojas E.

Genotoxic studies of vanadium pentoxide (V_2O_5) in male mice. II. Effects in several mouse tissues. Teratogenesis, carcinogenesis, and. Mutagenesis. 1999;**19**:243-255. DOI: 10.1002/(sici)1520-6866(1999)19:4<243::aid-tcm1>3.0.co;2-j

[16] Rojas-Lemus M, Altamirano-Lozano MA, Fortoul TI. Sex differences in blood genotoxic and cytotoxic effects as a consequence of vanadium inhalation: Micronucleus assay evaluation. Journal of Applied Toxicology. 2014;**34**:258-264. DOI: 10.1002/jat.2873

[17] Mitra S, Izumi T, Boldolgh I, Bhadak KK, Hill JW, Hazra TK. Choreography of oxidative damage and repair in mammalian genomes. Free Radical Biology and Medicine. 2002;**33**:15-28. DOI: 10.1016/s0891-5849(02)00819-5

[18] Léonard A, Gerber GB. Mutagenicity, carcinogenicity and teratogenicity of vanadium compounds. Mutation Research. 1994;**317**:81-88. DOI: 10.1016/0165-1110(94)90013-2

[19] Shlomovitz I, Speir M, Gerlic M. Flipping the dogma-phosphatidylserine in non-apoptotic cell death. Cell Communication and Signaling: CCS. 2019;**17**:139. DOI: 10.1186/s12964-019-0437-0

[20] Trevino S, Diaz A, Sanchez-Lara E, Sanchez-Gaytan BL, Perez-Aguilar JM, Gonzalez-Vergara E. Vanadium in biological action: Chemical, pharmacological aspects, and metabolic implications in diabetes mellitus. Biological Trace Element Research. 2019;**188**:68-98. DOI: 10.1007/s12011-018-1540-6

[21] Capella MA, Capella LS, Valente RC, Gefe M, Lopes AG. Vanadate-induced cell death is dissociated from H_2O_2 generation. Cell Biology and Toxicology. 2007;**23**:413-420. DOI: 10.1007/s10565-007-9003-4

[22] Guerrero-Palomo G, Rendon-Huerta EP, Montaño LF, Fortoul TI. Vanadium compounds and cellular death mechanisms in the A549 cell line: The relevance of the compound valence. Journal of Applied Toxicology. 2019;**39**:540-552. DOI: 10.1002/jat.3746

[23] Balaji B, Balakrishnan B, Perumalla S, Karande AA, Chakravarty AR. Photocytotoxic oxovanadium(IV) complexes of ferrocenyl-terpyridine and acetylacetonate derivatives. European Journal of Medicinal Chemistry. 2015;**92**:332-341. DOI: 10.1016/j.ejmech.2015.01.003

[24] Zhang Y, Wang L, Zeng K, Wang K, Yang X. Vanadyl complexes discriminate between neuroblastoma cells and primary neurons by inducing cell-specific apoptotic pathways. Journal of Inorganic Biochemistry. 2018;**188**:76-87. DOI: 10.1016/j.jinorgbio.2018.08.005

[25] Cunha-de Padua MM, SuterCorreia Cadena SM, de Oliveira Petkowicz CL, Martinez GR, Merlin-Rocha M, Merce AL, et al. Toxicity of native and oxovanadium (IV/V) galactomannan complexes on HepG2 cells is related to impairment of mitochondrial functions. Carbohydrate Polymers. 2017;**173**:665-675. DOI: 10.1016/j.carbpol.2017.06.027

[26] Naso LG, Lezama L, Rojo T, Etcheverry SB, Valcarcel M, Roura M, et al. Biological evaluation of morin and its new oxovanadium(IV) complex as antioxidant and specific anti-cancer agents. Chemico-Biological Interactions. 2013;**206**:289-301. DOI: 10.1016/j.cbi.2013.10.006

[27] Kowalski S, Wyrzykowski D, Hac S, Rychlowski M, Radomski MW, Inkielewicz-Stepniak I. New oxidovanadium(IV) coordination

complex containing 2-methylnitrilotriacetate ligands induces cell cycle arrest and autophagy in human pancreatic ductal adenocarcinoma cell lines. International Journal of Molecular Sciences. 2019;**20**(2);261. DOI: 10.3390/ijms20020261

[28] Wang J, Huang X, Zhang K, Mao X, Ding X, Zeng Q, et al. Vanadate oxidative and apoptotic effects are mediated by the MAPK-Nrf2 pathway in layer oviduct magnum epithelial cells. Metallomics. 2017;**9**:1562-1575. DOI: 10.1039/c7mt00191f

[29] Chandra AK, Ghosh R, Chatterjee A, Sarkar M. Protection against vanadium-induced testicular toxicity by testosterone propionate in rats. Toxicology Mechanisms and Methods. 2010;**20**:306-315. DOI: 10.3109/15376516.2010.485623

[30] Fortoul TI, Rodriguez-Lara V, González-Villalva A, Rojas-Lemus M, Cano-Gutiérrez G, Ustarroz-Cano M, et al. Inhalation of vanadium pentoxide and its toxic effects in a mouse model. Inorganica Chimica Acta. 2014;**420**:8-15

[31] Morgan AM, El-Tawil OS. Effects of ammonium metavanadate on fertility and reproductive performance of adult male and female rats. Pharmacological Research. 2003;**47**:75-85. DOI: 10.1016/s1043-6618(02)00241-4

[32] Aprioku JS. Pharmacology of free radicals and the impact of reactive oxygen species on the testis. Journal of Reproduction and Infertility. 2013;**14**:158-172

[33] Vijaya Bharathi B, Jaya Prakash G, Krishna KM, Ravi Krishna CH, Sivanarayana T, Madan K, et al. Protective effect of alpha glucosyl hesperidin (G-hesperidin) on chronic vanadium induced testicular toxicity and sperm nuclear DNA damage in male Sprague Dawley rats. Andrologia. 2015;**47**(5):568-578. DOI: 10.1111/and.12304

[34] Chandra AK, Ghosh R, Chatterjee A, Sarkar M. Amelioration of vanadium-induced testicular toxicity and adrenocortical hyperactivity by vitamin E acetate in rats. Molecular and Cellular Biochemistry. 2007a;**306**:189-200. DOI: 10.1007/s11010-007-9569-4

[35] Chandra AK, Ghosh R, Chatterjee A, Sarkar M. Effects of vanadate on male rat reproductive tract histology, oxidative stress markers and androgenic enzyme activities. Journal of Inorganic Biochemistry. 2007b;**101**:944-956. DOI: 10.1016/j.jinorgbio.2007.03.003

[36] Lu J, Wang Z, Cao J, Chen Y, Dong Y. A novel and compact review on the role of oxidative stress in female reproduction. Reproductive Biology and Endocrinology. 2018;**16**:80. DOI: 10.1186/s12958-018-0391-5

[37] Shrivastava S, Joshi D, Bhadauria M, Shukla S, Mathur R. Cotherapy of tiron and selenium against vanadium induced toxic effects in lactating rats. Iranian Journal of Reproductive Medicine. 2011;**9**:229-238

[38] Rinaldi M, Micali A, Marini H, Adamo E, Puzzolo D, Pisani A, et al. Cadmium organ toxicity and therapeutic approaches: A review on brain, kidney and testis damage. Current Medicinal Chemistry. 2017;**24**:3879-3893. DOI: 10.2174/0929867324666170801101448

[39] Orr S, Bridges C. Chronic kidney disease and exposure to nephrotoxic metals. International Journal of Molecular Sciences. 2017;**18**:1039. DOI: 10.3390/ijms18051039

[40] González-Villalva A, Colín-Barenque L, Bizarro-Nevares P, Rojas-Lemus M, Rodríguez-Lara V, García-Peláez I, et al. Pollution by

metals: Is there a relationship in glycemic control? Environmental Toxicology and Pharmacology. 2016;**46**:337-343. DOI: 10.1016/j.etap.2016.06.023

[41] Wilk A, Szypulska-Koziarska D, Wiszniewska B. The toxicity of vanadium on gastrointestinal, urinary and reproductive system, and its influence on fertility and fetuses malformations. Postępy Higieny i Medycyny Doświadczalnej. 2017;**71**:850-859. DOI: 10.5604/01.3001.0010.4783

[42] Boulassel B, Sadeg N, Roussel O, Perrin M, Belhadj-Tahar H. Fatal poisoning by vanadium. Forensic Science International. 2011;**206**:79-81. DOI: 10.1016/j.forsciint.2010.10.027

[43] Liu J, Cui H, Liu X, Peng X, Deng J, Zuo Z, et al. Dietary high vanadium causes oxidative damage-induced renal and hepatictoxicity in broilers. Biological Trace Element Research. 2012;**145**:189-200. DOI: 10.1007/s12011-011-9185-8

[44] Roy S, Majumdar S, Singh AK, Ghosh B, Ghosh N, Manna S, et al. Synthesis, characterization, antioxidant status, and toxicity study of vanadium-rutin complex in Balb/c mice. Biologial Trace Elements Research. 2015;**166**:183-200. DOI: 10.1007/s12011-015-0270-2

[45] Espinosa-Zurutuza M, González-Villalva A, Albarrán-Alonso JC, Colín Barenque L, Bizarro-Nevares P, Rojas-Lemus M, et al. Oxidative stress as a mechanism involved in kidney damage after subchronic exposure to vanadium inhalation and oral sweetened beverages in a mouse model. International Journal of Toxicology. 2018;**37**:45-52. DOI: 10.1177/1091581817745504

[46] Marouane W, Soussi A, Murat JC, Bezzine S, El Feki A. The protective effect of Malva sylvestris on rat kidney damaged by vanadium. Lipids in Health and Disease. 2011;**10**:65. DOI: 10.1186/1476-511X-10-65

[47] Scibior A, Golebiowska D, Adamczyk A, Niedfwiecka I, Fornal E. The renal effects of vanadate exposure: Potential biomarkers and oxidative stress as a mechanism of functional renal disorders-preliminary studies. BioMed Research International. 2014;**2014**:740105. DOI: 10.1155/2014/740105

[48] Parkin J, Cohen B. An overview of the immune system. Lancet. 2001;**357**:1777-1789. DOI: 10.1016/S0140-6736(00)04904-7

[49] Piñon-Zarate G, Rodriguez-Lara V, Rojas-Lemus M, Martinez-Pedraza M, Gonzalez-Villalva A, Mussali-Galante P, et al. Vanadium pentoxide inhalation provokes germinal center hyperplasia and suppressed humoral immune response. Journal of Immunotoxicology. 2008;**5**:115-122. DOI: 10.1080/15476910802085749

[50] Ustarroz-Cano M, López-Ángel M, López-Valdez N, García-Peláez I, Fortoul TI. The Effect of Atmospheric Pollution on the Thymus. Rijeka, Croatia: IntechOpen; 2019. DOI: 10.5772/intechopen.87027

[51] Usende IL, Olopade JO, Emikpe BO, Oyagbemi AA, Adedapo AA. Oxidative stress changes observed in selected organs of African giant rats (*Cricetomys gambianus*) exposed to sodium metavanadate. International Journal of Veterinary Science and Medicine. 2018;**6**:80-89. DOI: 10.1016/j.ijvsm.2018.03.004

[52] Tunali S, Yanardag R. Effect of vanadyl sulfate on the status of lipid parameters and on stomach and spleen tissues of streptozotocin-induced diabetic rats. Pharmacological Research. 2006;**53**:271-277. DOI: 10.1016/j.phrs.2005.12.004

[53] Bataller R, Brenner DA. Liver fibrosis. Journal of Clinical Investigation. 2005;**115**:209-218. DOI: 10.1172/JCI200524282.The. 2005

[54] Soares SS, Gutiérrez-Merino C, Aureliano M. Decavanadate induces mitochondrial membrane depolarization and inhibits oxygen consumption. Journal of Inorganic Biochemistry. 2007;**101**:789-796. DOI: 10.1016/j.jinorgbio.2007.01.012

[55] Rivas-García L, Quiles JL, Varela LA, Arredondo M, Lopez P, Dieguez AR, et al. In vitro study of the protective effect of manganese against vanadium-mediated nuclear and mitochondrial DNA damage. Food and Chemical Toxicology. 2019;**2019**:110900. DOI: 10.1016/j.fct.2019.110900

[56] Cano-Gutiérrez G, Acevedo NS, Santamaria A, Altamirano LM, Cano RM, Fortoul TI. Hepatic megalocytosis due to vanadium inhalation: Participation of oxidative stress. Toxicology and Industrial Health. 2012;**28**:353-360. DOI: 10.1177/0748233711412424

[57] Shoham DA, Durazo-Arvizu R, Kramer H, Luke A, Vopputuri S, Kshirsagar A, et al. Sugary soda consumption and albuminuria: Results from the national health and nutrition examination survey 1999-2004. PLoS One. 2008;**3**:e3431. DOI: 10.1371/journal.pone.0003431

[58] Vidale S, Campana C. Ambient air pollution and cardiovascular diseases: From bench to bedside. European Journal of Preventive Cardiology. 2018;**25**:818-825. DOI: 10.1177/2047487318766638

[59] Ye D, Klein M, Mulholland J, Russell A, Weber R, Edgerton E, et al. Estimating acute cardiovascular effects of ambient PM2.5 metals. Environmental Health Perspectives. 2018;**126**:027007. DOI: 10.1289/EHP2182

[60] Montiel-DávalosA,González-VillavaA, Rodriguez-Lara V, Montaño LF, Fortoul TI, López-Marure R. Vanadium pentoxide induces activation and death of endothelial cells. Journal of Applied Toxicology. 2012;**32**:26-33. DOI: 10.1002/jat.1695

[61] González-Villalva A, Fortoul TI, Avila-Costa MR, Piñón-Zárate G, Rodríguez Lara V, Martínez-Levy G, et al. Thrombocytosis induced in mice after subacute and subchronic V_2O_5 inhalation. Toxicology and Industrial Health. 2006;**22**:113-116. DOI: 10.1191/0748233706th250oa

[62] Fortoul TI, Gonzalez-Villalva A, Piñón-Zarate G, Rodriguez V, Montaño LF. Ultrastructural megakaryocyte modifications after vanadium inhalation in spleen and bone marrow. Journal of Electron Microscopy. 2009;**58**:375-380. DOI: 10.1093/jmicro/dfp031

[63] Fortoul TI, Piñón-Zárate G, Díaz-Bech ME, González-Villalva A, Mussali-Galante P, Rodríguez Lara V, et al. Spleen and bone marrow megakaryocytes as targets for inhaled vanadium. Histology and Histopathology. 2008;**23**:1321-1326. DOI: 10.14670/HH-23.1321

[64] González-Villalva A, Piñón-Zárate G, De la Peña-Díaz A, Flores-García M, Bizarro-Nevares P, Rendón-Huerta Erika P, et al. The effect of vanadium on platelet function. Environmental Toxicology and Pharmacology. 2011;**32**:447-456. DOI: 10.1016/j.etap.2011.08.010

[65] Fortoul TI, Rojas-Lemus M, Rodriguez-Lara V, Gonzalez-Villalva A, Ustarroz-Cano M, Cano-Gutierrez G, et al. Overview of environmental and occupational vanadium exposure and associated health outcomes: An article based on a presentation at the 8th international symposium on vanadium chemistry, biological chemistry, and toxicology;

Washington DC, August 15-18 2012. Journal of Immunotoxicology. 2014;**11**:13-18. DOI: 10.3109/1547691X.2013.789940

[66] Kulkarni A, Santosh Kumar G, Kaur J, Tikoo K. A comparative study of the toxicological aspects of vanadium pentoxide and vanadium oxide nanoparticles. Inhalation Toxicology. 2014;**26**:772-788. DOI: 10.3109/08958378.2014.960106

[67] López-Valdez N, Guerrero G, Rojas-Lemus M, Bizarro-Nevares P, Gonzalez-Villalva A, Ustarroz-Cano M, et al. The role of the non-ciliated bronchiolar cell in the tolerance to inhaled vanadium of the bronchiolar epithelium. Histology and Histopathology. 2019:18165. DOI: 10.14670/HH-18-165

[68] Wang L, Medan D, Mercer R, Overmiller D, Leornard S, Castranova V, et al. Vanadium-induced apoptosis and pulmonary inflammation in mice: Role of reactive oxygen species. Journal of Cellular Physiology. 2003;**195**:99-107. DOI: 10.1002/jcp.10232

[69] Zitka O, Skalickova S, Gumulec J, Masarik M, Adam V, Hubalek J, et al. Redox status expressed as GSH:GSSG ratio as a marker for oxidative stress in paediatric tumour patients. Oncology Letters. 2012;**4**:1247-1253. DOI: 10.3892/ol.2012.931

[70] Schuler D, Chevalier HJ, Merker M, Morgenthal K, Ravanat JL, Sagelsdorff M, et al. First steps towards an understanding of a mode of carcinogenic action for vanadium pentoxide. Journal of Toxicologic Pathology. 2011;**24**:149-162. DOI: 10.1293/tox.24.149

[71] Oluwabusayo RF, Snyder AM, Peters DG, Funmilayo O, Connor JR, Olopade JO. Brain metal distribution and neuro-inflammatory profiles after chronic vanadium administration and withdrawal in mice. Frontiers in Neuroanatomy. 2017;**11**:58. DOI: 10.3389/fnana.2017.00058

[72] Avila-Costa MR, Montiel-Flores E, Colin-Barenque L, Ordoñez JL, Gutierrez AL, Niño-Cabrera HG, et al. Nigrostriatal modifications after vanadium inhalation: An immunocytochemical and cytological approach. Neurochemical Research. 2004;**29**:1365-1369. DOI: 10.1023/b:nere.0000026398.86113.7d

[73] Avila-Costa MR, Colín BL, Zepeda RA, Antuna S, Saldivar L, Espejel G, et al. Ependymal epithelium disruption after vanadium pentoxide inhalation: A mice experimental model. Neuroscience Letters. 2005;**381**:21-25. DOI: 10.1016/j.neulet.2005.01.072

[74] Li H, Zhou D, Zhang Q, Feng C, Zheng W, He K, et al. Vanadium exposure-induced neurobehavioral alterations among Chinese workers. Neurotoxicology. 2013;**36**:49-54. DOI: 10.1016/j.neuro.2013.02.008

[75] Folarin O, Olopade F, Onwuka S, Olopade J. Memory deficit recovery after chronic vanadium exposure in mice. Oxidative Medicine and Cellular Longevity. 2016;**2016**:4860582. DOI: 10.1155/2016/4860582

[76] Afeseh Ngwa H, Kanthasamy A, Anantharam V, Song C, Witte T, Houk R, et al. Vanadium induces dopaminergic neurotoxicity via protein kinase Cdelta dependent oxidative signaling mechanisms: Relevance to etiopathogenesis of Parkinson's disease. Toxicology and Applied Pharmacology. 2009;**240**:273-285. DOI: 10.1016/j.taap.2009.07.025

[77] Halliwell B, Gutteridge JM. Oxygen toxicity, oxygen radicals, transition metals and disease. Biochemistry Journal. 1984;**219**:1-14. DOI: 10.1042/bj2190001

[78] Carr AC, Frei B. Chapter 9: Vitamin C and cardiovascular diseases. In: Cadenas E, Packer L, editors. Handbook of Antioxidants. 2nd ed. New York, NY; 2001. pp. 75-84

[79] Enstrom JE. Chapter 16: Epidemiology and clincial aspects of ascorbate and cancer. In: Cadenas E, Packer L, editors. Handbook of Antioxidants. 2nd ed. New York, NY; 2001. pp. 167-187

[80] Jones MM, Basinger MA. Chelate antidotes for sodium vanadate and vanadyl sulfate intoxication in mice. Journal of Toxicology and Environmental Health. 1983;**12**:749-756. DOI: 10.1080/15287398309530466

[81] Domingo JL, Llobet JM, Corbella J. Protection of mice against the lethal effects of sodium metavanadate: A quantitative comparison of a number of chelating agents. Toxicology Letters. 1985;**26**:95-99. DOI: 10.1016/0378-4274(85)90151-1

[82] Domingo JL, Gomez M, Llobet JM, Corbella J. Chelating agents in the treatment of acute vanadyl sulphate intoxication in mice. Toxicology. 1990;**62**:203-211. DOI: 10.1016/0300-483x(90)90110-3

[83] Boldyrev AA, Giancarlo A, Wim D. Physiology and pathophysiology of carnosine. Physiological Reviews. 2013;**93**:1803-1845. DOI: 10.1152/physrev.00039.2012

[84] Colín-Barenque L, Bizarro NP, González VA, Pedraza CJ, Medina-Campos O, Jimenez MR, et al. Neuroprotective effect of carnosine in the olfactory bulb after vanadium inhalation in a mouse model. International Journal of Experimental Pathology. 2018;**99**:180-188. DOI: 10.1111/iep.12285

[85] Valavanidis A, Vlachogianni T, Flotakis K, Lloridas S. Pulmonary oxidative stress, inflammation and cancer: Respirable particulate matter, fibrous dusts and ozone as major causes of lung carcinogenesis through reactive oxygen species mechanisms. International Journal of Environmental Research and Public Health. 2013;**10**:3886-3907. DOI: 10.3390/ijerph10093886

[86] Li Y, Vitamin C. Chapter 20. In: Yumbo L, editor. Antioxidants in Biology and Medicine: essentials, advances and clinical applicarions. New York: Nova Science Publishers, Inc; 2011. pp. 265-279. ISBN 13-9781611225020

Chapter 7

The w/w^+ Somatic Mutation and Recombination Test (SMART) of *Drosophila melanogaster* for Detecting Antigenotoxic Activity

Isabel Gaivão, João Ferreira and Luisa María Sierra

Abstract

Genotoxicological studies are emerging as fundamental for knowing the hazards to our genome, to our health. *Drosophila melanogaster* is one of the preferable organisms for toxicological research considering its metabolic similarities (viz. on dietary input, xenobiotic metabolizing system, antioxidant enzymes and DNA repair systems) to mammals. Accordingly, somatic mutation and recombination tests (SMARTs) of *D. melanogaster* are fast and low-cost in vivo assays that have shown solid results evaluating genotoxicity. The w/w^+ SMART uses the *white* (w) gene as a recessive marker to monitor the presence of mutant ommatidia (eye units), indicating the occurrence of point mutations, deletions, mitotic recombination or/and nondisjunction. Additionally, several studies used SMARTs to assess antigenotoxicity, with some using the w/w^+ SMART. We reviewed the state of the art of the w/w^+ SMART used for antigenotoxicity analysis, focusing on published results, aiming to contribute to the conception of a reliable protocol in antigenotoxicity. As such, genotoxic agents with known action mechanisms, as streptonigrin (oxidative stress inducer), were used as a genotoxic insult for proving the antigenotoxic effects of natural substances (e.g. seaweeds), demonstrating the presence of antimutagens in their composition. These antigenotoxicity studies are crucial for promoting preventive measures against environmental genotoxics that affect humans daily.

Keywords: genotoxicity test, w/w^+ SMART, eye-spot test, *Drosophila melanogaster*, streptonigrin, genotoxic agent, oxidative stress, DNA damage, ROS inhibition, antigenotoxicity, antimutagens, dietary antioxidants

1. Introduction

The environmental emergency is largely related to environmental toxicology. Each day, new molecules are synthesized, or natural molecules are intensively produced that enter in ecosystems and affect them at all levels. Nowadays there are circulating in living organisms thousands of substances that did not exist 100 years ago, with somewhat unpredictable consequences. As such, more than 159 million chemical substances are registered in the Chemical Abstracts Service (CAS), with

IntechOpen

approximately 4000 new substances being registered daily [1]. As a controlling measure, the EU Commission created, in 2004, a network (NORMAN network) of laboratories, research centres and organizations for monitoring the emerging environmental substances [1].

Environmental toxicology encompasses exposure to toxic substances whether through the air we breathe, the food we eat, the water we drink and the clothes we wear or through the skin, cosmetics, etc. There is also radiation exposure, which also has harmful effects, and is much more problematic today than some years ago. The planet is poisoned, affecting the air, the water, the soil and the food we produce, which causes serious problems to human health and ecosystems. It is hoped that worldwide awareness of this reality will be achieved, and the focus of humanity's greatest concerns will be on the cleansing of the planet by eliminating or at least greatly reducing the produced toxic agents.

This whole problem greatly affects DNA, causing DNA damage (genotoxicity), affecting DNA repair mechanisms and causing mutations when damage is not properly repaired. In the short term, this genome instability leads to diseases such as cancer, degenerative diseases, fertility decrease and other problems. In the long term, we may see the emergence of new diseases due to new mutations in the germ line, which, if recessive, may take several generations until there is a chance of homozygosis, where rare diseases may arise. All combined may affect the life expectancy of several species, causing an environmental collapse. Preventive strategies are indispensable to reduce the heavy burden on national healthcare systems and families. The most effective is a healthy lifestyle including diet, as an antigenotoxic diet reduces DNA damage and all the associated diseases. Antigenotoxic activities include inactivation of genotoxic compounds, by several mechanisms and increasing repair capacity, decreasing the effectiveness of a genotoxic. While DNA damage is clearly implicated as the initiating event in most cancers, the link is not a simple one. Most damage is removed by repair enzymes before it can interfere with the process of DNA replication and introduce mutations. Given a carcinogenic exposure, the individual variation in the capacity for DNA repair is therefore likely to be an important factor in determining cancer risk.

Over the years, many investigations in DNA damage and DNA repair mechanisms were made, in vitro and in vivo, aiming to know our environment and thus identifying the harmful compounds to our genome, to our health, leading to preventive actions such as prohibiting the commercialization of certain drugs, construction materials, foods and drinks. Genotoxicological studies using cell cultures and animals are essential for increasing human's wellbeing, since they display solid results in showing the genotoxicity of compounds and should be standardized (with optimal test conditions) for increasing their reproducibility and precision.

2. *Drosophila melanogaster* in toxicological research

Drosophila melanogaster is currently being used as one of the preferable organisms for toxicological research [2]. According to current knowledge, the use of *D. melanogaster* as a model organism respects the principles of animal welfare (3Rs), since ethical matters do not urge when using this organism [2, 3]. Considering the metabolic pathways responsible for dietary input (including nutrient uptake, digestion, absorption, storage and metabolism) [4], the xenobiotic metabolizing system, the antioxidant enzymes and the DNA repair systems of *D. melanogaster*, which are analogous to those of mammals, *D. melanogaster* emerges as an optimal replacer of higher animals in toxicological studies [2, 5]. Furthermore, contrasting with in vitro methods, *D. melanogaster* has the advantage of enabling a more solid extrapolation at the organism level [3].

D. melanogaster exposure to toxic agents leads to the alteration of simple life traits, which are perturbed negatively, such as development time, number of eclosed individuals, sex ratio, adult body size, fertility and others [6, 7]. These life traits can be assessed as a way of measuring the toxicological effects of a given drug, food, drink and so on. However, as science progresses and hazards are targeted in a more specific way, genotoxicological studies with *D. melanogaster* were developed, aiming to identify environmental hazards inducing damages to genome, *i.e.* genotoxic agents. In this way, genotoxicological studies with *D. melanogaster* deal with the assessment of changes in genetic material through various assays, such as germ line mutation assays, somatic mutation assays, the chromosomal aberration assay, the micronucleus test, the comet assay and DNA sequence-based assays, among others. In particular, somatic mutation and recombination tests (SMARTs) have proven to be a good tool for detecting a broad range of genetic alterations quickly and inexpensively [2, 8].

2.1 Somatic mutation and recombination tests of *D. melanogaster*

The somatic mutation and recombination tests of *D. melanogaster* have shown excellent results in assessing the genotoxicity of several and diversified compounds in somatic cells. Originally, in the 1980s, the SMART could be performed by four different assays, but only two of them made it through to the present day: the wing-spot test and the eye-spot test (or w/w^+ SMART) [9]. The wing-spot test was firstly described by Graf and Würgler [10] and the w/w^+ SMART by Würgler and Vogel [11], with both showing high values of sensitivity, specificity and accuracy.

Briefly, in the late embryogenesis, larval structures are set, and groups of diploid cells of undifferentiated epithelium, imaginal discs, are formed in the embryo [12]. Then, upon the ending of the larval stages, pupa emerges, and metamorphosis takes place upon systemic hormonal regulation, with the histolysis of the larval organs and differentiation of the imaginal discs into adult structures [13, 14]. Accordingly, the exposure of imaginal discs to genotoxic agents may lead to genetic alterations (the product of DNA damage) capable of being transmitted to daughter cells upon mitosis. These genetic alterations can be phenotypically manifested in the adults in structures such as the wings and the eyes, which can be assessed according to the wing-spot test and the eye-spot test, respectively. The loss of heterozygosity (LOH) for specific genetic markers in heterozygous individuals allows the quantification of DNA damage/level of genotoxicity in the adult tissues by visual scoring [9, 15].

Between the two types of SMART currently used, from the practical point of view, the w/w^+ SMART can be assayed with six different strains, as firstly shown by Vogel and Nivard [16], contrasting with only two strains available for the wing-spot one; in the w/w^+ SMART, a standardized genotoxic agent, inducing a high genotoxicity without toxic effects, streptonigrin (further focused on the chapter) [17], is available and has proved its effectiveness. Nevertheless, since the wing-spot test allows the visual scoring of wings over time, considering that wings are mounted/preserved on slides, opposite from what happens in the w/w^+ SMART, where eyes have to be analysed quickly since no preserving actions are available (time limited scoring), a greater number of studies have been performed using the wing-spot test (**Table 1**). Henceforward, as a measure of further exploring the potential of this test and increasing its number of studies, the w/w^+ SMART will be focused.

Reference	SMART type	Genotoxic agent	Substance tested as antigenotoxic	Response
Abraham [18]	Wing-spot	Cyclophosphamide (CPH) Diethylnitrosamine (DEN) Mitomycin C (MMC) Procarbazine (PRO) Urethane (URE)	Coffee	+ + + – +
Alaraby et al. [19]	Wing-spot	Potassium dichromate (PD)	CeO_2 NPs Cerium sulphate	+
Alaraby et al. [20]	Wing-spot	Potassium dichromate (PD) Ethyl methanesulfonate (EMS) Potassium dichromate (PD) Ethyl methanesulfonate (EMS)	CuO NPs Copper oxide	+ +
Amkiss et al. [21]	Eye-spot	Methyl methanesulfonate (MMS)	Fennel plant fruit extracts	+
Anter et al. [22]	Wing-spot	Hydrogen peroxide	Virgin Olive oil Triolein Tyrosol Squalene	+ + + +
Anter et al. [23]	Wing-spot	Hydrogen peroxide	Red table grapes	+
Anter et al. [24]	Wing-spot	Hydrogen peroxide	Phenols: apigenin, bisabolol, protocatechuic acid	+ + +
Aydemir et al. [25]	Wing-spot	Fotemustine	Amifostine	+
Cápiro et al. [26]	Eye-spot	Methyl methanesulfonate (MMS) Ethylnitrosourea (ENU) Juglone (JG) Dimethylbenz(a)anthracene (DMBA)	*Cymbopogon citratus*	+ + + +
Demir and Marcos [27]	Wing-spot	Potassium dichromate	Boron nitride nanotubes	+
De Rezende et al. [28]	Wing-spot	Doxorubicin (DXR)	Grape seed proanthocyanidins	+
De Rezende et al. [29]	Wing-spot	Doxorubicin (DXR)	Dibenzylbutyrolactolic lignan(–)-cubebin	+/–
Drosopoulou et al. [30]	Wing-spot	Mitomycin C (MMC)	Chios mastic products: verbenone α-terpineol linalool trans-pinocarveol	+ + + –
El Hamss et al. [31]	Wing-spot	Urethane (URE)	Turmeric	+
Fernandes et al. [32]	Wing-spot	Doxorubicin (DXR) Benzo(a)pyrene (B(a)P)	Vitexin	+ +
Fernandez-Bedmar and Alonso-Moraga [33]	Wing-spot	Hydrogen peroxide	Green sweet pepper Red sweet pepper Green hot pepper Red hot pepper Capsaicin Capsanthin Lutein	+ + – + + + +

Reference	SMART type	Genotoxic agent	Substance tested as antigenotoxic	Response
Fernández-Bedmar et al. [34]	Wing-spot	Hydrogen peroxide	Citrus juices Hesperidin Limonene	+ + +
Fernandez-Bedmar et al. [35]	Wing-spot	Hydrogen peroxide	Tomato Lycopene	+ +
Fernández-Bedmar et al. [36]	Wing-spot	Hydrogen peroxide	Garlic Onion Diallyl disulphide Dipropyl disulphide	+ + + +
Ferreira et al. [3]	Eye-spot	Streptonigrin (SN)	*Grateloupia turuturu* *Porphyra umbilicalis*	+ +
Graf et al. [37]	Wing-spot	Urethane (URE) Methyl urea + sodium nitrite	Instant coffee Ascorbic acid Catechin	+ + +
Guterres et al. [38]	Wing-spot	Doxorubicin (DXR)	*Momordica charantia*: aerial parts Fruit	– +
Idaomar et al. [39]	Wing-spot	Urethane (URE)	Essential oils from: *Helichrysum italicum*, *Ledum groenlandicum*, *Ravensara aromatica*	+ + +
Kylyc and Yesilada [40]	Wing-spot	Mitomycin C (MMC)	Dried mycelia from: *Trametes versicolor* *Pleurotus ostreatus*	+ +
Laohavechvanich et al. [41]	Wing-spot	Urethane (URE)	Bird pepper Red chili spur pepper Green bell pepper Green sweet pepper	+ + + +
Lozano-Baena et al. [42]	Wing-spot	Hydrogen peroxide	*Brassica carinata* Sinigrin	+ +
Marques et al. [43]	Eye-spot	Streptonigrin (SN)	*Ulva rigida* *Fucus vesiculosus* *Gracilaria* species	+ + +
Martinez-Valdivieso et al. [44]	Wing-spot	Hydrogen peroxide	Lutein β-Carotene Zeaxanthin Dehydroascorbic acid Yellow zucchini Light green zucchini	+ + + + + +
Mateo-Fernandez et al. [45]	Wing-spot	Hydrogen peroxide	Caramel color class IV	+
Merinas-Amo et al. [46]	Wing-spot	Hydrogen peroxide	Choline	+
Mezzoug et al. [47]	Wing-spot	Urethane (URE)	*Origanum compactum* essential oil	+
Niikawa et al. [48]	Wing-spot	Mitomycin C (MMC)	Salicylic acid Salicyluric acid Gentisic acid Gentisuric acid 2,3-Dihydroxybenzoic acid	– + + + +

Reference	SMART type	Genotoxic agent	Substance tested as antigenotoxic	Response
Niikawa et al. [49]	Wing-spot	Mitomycin C (MMC)	Salicylic acid	–
			Salicyluric acid	+
			Gentisic acid	+
			Gentisuric acid	+
			2,3-Dihydroxybenzoic acid	+
Oliveira et al. [50]	Wing-spot	Doxorubicin (DXR)	Metformin	+
Orsolin et al. [51]	Wing-spot	Doxorubicin (DXR)	Simvastatin	+
Pádua et al. [52]	Wing-spot	Mitomycin C (MMC)	*Terminalia actinophylla* extracts	+
		Ethyl methanesulfonate (EMS)		+
Patenkovic et al. [53]	Wing-spot	Methyl methanesulfonate (MMS)	Sage tea	+
Patenkovic et al. [54]	Wing-spot	Methyl methanesulfonate (MMS)	Gentian tea	–
Prakash et al. [55]	Wing-spot	Ethyl methanesulfonate (EMS)	Caffeine	+
Prakash et al. [56]	Wing-spot	Methyl methanesulfonate (MMS)	*Dioscorea pentaphylla*	+
Rizki et al. [57]	Wing-spot	Potassium dichromate (PD)	Sodium selenite	+
Romero-Jiménez et al. [58]	Wing-spot	Hydrogen peroxide	*Matricaria chamomilla*	+
			Tilia cordata	+
			Mentha piperita	+
			Mentha pulegium	+
			Uncaria tomentosa	+
			Valeriana officinalis	+
Sarıkaya et al. [59]	Wing-spot	Ethyl methanesulfonate (EMS)	Boron	+
Savić et al. [60]	Wing-spot	Methyl methanesulfonate (MMS)	Royal Sun Agaricus extract	–
Sukprasansap et al. [61]	Wing-spot	Urethane (URE)	Eggplants	+
Taira et al. [62]	Wing-spot	2-AAF	*Agrocybe cylindracea*	+
		Aflatoxin B1	*Lentinula edodes*	+
		DMBA	*Pleurotus ostreatus*	+
		IQ		+
		MeIQx		+
		MNU		+
		NDMA		+
		4NQO		+
		2-AAF		-
		Aflatoxin B1		+
		DMBA		–
		IQ		–
		MeIQx		–
		MNU		+
		NDMA		+
		4NQO		+
		2-AAF		+
		Aflatoxin B1		+
		DMBA		+
		IQ		+
		MeIQx		+
		MNU		+

Reference	SMART type	Genotoxic agent	Substance tested as antigenotoxic	Response
		NDMA 4NQO		+ +
Tasset-Cuevas et al. [63]	Wing-spot	Hydrogen peroxide	Borage seed oil Gamma linolenic acid	+ +
Toyoshima et al. [64]	Wing-spot	Sun and UV light	Sunscreens: SPF 20 SPF 40 SPF 60	+ + +
Valadares et al. [65]	Wing-spot	Doxorubicin (DXR)	Propolis (water extracts)	+
Valente et al. [66]	Eye-spot	Streptonigrin (SN)	Thalassotherapy products	+

The type of test, wing- or eye-spot, the used genotoxic agents, as well as the information about the antigenotoxic potential of the tested substances (response: + antigenotoxic activity; – no antigenotoxic activity or synergistic genotoxic activity) is presented.

Table 1.
Published studies focusing the antigenotoxic evaluation of several types of chemicals, nanoparticles and plants/seaweeds/seeds/oils using somatic mutation and recombination tests (SMARTs).

3. w/w^+ SMART (eye-spot test)

D. melanogaster presents two symmetrically positioned eyes in its head. Each eye consists of repeated hexagonal arrays of approximately 750–800 ommatidia (eye units formed upon differentiation of imaginal discs), homogenous in size and regularly spaced, with each ommatidium being constituted by 14 cells (8 photoreceptor cells, 4 cone cells and 2 primary pigment cells) [67]. Between each two ommatidia, six secondary pigment cells, three tertiary pigment cells and three mechanosensory bristle complexes are present [67]. The adult eye of *D. melanogaster* is particularly used in toxicological assays since subtle defects in ommatidia development are amplified, by mitosis, several hundred times in the eye [68]. Therefore, it is quite simple to detect genetic alterations changing its pigmentation.

The basis of the w/w^+ SMART is the *white* (w) gene located at the position 1.5 of the X chromosome. This gene is used as a recessive genetic marker to monitor the presence of mutant ommatidia/spots, indicating the occurrence of LOH by deletions, point mutations, mitotic/somatic recombination (the most frequent) or/and nondisjunction (chromosome losses) in somatic cells (**Figures 1** and **2**) [9, 16]. These genetic events are known to display a significant role in the induction of carcinogenesis [69]. Accordingly, when wild-type females (w^+/w^+; red eyes) are crossed with white-eyed males (w/Y; eyes without pigmentation), or vice versa (w/w with w^+/Y), a heterozygous offspring is developed for females (w^+/w; red eyes). However, if the offspring is exposed to genotoxic agents in its development phase, the presence of white/mutant phenotype spots in the red eyes may occur (**Figures 1** and **2**). In addition, when crossing wild-type females with white-eyed males, males' eyes can also be analysed, although somatic recombination should not be considered in this case [9]. The difference between females and males scoring will provide quantitative information on somatic recombination [9].

Moreover, Vogel and Nivard [69, 70] designed a more refined, as well as time-consuming, version of the w/w^+ SMART, which allows the detection of chromosomal aberrations in late larval stages. However, and according to Marcos and Sierra [9], the ratio of results obtained/time consumption is low in comparison with the

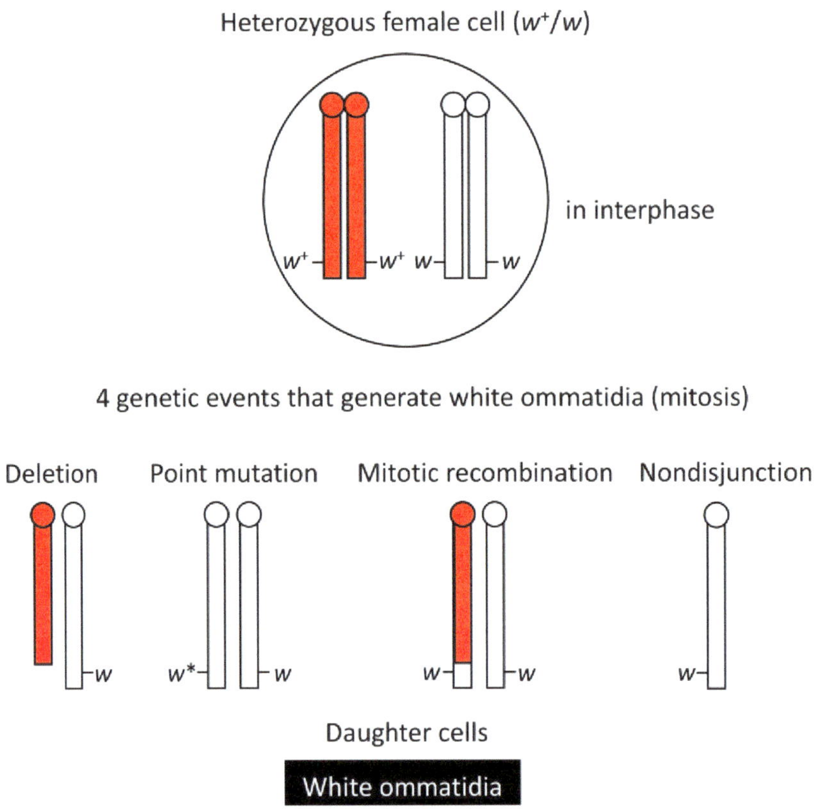

Figure 1.
Scheme of the possible four types of genetic alterations that generate white ommatidia in a heterozygous D. melanogaster *female for the white (w) gene. In the scheme, the heterozygous female cell has two X chromosomes with two chromatids each (duplicated DNA in interphase) and daughter cells have two X chromosomes but only one chromatid each (except for nondisjunction). The X chromosomes in red carry the w^+ allele (dominant) and those in white carry the w allele (recessive), however there are a few exceptions that will be described below. The position of the alleles in the X chromosomes is represented in a purely illustrative, non-exact way. w^* is a mutated wild-type expressing white phenotype. In the development phase of a heterozygous female for the w gene (w^+/w), genetic alterations may be induced in the imaginal discs and, upon cell division, daughter cells with mutant/white phenotype ommatidia may appear. The genetic alterations that cause mutant phenotypes are: deletion in one X chromosome including the white locus (in the wild-type allele); point mutation in the wild-type allele by substitution, insertion, or deletion; mitotic recombination between chromatids of the homologous X chromosomes, that replaces the wild-type locus by a mutant locus; nondisjunction, that causes the loss of the chromosome with the wild-type allele.*

original version of the assay, making it less efficient in the laboratorial routine. Thus, the original version of the assay continues to be the main choice when performing w/w^+ SMART.

3.1 Antigenotoxicity with w/w^+ SMART

w/w^+ SMART was, in its original concept, used for the genotoxicological evaluation of several chemical agents, directed to unveiling the action mechanisms behind their genotoxic activities [17, 71–73]. As such, alkylating agents, such as methyl methanesulfonate (MMS), ethyl methanesulfonate (EMS) and ethylnitrosourea (ENU), are between the chemicals that induce a great number of mutant ommatidia in *D. melanogaster* [72]. Even so, and considering the study from Gaivão and Sierra [17], a quinone-based antibiotic, streptonigrin (SN), showed its potential to induce a great level of genotoxicity (increased number of mutant

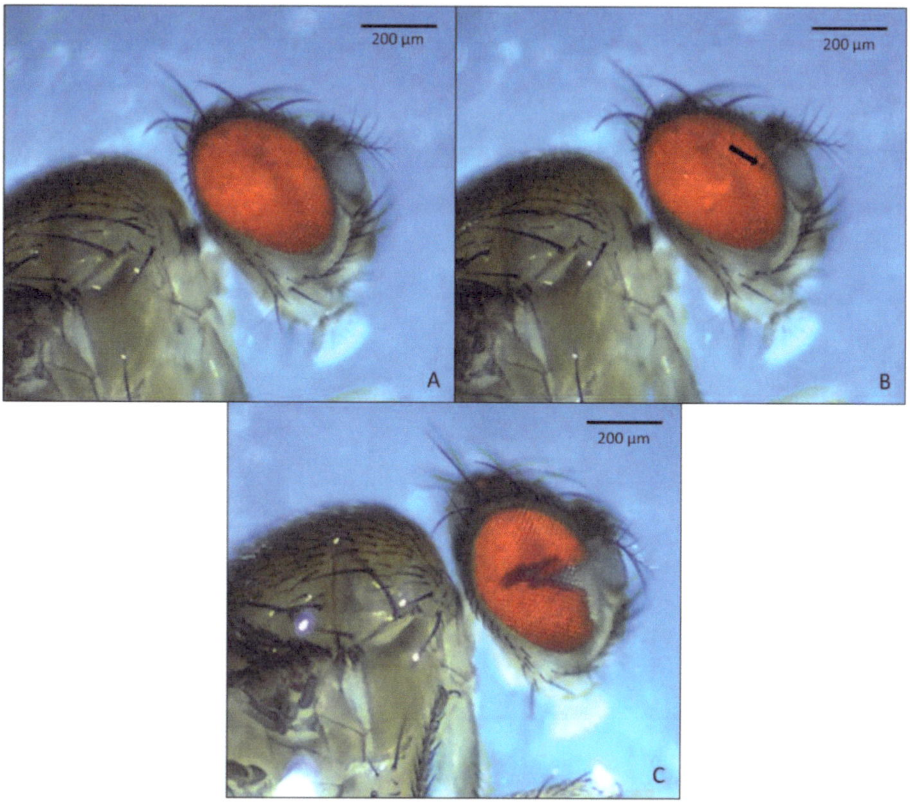

Figure 2.
Wild-type eyes of D. melanogaster *(females) at the stereoscopic microscope (80× magnification). (A) An eye without mutant spots, (B) an eye with a dark spot affecting one to two ommatidium(a) (marked by a black arrow) and (C) an eye with a spot affecting innumerable ommatidia. White mutant spots appear as black when surrounded by pigmented/red ommatidia.*

ommatidia) without toxic effects (at 20 μM) in the *w*/*w*⁺ SMART, making it a suitable genotoxic insult for this assay. SN, in the presence of certain metal cations (Zn^{2+}, Cu^{2+}, Fe^{2+}, Mn^{2+}, Cd^{2+} and/or Au^{2+}), binds to DNA establishing SN-metal-DNA complexes, known as DNA adducts [74–76] (**Figure 3**). Upon the binding, the quinone reduces, via one or two e^- (NADH as a cofactor), producing a semiquinone or a hydroquinone, respectively. Semiquinone reacting with O_2 leads to the production of O_2^- and quinone regeneration. Hydroquinone can lead to the production of H_2O_2, while quinone is regenerated (**Figure 3**). In consequence, OH can be produced by the Fenton reaction ($H_2O_2 + Fe^{2+} \rightarrow OH + OH^- + Fe^{3+}$) and by the Haber-Weiss reaction ($O_2^- + H_2O_2 \rightarrow OH + OH^- + O_2$), leading to oxidative stress [74–76]. The production of reactive oxygen species (ROS), and the prolonged SN linkage to DNA, can lead to the inhibition of DNA (and RNA) synthesis, induce unscheduled DNA synthesis, promote DNA strand breaks as well as inhibit topoisomerase II [77]. Chromosomal aberrations may occur upon mutagenic events, creating genomic instability that can culminate into carcinogenic events [76] (**Figure 3**).

Among the processes related to genotoxicity, with an increased relevance in the last years, the analysis of antigenotoxicity is probably the most important one. The search for antigenotoxic agents that could prevent or counteract the harmful consequences of the exposure to DNA damaging agents has increased exponentially lately [78–80]. Since most of the possible antigenotoxic agents are components of natural products that could be included in the diet, the analysis of their properties

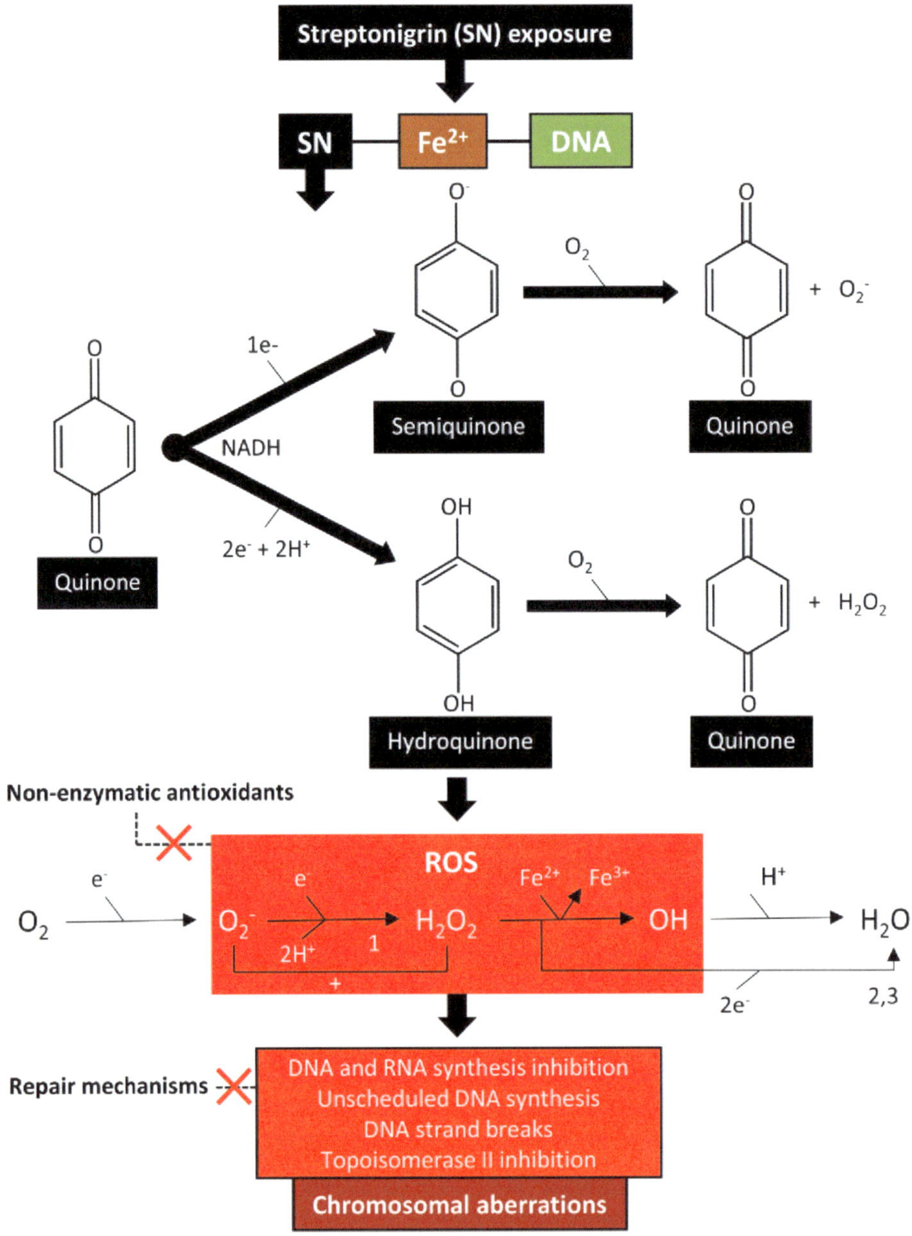

Figure 3.
Simplistic scheme of the genotoxic activity of streptonigrin (SN) on an animal cell. Cell exposure to SN leads to the formation of DNA adducts [SN + metal cation (such as Fe^{2+}) + DNA]. SN's quinone groups are reduced (NADH as a cofactor) to semiquinone and hydroquinone that, in the presence of O_2, lead to the formation of O_2^- and H_2O_2, respectively, both with quinone regeneration (vicious cycle). Thus, by chemical reactions (such as the Fenton and Haber-Weiss ones), OH is produced, the most severe reactive oxidative species (ROS). In this case, the antioxidants (endogenous enzymatic and non-enzymatic, and dietary inputs) are not capable of avoiding excessive ROS formation and progression, as well as communicating to repair mechanisms for repairing the induced genetic damages that may lead to chromosomal aberrations. (1) Superoxide dismutase (SOD); (2) catalase (CAT); (3) glutathione peroxidases.

should be performed in in vivo experiments. As so, *Drosophila* fulfils all the requirements for this analysis, specifically when using SMARTs. In fact, there are numerous published studies using *D. melanogaster* in antigenotoxicity analyses, and most of them are using SMARTs, especially with the wing-spot test (**Table 1**).

Focusing on the *w*/*w*+ SMART performed for antigenotoxicity testing, there are a few studies evaluating the antigenotoxic potential of lemongrass extracts [26]; fennel plant fruit extracts [21]; red, green and brown seaweeds [3, 43]; and thalassotherapy products (containing seaweeds) [66].

Ferreira and Marques [3] and Marques and Ferreira [43] studied the exposure of *D. melanogaster* [*Oregon-K* (*OK*) strain] to a chronic treatment (from egg to adult eclosion) with media (Formula 4-24® Instant Drosophila Medium) supplemented with red, green or brown seaweeds and SN (at 20 μM). Reductions in the number of mutant ommatidia were shown in individuals cotreated with seaweed and SN in relation to the positive control. Thus, protective properties of seaweeds were exerted against the genotoxic insult of SN, demonstrating antigenotoxic potential. Even more, some species displayed antigenotoxic effects against the spontaneous genotoxicity (without SN insult) of *D. melanogaster*. The authors also refer the possible phytochemicals acting as antimutagens that include vitamins, phenolic compounds, pigments and polysaccharides. These phytochemicals, which may promote their action in a synergetic way, may inhibit ROS triggered by SN activity, acting as dietary antioxidants [3] (**Figure 3**). Their mechanisms of action may include ROS scavenging, donation of electrons and/or protons to endogenous enzymatic and/or non-enzymatic antioxidants for converting ROS to H_2O and/or chelating metal ions responsible for producing OH (Fenton reaction inhibition) [34, 81]. In line, using the same conditions, Valente and Borges [66] showed the antigenotoxicity of thalassotherapy products (with seaweeds) against SN. Once more, the potential of seaweeds as dietary antioxidants/antimutagens, as well as the potential of SN as an optimal inducer of chromosomal aberrations quantifiable by the SMART, was demonstrated. Longevity-promoting properties were also displayed upon seaweed supplementation which, according to free radical and mitochondrial theories of ageing, may be a collateral effect of the dietary antioxidants that modulate the enzymatic antioxidants and exert direct antioxidant-scavenging actions [3, 66].

MMS (at 1 mM) was used as a genotoxic insult against a fennel plant fruit aqueous extract [21]. The positive control showed a great number of induced mutant ommatidia, proving the results from Vogel and Nivard [72], and the fennel extract showed antigenotoxic activity against MMS. According to the authors, and considering the mutagenic activity of MMS, an alkylating agent, consisting of direct interactions with DNA bases that induce mutagenic events, fennel may possess antimutagens that interact directly with the methyl radical groups of MMS and inactivate them in such a manner that they cannot bind to DNA as effectively to induce their mutagenic activity. The antimutagenic properties displayed by fennel may be related to components of its essential oil [21]. In a similar way, Cápiro and Sánchez-Lamar [26] demonstrated the antigenotoxic potential of lemongrass decoction extracts against different genotoxics, MMS, ENU, juglone (JG) and dimethylbenz(a)anthracene (DMBA), that exhibit different mechanisms of action. According to the authors, the lemongrass extract modulated the genotoxic action of the alkylating agents MMS and ENU by interacting with them directly or/and with their mutagenic derivatives. Regarding JG, a naphthoquinone that induces ROS production in an analogous way to SN, damages were reduced upon exposure to the decoction extract by probably inhibiting ROS production, by sequestrating/inhibiting ROS activity or/and activating intracellular defence mechanisms. For DMBA, as it needs metabolic activation by microsomal enzymes, the extract may have interfered with the microsomal enzymatic system for avoiding DMBA activation. Overall, lemongrass extract acted as an antimutagen in the protection of DNA.

In fact, SMART can be assayed using different test conditions, including the *D. melanogaster* strain (OK strain has potential for genotoxicity testing; presents high susceptibility to ROS, mainly due to a low activity of antioxidant enzymes, being more sensitive to increase its antioxidant status upon intake of dietary antioxidants [3, 73]), treatment method (chronic or acute and pre-, co- and post-treatments), genotoxic agent (should always be chosen among those with a known mechanism of action; an example is SN) and sample size. For more details on the methodological approaches of SMARTs, see the protocol from Marcos and Sierra [9].

4. Conclusions

In vitro and especially in vivo genotoxicity testing of substances such as foods, drinks, drugs and herbicides is fundamental for increasing humans' knowledge on the hazards that we may be exposed to. In this way, upon the identification of a substance/compound as genotoxic, priorities should be focused on avoiding this genotoxic or, at least, when the exposure is unavoidable, preventing our metabolism from damages to DNA that can culminate in mutagenic events and, in a later stage, on carcinogenesis. Upon in vitro testing, in vivo genotoxicological assays, such as w/w^+ SMART in *D. melanogaster*, are great tools for evaluating the antigenotoxic potential of a given substance/compound, considering optimal test conditions. The ultimate objective of these tests is to promote the dietary intake of antimutagens, since they are essential for reinforcing our metabolic defences towards genotoxic events, especially the ones that may be produced by strong exogenous agents. Foods, teas, nutraceuticals and others who are richly composed of dietary antimutagens should be of daily intake, considering that there is an increasing threat of new chemical substances with genotoxic potential every day.

Acknowledgements

This work was supported by the project UIDB/CVT/00772/2020, which was supported by the Portuguese Science and Technology Foundation (FCT), and by the Gobierno del Principado de Asturias (Oviedo, Spain) through Plan de Ciencia, Tecnología e Innovación (PCTI), co-financed by FEDER funds (Ref. FC-GRUPIN-IDI/2018/000242) and by the Ministerio de Economia y Competitividad (MINECO) of Spain under the Project CTQ2016-80060-C2-1R.

Conflict of interest

The authors declare no conflict of interest.

Author details

Isabel Gaivão[1*], João Ferreira[1,2] and Luisa María Sierra[3]

1 Department of Genetics and Biotechnology and Animal and Veterinary Research Centre (CECAV), University of Trás-os-Montes and Alto Douro (UTAD), Vila Real, Portugal

2 Centre for the Research and Technology of Agro-Environmental and Biological Sciences (CITAB), UTAD, Vila Real, Portugal

3 Department of Functional Biology, Genetics Area, Oncology University Institute (IUOPA) and Institute of Sanitary Research of Asturias (ISPA), University of Oviedo, Spain

*Address all correspondence to: igaivao@utad.pt

References

[1] Dulio V, Bv B, Brorström-Lundén E, Harmsen J, Hollender J, Schlabach M, et al. Emerging pollutants in the EU: 10 years of NORMAN in support of environmental policies and regulations. Environmental Sciences Europe. 2018; **30**(5):1-13. DOI: 10.1186/s12302-018-0135-3

[2] Mishra N, Srivastava R, Agrawal UR, Tewari RR. An insight into the genotoxicity assessment studies in dipterans. Mutation Research. 2017;**773**: 220-229. DOI: 10.1016/j.mrrev.2016.10.001

[3] Ferreira J, Marques A, Abreu MH, Pereira R, Rego A, Pacheco M, et al. Red seaweeds *Porphyra umbilicalis* and *Grateloupia turuturu* display antigenotoxic and longevity-promoting potential in *Drosophila melanogaster*. European Journal of Phycology. 2019;**54**(4):519-530. DOI: 10.1080/09670262.2019.1623926

[4] Lemaitre B, Miguel-Aliaga I. The digestive tract of *Drosophila melanogaster*. Annual Review of Genetics. 2013;**47**:377-404. DOI: 10.1146/annurev-genet-111212-133343

[5] Holmes AM, Creton S, Chapman K. Working in partnership to advance the 3Rs in toxicity testing. Toxicology. 2010;**267**(1-3):14-19. DOI: 10.1016/j.tox.2009.11.006

[6] Neethu BK, Babu YR, Harini BP. Enriched nutrient diet shortens the developmental time—A transgenerational effect in *Drosophila sulfurigaster sulfurigaster*. *Drosophila* Information Service. 2013;**96**:98-102

[7] Güler P, Ayhan N, Koşukcu C, Önder BŞ. The effects of larval diet restriction on developmental time, preadult survival, and wing length in *Drosophila melanogaster*. Turkish Journal of Zoology. 2015;**39**:395-403. DOI: 10.3906/zoo-1305-42

[8] Stamenković-Radak M, Andjelković M. Studying genotoxic and antimutagenic effects of plant extracts in *Drosophila* test systems. Botanica Serbica. 2016;**40**(1):21-28. DOI: 10.5281/zenodo.48854

[9] Marcos R, Sierra LM, Gaivão I. The SMART assays of *Drosophila*: Wings and eyes as target tissues. In: Sierra LM, Gaivão I, editors. Genotoxicity and DNA Repair: A Practical Approach. New York: Humana Press; 2014. pp. 283-295

[10] Graf U, Würgler FE, Katz AJ, Frei H, Juon H, Hall CB, et al. Somatic mutation and recombination test in *Drosophila melanogaster*. Environmental Mutagenesis. 1984;**6**(2):153-188. DOI: 10.1002/em.2860060206

[11] Würgler EE, Vogel EW. *In vivo* mutagenicity testing using somatic cells of *Drosophila melanogaster*. In: Serres FJd, editor. Chemical Mutagens, Principles and Methods for Their Detection. 10. New York: Plenum Press; 1986. p. 1-72

[12] Gilbert SF, Barresi JF. Developmental Biology. 11th ed. Sunderland, Massachusetts, USA: Sinauer Associates, Inc.; 2016

[13] Kumar JP. Building an ommatidium one cell at a time. Developmental Dynamics. 2012;**241**(1):136-149. DOI: 10.1002/dvdy.23707

[14] Tyler MS. Developmental Biology: A Guide for Experimental Study. 3.1 ed. Sunderland, Massachusetts, USA: Sinauer Assoc., Inc.; 2010

[15] Vlastos D, Drosopoulou E, Efthimiou I, Gavriilidis M, Panagaki D, Mpatziou K, et al. Genotoxic and antigenotoxic assessment of chios mastic oil by the *in vitro* micronucleus test on human lymphocytes and the *in vivo* wing somatic test on *Drosophila*.

PLoS One. 2015;**10**(6):e0130498. DOI: 10.1371/journal.pone.0130498

[16] Vogel EW, Nivard MJM, Zijlstra JA. Variation of spontaneous and induced mitotic recombination in different *Drosophila* populations: A pilot study on the effects of polyaromatic hydrocarbons in six newly constructed tester strains. Mutation Research. 1991; **250**:291-298. DOI: 10.1016/0027-5107(91)90184-p

[17] Gaivão I, Sierra LM, Comendador MA. The *w/w*+ SMART assay of *Drosophila melanogaster* detects the genotoxic effects of reactive oxygen species inducing compounds. Mutation Research. 1999;**440**:139-145. DOI: 10.1016/S1383-5718(99)00020-0

[18] Abraham SK. Antigenotoxicity of coffee in the *Drosophila* assay for somatic mutation and recombination. Mutagenesis. 1994;**9**:383-386. DOI: 10.1093/mutage/9.4.383

[19] Alaraby M, Hernández A, Annangi B, Demir E, Bach J, Rubio L, et al. Antioxidant and antigenotoxic properties of CeO_2 NPs and cerium sulphate: Studies with *Drosophila melanogaster* as a promising *in vivo* model. Nanotoxicology. 2015;**9**(6): 749-759. DOI: 10.3109/17435390.2014.976284

[20] Alaraby M, Hernández A, Marcos R. Copper oxide nanoparticles and copper sulphate act as antigenotoxic agents in *Drosophila melanogaster*. Environmental and Molecular Mutagenesis. 2017;**58**(1): 46-55. DOI: 10.1002/em.22068

[21] Amkiss S, Dallouh A, Idaomar M, Amkiss B. Genotoxicity and anti-genotoxicity of fennel plant (*Foeniculum vulgare* Mill) fruit extracts using the somatic mutation and recombination test (SMART). African Journal of Food Science. 2013;7(8):193-197. DOI: 10.5897/AJFS2013.0999

[22] Anter J, Campos-Sánchez J, Hamss RE, Rojas-Molina M, Muñoz-Serrano A, Analla M, et al. Modulation of genotoxicity by extra-virgin olive oil and some of its distinctive components assessed by use of the *Drosophila* wing-spot test. Mutation Research. 2010; **703**(2):137-142. DOI: 10.1016/j.mrgentox.2010.08.012

[23] Anter J, de Abreu-Abreu N, Fernandez-Bedmar Z, Villatoro-Pulido M, Alonso-Moraga A, Munoz-Serrano A. Targets of red grapes: Oxidative damage of DNA and leukaemia cells. Natural Product Communications. 2011; **6**(1):59-64

[24] Anter J, Romero-Jimenez M, Fernandez-Bedmar Z, Villatoro-Pulido M, Analla M, Alonso-Moraga A, et al. Antigenotoxicity, cytotoxicity, and apoptosis induction by apigenin, bisabolol, and protocatechuic acid. Journal of Medicinal Food. 2011;**14**(3): 276-283. DOI: 10.1089/jmf.2010.0139

[25] Aydemir N, Sevim N, Celikler S, Vatan O, Bilaloglu R. Antimutagenicity of amifostine against the anticancer drug fotemustine in the *Drosophila* somatic mutation and recombination (SMART) test. Mutation Research. 2009;**679**(1-2):1-5. DOI: 10.1016/j.mrgentox.2009.08.005

[26] Cápiro N, Sánchez-Lamar A, Baluja L, Sierra LM, Comendador MA. Efecto de la Concentración de Cymbopogon Citratus (Dc) Stapf. Sobre la Genotoxicidad de Mutágenos Modelos, en el Ensayo Smart de Ojos W/W+ de *Drosophila melanogaster*. Revista CENIC Ciencias Biológicas. 2005:36

[27] Demir E, Marcos R. Antigenotoxic potential of boron nitride nanotubes. Nanotoxicology. 2018;**12**(8):868-884. DOI: 10.1080/17435390.2018.1482379

[28] De Rezende AA, Graf U, Guterres Zda R, Kerr WE, Spano MA. Protective effects of proanthocyanidins of grape

(*Vitis vinifera* L.) seeds on DNA damage induced by doxorubicin in somatic cells of *Drosophila melanogaster*. Food and Chemical Toxicology. 2009;**47**(7): 1466-1472. DOI: 10.1016/j.fct.2009.03.031

[29] De Rezende AA, Silva ML, Tavares DC, Cunha WR, Rezende KC, Bastos JK, et al. The effect of the dibenzylbutyrolactolic lignan (−)-cubebin on doxorubicin mutagenicity and recombinogenicity in wing somatic cells of *Drosophila melanogaster*. Food and Chemical Toxicology. 2011;**49**(6): 1235-1241. DOI: 10.1016/j.fct.2011.03.001

[30] Drosopoulou E, Vlastos D, Efthimiou I, Kyrizaki P, Tsamadou S, Anagnostopoulou M, et al. *In vitro* and *in vivo* evaluation of the genotoxic and antigenotoxic potential of the major Chios mastic water constituents. Scientific Reports. 2018;**8**:12200. DOI: 10.1038/s41598-018-29810-y

[31] El Hamss R, Analla M, Campos-Sanchez J, Alonso-Moraga A, Munoz-Serrano A, Idaomar M. A dose dependent anti-genotoxic effect of turmeric. Mutation Research. 1999; **446**(1):135-139. DOI: 10.1016/s1383-5718(99)00140-0

[32] Fernandes LM, Da Rosa Guterres Z, Almeida IV, Vicentini VEP. Genotoxicity and antigenotoxicity assessments of the flavonoid vitexin by the *Drosophila melanogaster* somatic mutation and recombination test. Journal of Medicinal Food. 2017;**20**(6): 601-609. DOI: 10.1089/jmf.2016.0149

[33] Fernandez-Bedmar Z, Alonso-Moraga A. *In vivo* and *in vitro* evaluation for nutraceutical purposes of capsaicin, capsanthin, lutein and four pepper varieties. Food and Chemical Toxicology. 2016;**98**(Pt B):89-99. DOI: 10.1016/j.fct.2016.10.011

[34] Fernández-Bedmar Z, Anter J, Cruz-Ares SL, Muñoz-Serrano A, Alonso-Moraga Á, Pérez-Guisado J. Role of citrus juices and distinctive components in the modulation of degenerative processes: Genotoxicity, antigenotoxicity, cytotoxicity, and longevity in *Drosophila*. Journal of Toxicology and Environmental Health. 2011;**74**(15-16):1052-1066. DOI: 10.1080/15287394.2011.582306

[35] Fernandez-Bedmar Z, Anter J, Alonso Moraga A. Anti/genotoxic, longevity inductive, cytotoxic, and clastogenic-related bioactivities of tomato and lycopene. Environmental and Molecular Mutagenesis. 2018;**59**(5): 427-437. DOI: 10.1002/em.22185

[36] Fernández-Bedmar Z, Demyda-Peyrás S, Merinas-Amo T, Del Río-Celestino M. Nutraceutic potential of two *Allium* species and their distinctive organosulfur compounds: A multi-assay evaluation. Foods. 2019;**8**(6):222. DOI: 10.3390/foods8060222

[37] Graf U, Abraham SK, Guzman-Rincon J, Würgler FE. Antigenotoxicity studies in *Drosophila melanogaster*. Mutation Research. 1998;**402**:203-209. DOI: 10.1016/S0027-5107(97)00298-4

[38] Guterres ZR, Zanetti TA, Sennes-Lopes TF, Da Silva AF. Genotoxic and antigenotoxic potential of *Momordica charantia* Linn (Cucurbitaceae) in the wing spot test of *Drosophila melanogaster*. Journal of Medicinal Food. 2015;**18**(10):1136-1142. DOI: 10.1089/jmf.2014.0099

[39] Idaomar M, El Hamss R, Bakkali F, Mezzoug N, Zhiri A, Baudoux D, et al. Genotoxicity and antigenotoxicity of some essential oils evaluated by wing spot test of *Drosophila melanogaster*. Mutation Research. 2002;**513**(1):61-68. DOI: 10.1016/S1383-5718(01)00287-X

[40] Kylyc A, Yesilada E. Preliminary results on antigenotoxic effects of dried mycelia of two medicinal mushrooms in *Drosophila melanogaster* somatic

mutation and recombination test. International Journal of Medicinal Mushrooms. 2013;**15**(4):415-421. DOI: 10.1615/intjmedmushr.v15.i4.90

[41] Laohavechvanich P, Kangsadalampai K, Tirawanchai N, Ketterman AJ. Effect of different Thai traditional processing of various hot chili peppers on urethane-induced somatic mutation and recombination in *Drosophila melanogaster*: Assessment of the role of glutathione transferase activity. Food and Chemical Toxicology. 2006;**44**(8):1348-1354. DOI: 10.1016/j.fct.2006.02.013

[42] Lozano-Baena M-D, Tasset I, Obregón-Cano S, Haro-Bailon A, Muñoz-Serrano A, Alonso-Moraga Á. Antigenotoxicity and tumor growing inhibition by leafy *Brassica carinata* and sinigrin. Molecules. 2015;**20**(9):15748-15765. DOI: 10.3390/molecules200915748

[43] Marques A, Ferreira J, Abreu MH, Pereira R, Rego A, Serôdio J, et al. Searching for antigenotoxic properties of marine macroalgae dietary supplementation against endogenous and exogenous challenges. Journal of Toxicology and Environmental Health. Part A. 2018;**81**(18):939-956. DOI: 10.1080/15287394.2018.1507856

[44] Martinez-Valdivieso D, Font R, Fernandez-Bedmar Z, Merinas-Amo T, Gomez P, Alonso-Moraga A, et al. Role of zucchini and its distinctive components in the modulation of degenerative processes: Genotoxicity, anti-genotoxicity, cytotoxicity and apoptotic effects. Nutrients. 2017;**9**(7). DOI: 10.3390/nu9070755

[45] Mateo-Fernandez M, Alves-Martinez P, Del Rio-Celestino M, Font R, Merinas-Amo T, Alonso-Moraga A. Food safety and nutraceutical potential of caramel colour class IV using *in vivo* and *in vitro* assays. Foods. 2019;**8**(9). DOI: 10.3390/foods8090392

[46] Merinas-Amo T, Tasset-Cuevas I, Diaz-Carretero AM, Alonso-Moraga A, Calahorro F. Role of choline in the modulation of degenerative processes: *In vivo* and *in vitro* studies. Journal of Medicinal Food. 2017;**20**(3):223-234. DOI: 10.1089/jmf.2016.0075

[47] Mezzoug N, Elhadri A, Dallouh A, Amkiss S, Skali NS, Abrini J, et al. Investigation of the mutagenic and antimutagenic effects of *Origanum compactum* essential oil and some of its constituents. Mutation Research. 2007;**629**(2):100-110. DOI: 10.1016/j.mrgentox.2007.01.011

[48] Niikawa M, Nakamura T, Nagase H. Effect of cotreatment of aspirin metabolites on mitomycin C-induced genotoxicity using the somatic mutation and recombination test in *Drosophila melanogaster*. Drug and Chemical Toxicology. 2006;**29**(4):379-396. DOI: 10.1080/01480540600820528

[49] Niikawa M, Shin S, Nagase H. Suppressive effect of post- or pre-treatment of aspirin metabolite on mitomycin C-induced genotoxicity using the somatic mutation and recombination test in *Drosophila melanogaster*. Biomedicine & Pharmacotherapy. 2007;**61**(2-3):113-119. DOI: 10.1016/j.biopha.2006.07.094

[50] Oliveira VC, Constante SAR, Orsolin PC, Nepomuceno JC, De Rezende AAA, Spano MA. Modulatory effects of metformin on mutagenicity and epithelial tumor incidence in doxorubicin-treated *Drosophila melanogaster*. Food and Chemical Toxicology. 2017;**106**(Pt A):283-291. DOI: 10.1016/j.fct.2017.05.052

[51] Orsolin PC, Silva-Oliveira RG, Nepomuceno JC. Modulating effect of simvastatin on the DNA damage induced by doxorubicin in somatic cells of *Drosophila melanogaster*. Food and Chemical Toxicology. 2016;**90**:10-17. DOI: 10.1016/j.fct.2016.01.022

[52] Pádua PFMR, Dihl RR, Lehmann M, Abreu BRR, Richter MF, Andrade HHR. Genotoxic, antigenotoxic and phytochemical assessment of *Terminalia actinophylla* ethanolic extract. Food and Chemical Toxicology. 2013;**62**:521-527. DOI: 10.1016/j.fct.2013.09.021

[53] Patenkovic A, Stamenkovic-Radak M, Banjanac T, Andjelkovic M. Antimutagenic effect of sage tea in the wing spot test of *Drosophila melanogaster*. Food and Chemical Toxicology. 2009;**47**:180-183. DOI: 10.1016/j.fct.2008.10.024

[54] Patenkovic A, Stamenkovic-Radak M, Nikolic D, Markovic T, Andelkovic M. Synergistic effect of *Gentiana lutea* L. on methyl methanesulfonate genotoxicity in the *Drosophila* wing spot test. Journal of Ethnopharmacology. 2013;**146**(2): 632-636. DOI: 10.1016/j.jep.2013.01.027

[55] Prakash G, Hosetti BB, Dhananjaya BL. Protective effect of caffeine on ethyl methanesulfonate-induced wing primordial cells of *Drosophila melanogaster*. Toxicology International. 2014;**21**(1):96-100. DOI: 10.4103/0971-6580.128814

[56] Prakash G, Hosetti BB, Dhananjaya BL. Antimutagenic effect of *Dioscorea pentaphylla* on genotoxic effect induced by methyl methanesulfonate in the *Drosophila* wing spot test. Toxicology International. 2014;**21**(3):258-263. DOI: 10.4103/0971-6580.155341

[57] Rizki M, Amrani S, Creus A, Xamena N, Marcos R. Antigenotoxic properties of selenium: Studies in the wing spot test in *Drosophila*. Environmental and Molecular Mutagenesis. 2001;**37**:70-75. DOI: 10.1002/1098-2280(2001)37:1<70::AID-EM1007>3.0

[58] Romero-Jiménez M, Campos-Sánchez J, Analla M, Muñoz-Serrano A, Alonso-Moraga A. Genotoxicity and anti-genotoxicity of some traditional medicinal herbs. Mutation Research. 2005;**585**(1-2):147-155. DOI: 10.1016/j.mrgentox.2005.05.004

[59] Sarıkaya R, Erciyas K, Kara MI, Sezer U, Erciyas AF, Ay S. Evaluation of genotoxic and antigenotoxic effects of boron by the somatic mutation and recombination test (SMART) on *Drosophila*. Drug and Chemical Toxicology. 2016;**39**:400-406. DOI: 10.3109/01480545.2015.1130719

[60] Savić T, Patenković A, Soković M, Glamoclija J, Andjelković M, van Griensven LJ. The effect of royal sun agaricus, *Agaricus brasiliensis* S. Wasser et al., extract on methyl methanesulfonate caused genotoxicity in *Drosophila melanogaster*. International Journal of Medicinal Mushrooms. 2011; **13**(4):377-385. DOI: 10.1615/intjmedmushr.v13.i4.80

[61] Sukprasansap M, Sridonpai P, Phiboonchaiyanan PP. Eggplant fruits protect against DNA damage and mutations. Mutation Research. 2019; **813**:39-45. DOI: 10.1016/j.mrfmmm.2018.12.004

[62] Taira K, Miyashita Y, Okamoto K, Arimoto S, Takahashi E, Negishi T. Novel antimutagenic factors derived from the edible mushroom *Agrocybe cylindracea*. Mutation Research. 2005; **586**(2):115-123. DOI: 10.1016/j.mrgentox.2005.06.007

[63] Tasset-Cuevas I, Fernández-Bedmar Z, Lozano-Baena MD, Campos-Sánchez J, de Haro-Bailón A, Muñoz-Serrano A, et al. Protective effect of borage seed oil and gamma linolenic acid on DNA: *In vivo* and *in vitro* studies. PLoS One. 2013;**8**(2):e56986. DOI: 10.1371/journal.pone.0056986

[64] Toyoshima M, Hosoda K, Hanamura M, Okamoto K, Kobayashi H, Negishi T. Alternative methods to

evaluate the protective ability of sunscreen against photo-genotoxicity. Journal of Photochemistry and Photobiology. B. 2004;**73**(1-2):59-66. DOI: 10.1016/j.jphotobiol.2003.09.005

[65] Valadares BL, Graf U, Spanó MA. Inhibitory effects of water extract of propolis on doxorubicin-induced somatic mutation and recombination in *Drosophila melanogaster*. Food and Chemical Toxicology. 2008;**46**(3): 1103-1110. DOI: 10.1016/j.fct.2007.11.005

[66] Valente N, Borges J, Baptista A, Gaivão I. Benefits of thalassotherapy in the Portuguese coast: A study in *Drosophila melanogaster*. In: Annual Portuguese Drosophila Meeting; Tomar, Portugal. 2014

[67] Lyer J, Wang Q, Le T, Imai Y, Srivastava A, Troisí BL, et al. Quantitative assessment of eye phenotypes for functional genetic studies using *Drosophila melanogaster*. G3: Genes|Genomes|Genetics. 2016;**6**: 1427-1437. DOI: 10.1534/g3.116.027060

[68] Gonzalez C. *Drosophila melanogaster*: A model and a tool to investigate malignancy and identify new therapeutics. Nature Reviews. Cancer. 2013;**13**:172-183. DOI: 10.1038/nrc3461

[69] Vogel EW, Nivard MJ. Parallel monitoring of mitotic recombination, clastogenicity and teratogenic effects in eye tissue of *Drosophila*. Mutation Research. 2000;**455**(1-2):141-153. DOI: 10.1016/s0027-5107(00)00067-1

[70] Vogel EW, Nivard MJ. A novel method for the parallel monitoring of mitotic recombination and clastogenicity in somatic cells *in vivo*. Mutation Research. 1999;**431**(1): 141-153. DOI: 10.1016/s0027-5107(99) 00198-0

[71] Vogel EW, Zijlstra JA. Mechanistic and methodological aspects of chemically induced somatic mutation and recombination in *Drosophila melanogaster*. Mutation Research. 1987; **182**:243-264. DOI: 10.1016/0165-1161 (87)90010-0

[72] Vogel EW, Nivard MJM. Performance of 181 chemicals in a *Drosophila* assay predominantly monitoring interchromosomal mitotic recombination. Mutagenesis. 1993;**8**(1): 57-81. DOI: 10.1093/mutage/8.1.57

[73] Gaivão I, Comendador MA. The *w/w*+ somatic mutation and recombination test (SMART) of *Drosophila melanogaster* for detecting reactive oxygen species: Characterization of 6 strains. Mutation Research. 1996;**360**:145-151. DOI: 10.1016/0165-1161(96)00003-9

[74] Donohoe TJ, Jones CR, Kornahrens AF, Barbosa LCA, Walport LJ, Tatton MR, et al. Total synthesis of the antitumor antibiotic (±)-streptonigrin: First-and second-generation routes for de novo pyridine formation using ring-closing metathesis. American Chemical Society. 2013;**78**: 12338-12350. DOI: 10.1021/jo402388f

[75] Troxell B, Xu H, Yang XF. *Borrelia burgdorferi,* a pathogen that lacks iron, encodes manganese-dependent superoxide dismutase essential for resistance to streptonigrin. The Journal of Biological Chemistry. 2012;**287**(23): 19284-19293. DOI: 10.1074/jbc.M112.344903

[76] Bolzán AD, Bianchi MS. Genotoxicity of streptonigrin: A review. Mutation Research. 2001;**488**:25-37. DOI: 10.1016/S1383-5742(00)00062-4

[77] Deepa PV, Akshaya AS, Solomon FDP. Anthracycline (epirubicin) induced mutation studies in *Drosophila melanogaster*. Drososphila Information Service. 2011;**94**:53-61

[78] López-Romero D, Izquierdo-Vega JA, Morales-González JA, Madrigal-Bujaidar

E, Chamorro-Cevallos G, Sánchez-Gutiérrez M, et al. Evidence of some natural products with antigenotoxic effects. Part 2: Plants, vegetables, and natural resin. Nutrients. 2018;**10**(12):1954. DOI: 10.3390/nu10121954

[79] Słoczyńska K, Powroźnik B, Pękala E, Waszkielewicz AM. Antimutagenic compounds and their possible mechanisms of action. Journal of Applied Genetics. 2014;**55**:273-285. DOI: 10.1007/s13353-014-0198-9

[80] Izquierdo-Vega JA, Morales-González JA, Sánchez-Gutiérrez M, Betanzos-Cabrera G, Sosa-Delgado SM, Sumaya-Martínez MT, et al. Evidence of some natural products with antigenotoxic effects. Part 1: Fruits and polysaccharides. Nutrients. 2017;**9**(2): 102. DOI: 10.3390/nu9020102

[81] Panieri E, Santoro MM. ROS homeostasis and metabolism: A dangerous liason in cancer cells. Cell Death & Disease. 2016;7(6):e2253. DOI: 10.1038/cddis.2016.105

Chapter 8

Current Trends and Future Perspectives of Antimutagenic Agents

Adel M. AbdelHakem and El-Shimaa M.N. Abdelhafez

Abstract

Mutation is the process leading to heritable changes in DNA caused mainly by internal and external factors. Recently, studies on mutagenic agents have been increased due to increasing in mutation-related disease. The antimutagenic effect is desired to prevent mutation on genes or to inactivate the mutagenic agent. It seems that the interest in antimutagenic substances displaying multiple mechanisms of action will be an important trend in the research and development of new antimutagenic compounds in the near future. Therefore, this chapter displays various possible mechanisms of action for antimutagenic agent and introduces different types of antimutagens, natural and synthetic, that are considered very important.

Keywords: mutagenesis, antimutagenic, mechanism, natural, synthetic, DNA

1. Introduction

Mutagenicity is the process of induction of permanent heritable changes in the DNA sequence of living systems [1]. It is caused mainly by the external factors, including chemical and physical agents, or can also occur spontaneously due to errors in DNA repair, replicationand recombination [2]. A number of mutagens have been recognized in our environment recently as many factors which modulate the toxic activities either in vitro or in vivo [3]. Agents contributing to mutagenesis in the environment could be from wide-spectrum applications of biocides in the agriculture, industrial sources, and other contaminants [3].

These mutagenic chemicals have severe drawbacks in humans such as cancer and various inherited diseases; therefore, it is important to detect such mutagenic agents precisely and rapidly and also look for solutions to combat them [2].

Natural occurring dietary antimutagens such as healthy protective foods such as fruits and vegetables could strongly counteract the deleterious effect of these mutagens [4]. Additionally, the World Health Organization (WHO) revealed that one-third of all cancer death incidences are preventable depending on the diet type especially health protective phytochemicals that provide an effective solution to these concerns [4]. The current chapter will present the mutagenic events and a brief compilation of the existing scientific findings either from dietary sources or synthetic agents that have the potential activity to combat the disorders caused by the mutagenic agents, putting in mind possible future perspectives and mechanism of antimutagenics [2].

2. Mechanisms of action

Several classes of antimutagenic compounds may be distinguished based on their mechanism of action as the following:

2.1 Antimutagens with antioxidant potency

Reactive oxygen species (ROS) are generated by many mutagens; therefore, the removal of reactive molecules is considered an important strategy in the process of antimutagenesis. It is reported that compounds with antioxidant propertiescan remove ROS before these molecules react with DNA, resulting in a mutation [5].

It was reported that the antigenotoxic effects of Lipoic acid (LA) (**Figure 1**) against mitomycin-C induced chromosomal aberrations, sister chromatid exchanges, and micronucleus formation was observed in human peripheral lymphocytes. Moreover, LA exhibits both anticlastogenic and antimutagenic activity [6].

2.2 Interaction with mutagen

A potential protective mechanism against mutagenesis is related to the direct chemical interaction between a mutagen and an antimutagenic compound before it induces DNA damage leading to the inhibition of their damaging activity. Sulfhydryl compounds, such as cysteine, can inactivate 3-chloro-4-(dichloromethyl)-5-hydroxy-2(5H)-furanone (MX) (**Figure 2**) [7].

2.3 Antimutagen as blocking agents

The mechanism of action for this type of antimutagenics is to prevent mutagenic compounds from reaching target sites such as nucleophilic bichalcophenes (**Figure 3**). They might be able to bind to DNA and, therefore, protect genetic materials from electrophilic mutagenic agents [8].

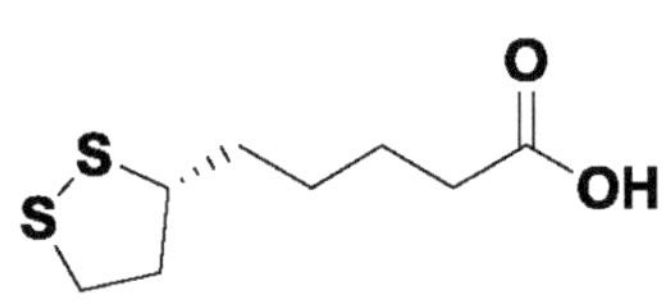

Figure 1.
Lipolic acid.

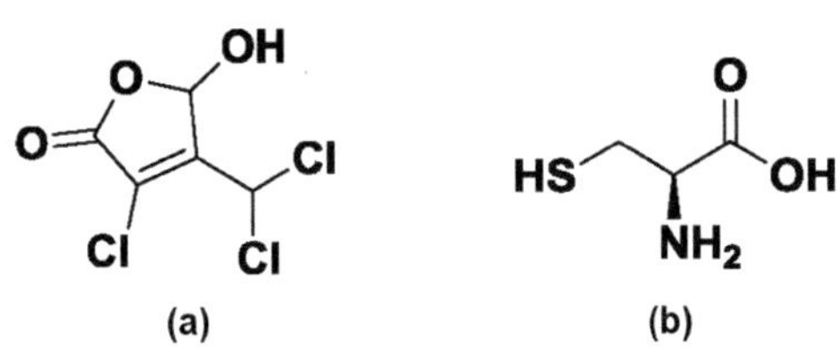

Figure 2.
(a) Mutagen (MX) and (b) antimutagen (cysteine).

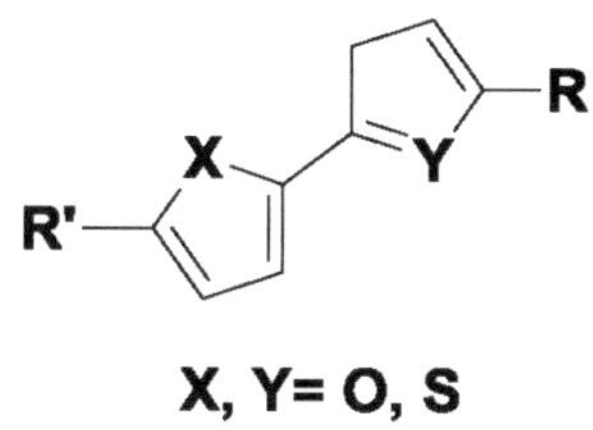

Figure 3.
Bichalcophene derivatives.

2.4 Multifunctionally acting antimutagens

Various antimutagenic agents work through multiple mechanisms affording protection against several mutagens. Noteworthy, the ability of compounds to affect mutagens simultaneously in varied ways significantly enhances antimutagenic effectiveness. Hence, searching for such multifunctionally acting antimutagens is of great importance [9].

2.5 Desmutagenesis

This way of preventing induced cellular mutagenesis depends on mutagens that are inactivated before they can attack the DNA in vitro [3].

2.6 Bio-antimutagenesis

Damaged DNAusually requires fixation steps (e.g., DNAreplication and/or repair) before it can be expressed as stable and heritable mutant genes. Hence this mechanism relates to interference with some aspects of cellular DNA fixation processes working on reducing genetic damage in DNA [3].

3. Antimutagenic agents

Antimutagenic agents are able to combat the disorders caused by mutagens [10]. This group of agents includes both natural and synthetic compounds categories [1].

3.1 Natural antimutagenic agents

The antimutagenic effect of natural sources was investigated due to certain compounds in them or due to whole extract.

3.1.1 Isolated compounds

3.1.1.1 Cinnamaldehyde

It is the first naturally occurring organic antimutagen [11]; it has been involved in screening and chemical studies of such biologically active substances [12]. Antimutagenic action is attributed to either by a selective killing effect of cells which have premutation lesion of DNA via inhibition of the errorprone SOS repair system, or by enhancement of the error-free DNA repair system (**Figure 4**) [13].

3.1.1.2 Punicalagin (PC) and ellagic acid (EA)

Punicalagin is an ellagitannin found in the fruit peel of *Punica granatum*. PC and EA (**Figure 5a, b**) had antioxidant and antigenotoxic properties which dose-dependently and markedly antagonized the effect of tested mutagens such as NaN_3, benzo[a]pyrene, 2-aminoflourine, and methyl methanesulfonate (EMS), with 90% mutagenicity inhibition [14].

3.1.1.3 Luteolin derivatives

Luteolin derivatives (luteolin 7-O-rutinoside, luteolin 7-O-glucoside, and luteolin 7-O-glucuronide) (**Figure 6**) are isolated from *Mentha longifolia* (L.) to evaluate the antimutagenic activities by using Ames *Salmonella* test (TA 1535 and TA1537 strains). The antimutagenic activity on TA1537 was 87.63, 84.03, and 67.77%, respectively. The antimutagenic activity of these compoundscan be due to

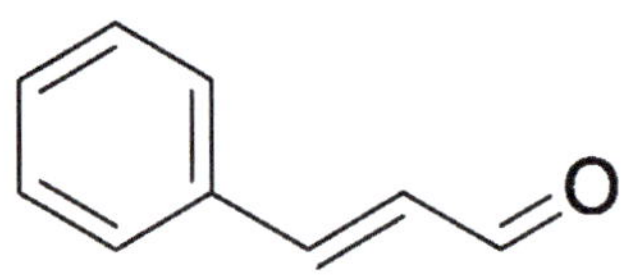

Figure 4.
Cinnamaldehyde.

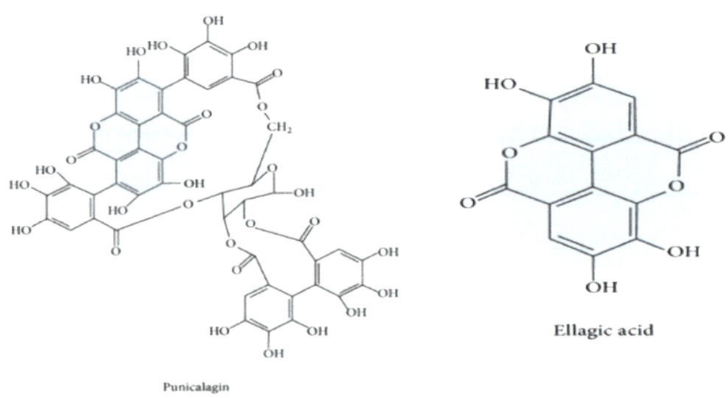

Figure 5.
(a) Punicalagin (b) ellagic acid.

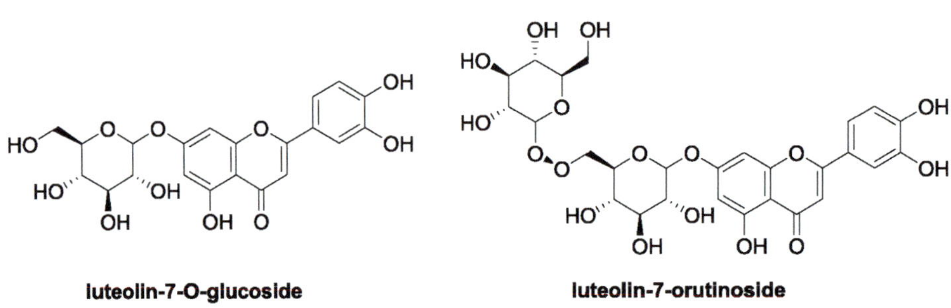

Figure 6.
Luteolin derivatives.

the inhibition capability by blocking 9-aminoacridine binding to DNA [15]. In addition, the inhibition effects against ethyl methanesulfonate may be related to the protection against DNA double-strand breaks or EMS alkylating action (**Figure 6**) [16].

3.1.1.4 Acetogenins

Annona crassiflora Mart. (AcM) is a Brazilian plant, *araticum*, which is widely used as a therapeutic medicine to treat several diseases such as rheumatism, diarrhea, and syphilis. Ethanolic extract were evaluated for antimutagenic and cytotoxic effects. The results indicated an antimutagenic activity of the AcM due to the presence of acetogenins (**Figure** 7) and other flavonoids [17].

3.1.1.5 Pinocembrin and cardamonin

Pinocembrin and cardamonin (**Figure 8**) are found in Sozuku (Chinese drug from dried seed of *Alpinia katsumadae* HAYATA). These compounds showed potent antimutagenic activity against 2-amino3,4-dimethylimidazo-[4,5-f] quinolone (MeIQ) mutagenesis in Ames test using the *S. typhimurium* TA100 and TA98 strains [18].

3.1.1.6 Harpagoside (HS)

It isa type of iridoid glycoside. HS (**Figure 9**) is considered as the main active component extracted from *Harpagophytumprocumbens* (HP) which is used as anti-inflammatory and analgesic particularly against painful osteoarthritis. The extract wastested to evaluate the antimutagenic activity of HS and HP against mutagenic activity of 1-nitropyrene (1-NPy) that is one of the most abundant nitro-polycyclic aromatic hydrocarbons particularly in diesel exhausts. The results showed that HS significantly reduced the mutagenicity of 1-NPy in pretreatment and particularly in co-treatment. Moreover, HP extract significantly reduced the genotoxicity [19].

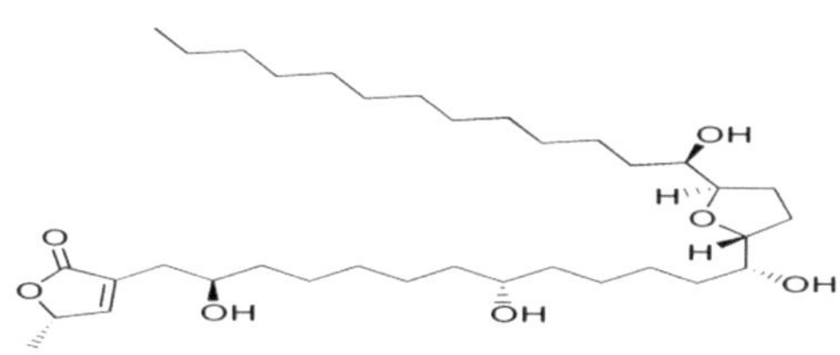

Figure 7.
Acetogenins.

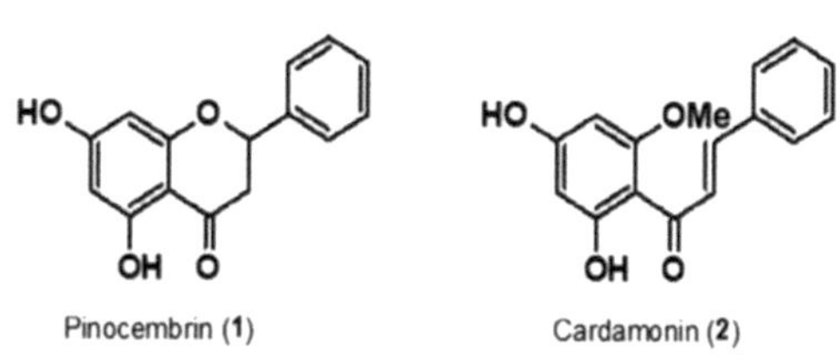

Figure 8.
Pinocembrin and cardamonin.

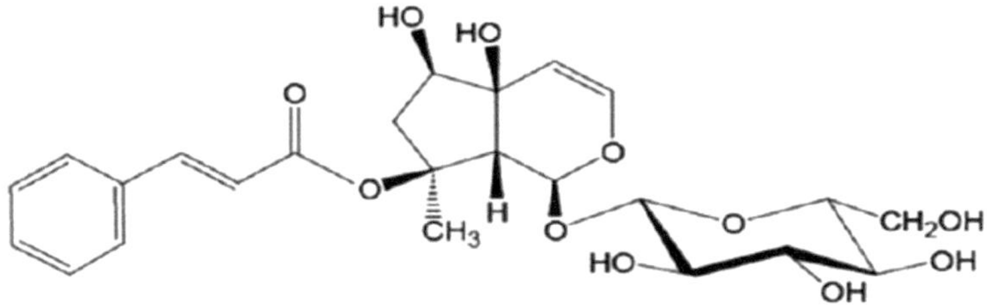

Figure 9.
Harpagoside (HS)

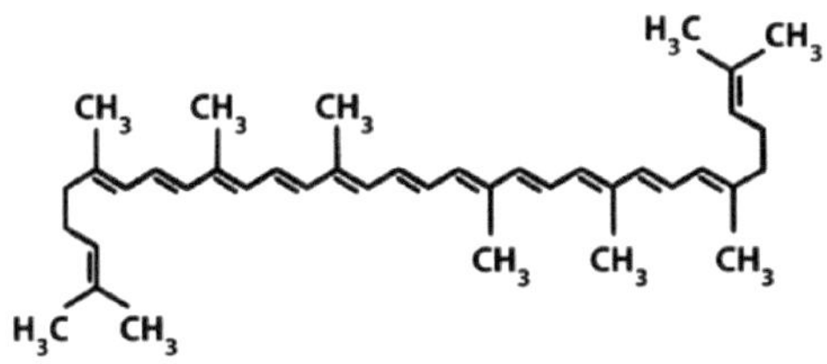

Figure 10.
Lycopene.

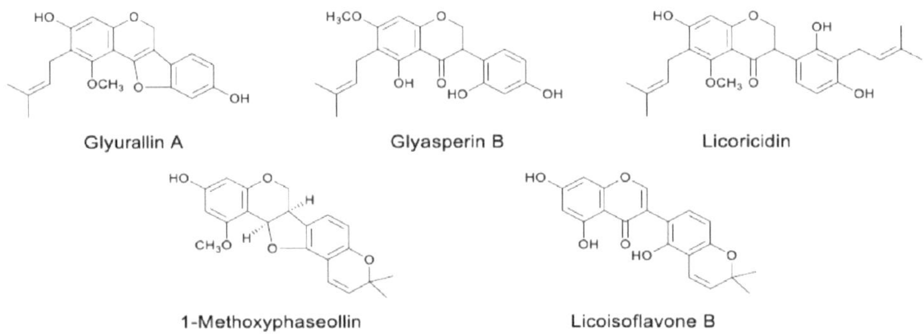

Figure 11.
Glycyrrhiza aspera root extract.

3.1.1.7 Lycopene

Natural oleoresin is rich in lycopene (**Figure 10**), which was obtained from two types of tomato (Zedona and Gironda). The antimutagenic activity of oleoresin was tested against aflatoxin B1 (AFB1), and both varieties had awfully high antimutagenic potential against AFB1 (60–66%) [20].

3.1.1.8 Compounds extracted from Glycyrrhiza aspera *root*

The powdered extract of *G. aspera* root was assayed for antimutagenic activity against N-methyl-N-nitrosourea (MNU) in S. typhimurium TA1535. Five components that were extracted by using ethanol which had antimutagenic activity against MNU were identified as glyurallin A, glyasperin B, licoricidin, 1-methoxyphaseollin, and licoisoflavone B (**Figure 11**). These components were demonstrated to possess an antigenotoxic effect against carcinogenic MNU. So this extract can be used to prevent DNA damage by N-nitrosamines for cancer chemoprevention [21].

3.1.2 Plant extract

3.1.2.1 Date palm *fruit aqueous extract*

It was found that *date palm* extract displays strong antimutagenic activity against ultraviolet (UV) radiation, and mitomycin C-induced mutagenesis, when it was analyzed using *E. coli* RNA polymerase β-based rifampicin resistance assay, but did not show any significant antimutagenesis against ethyl methane sulfonate (EMS) [22].

3.1.2.2 Maytenus ilicifolia *and* Peltastes peltatus *extract*

These two plants are both rich in compounds of the tanninand flavonoid groups and frequently employed in folk medicine. Antimutagenicity was determined against known mutagenic substances such as 4-oxide-1-nitroquinoline, NaN_3, aflatoxin B1, 2-aminofluorene and 2-aminoanthracene, and 2-nitrofluorene using the *Salmonella*/microsome assay. There was a significant decrease in mutagenicity for the tested extract by 75%.The mechanism of antimutagenicity of this extract is still under study [23].

3.1.2.3 Citrus limonum *fruit residues (CLFR)*

Aqueous and acidified methanol extracts of CLFR were evaluated for their total phenolic contents and antioxidant and antimutagenic activities. Antimutagenic potential of the extracts was done by Ames test. The results supported that the extracts from CLFR were mutagenically safe due to its high phenolic content which can act as antioxidant and anitmutagenic [24].

3.1.2.4 Mimosa tenuiflora *(MT) extract*

The genotoxic effect of MT was investigated by using both micronucleus test and Ames test in *Salmonella typhimurium* TA97, TA98, TA100, and TA102, respectively. The results showed that the extract did not induce mutations in any strain. Further studies of toxicity were performed to investigate the use of this plant in the treatment of diseases [25].

3.1.2.5 Albeofructus *(ADA) extract*

It is an extract of *Acanthopanax divaricatus* which possesses antimutagenic activity against direct-acting mutagenic agents through the rapid elimination of mutagenic compounds from the cells before the induction of genetic material damage [26].

3.1.2.6 Anemopsis californica *(AC)*

Although *A. californica* (AC) possesses therapeutic uses, so it could be useful for reducing genotoxic risk generating from ROS-agents exposure and provide protection against poly-cyclic aromatic hydrocarbons which are well known as premutagens and precarcinogens [27].

3.1.2.7 Citrus sinensis *and* Citrus latifolia

The essential oils of *Citrus sinensis* and *Citrus latifolia* showed antimycotic besides antimutagenic and antioxidant activity. Their main components are R-(+)-limonene, α-myrcene, β-thujene, and γ-terpinene [28].

3.1.2.8 Heterotheca inuloides *(HI) extract*

The methanolic extract of HI reduced the mutagenicity of benzo[a]pyrene, norfloxacin, and 2-aminoanthracene. The antigenotoxic properties could be due to the antioxidant properties of component into extract such as catenanes, sterols, polyacetylenes, triterpenes, sesquiterpenes, flavonoids, and flavonoid glycosides [29].

3.1.2.9 Extracts of Acacia salicina

Literatures revealed that this extract displayed potent antioxidant and antimutagenic activities [30]. Also chloroform extract showed antimutagenic effect against both direct- and indirect-acting mutagens, as the extract may act as a blocking agent that is capable of influencing the activities of enzymes engaged in the metabolism of mutagens and carcinogens. Moreover, the tested extract displayed the ability to react directly with the mutagens electrophilic metabolite sand was capable of protecting against oxidative DNA damage [30].

3.1.2.10 Wheat bran

It was reported that wheat bran provides antimutagenic effects that related to the presence of the antioxidant phytic acid. It was demonstrated that phytic acid may intercept carcinogenic azoxymethane, inhibiting it even before it can damage DNA. Moreover, antioxidants included in wheat bran are able tomodulate DNA repair enzymes [31].

3.1.2.11 Vegetables

Activity was displayed by beets, chives, horseradish, onions, rhubarb, and spinach. All cruciferous vegetables showed strong to moderate antimutagenic activities, except Chinese cabbage, which displayed weak activity. Moderate antimutagenicity was found in green beans and tomatoes, whereas weak activities in egg plant, garden cress, many types of lettuces, leeks, mangold, cucumber, pumpkin, radish, and summer squash. However, some vegetables such as *Asparagus*, carrots, fennel leaves, parsley, green pepper, and radishes were not found to display any antimutagenicity [32].

Antimutagenic activity of many vegetable juiceswere earlier studied againstmutagenicity induced by2-amino-3-methyl[4,5-f]-quinoline (IQ), 2-amino-3,4dimethylimidazo[4,5-f] quinoline (MeIQ) or 2-amino3,8-dimethylimidazo [4,5-f] quinoxaline (MeIQx) in S.typhimurium TA98 and TA100 [33].

3.1.2.12 Fruits

Current research all over the world has focused on health protectiveproperties of fruits including antimutagenic potential of different fruittypes and their cultivars. Concerning apple fruit, its antioxidant and radioprotective properties were found to be better correlated with its antimutagenic effect [34]. Recently, copaiba, an exotic

Brazilian fruit, possesses the antimutagenic potential of copaiba powder (dose of 100 mg/kg) showing great reduction of micronuclei [35].

3.1.2.13 Other sources

3.1.2.13.1 Ganoderma lucidum

Ganoderma lucidum was extracted with hot water (GLW) and then partially purified with crude glycoside extract (GLG) and crude polysaccharide extract (GLP). The extract was tested to evaluate the antioxidant and antimutagenic activity. The results showed that the extract has antimutagenic activity due to β-glucan content and antioxidant action due to the presence of high polyphenolic content [36].

3.1.2.13.2 Macro fungus

It was demonstrated that ethyl acetate extract of macro fungus showed the in vitro antimutagenic activity of *Phellinus rimosus*. The activity of the extract against direct-acting mutagens may result from the direct inactivation of mutagens. It is probable that, due to stimulation of the transmembrane export system in bacteria, mutagenic compounds are removed from the cells before they influence the DNA structure [37]. Additionally, in the case of doxorubicin (DXN), the extract of *P. rimosus* may affect the intercalation of mutagens to genetic material.

3.2 Synthetic antimutagenic agents

Synthetic antimutagens is another important trend in the area of antimutagenicity research.

3.2.1 Steroidal hormonal molecules

Bile acids have either a co- or an antimutagenic activity toward various direct- and indirect-acting mutagens [38]. It was reported that steroidal hormones could inhibit the genotoxicity of both direct- and indirect-acting mutagens [39]. For example, both ethinyl oestradiol and mestranol (**Figure 12**), which are synthetic derivatives of 3-estradiol largely used in contraceptive pills, are strong mutagenic inhibitors acting at nanomolar concentrations [39].

3.2.2 Gallic acid

It could act as a nucleophile to scavenge the electrophilic mutagens. It was implied that gallic acid (**Figure 13**) can bind or insert into the outer membrane

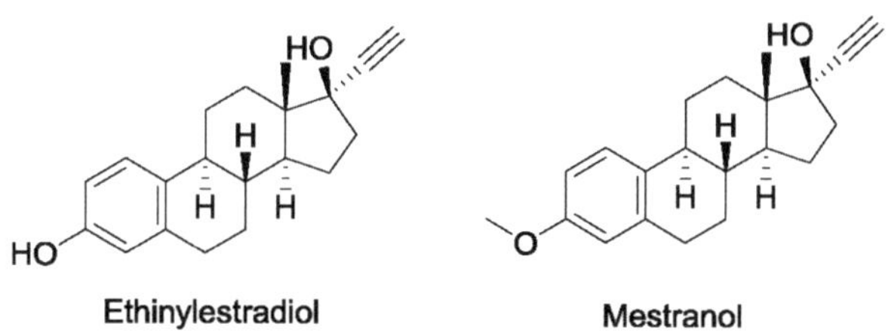

Figure 12.
Steroidal hormonal molecules

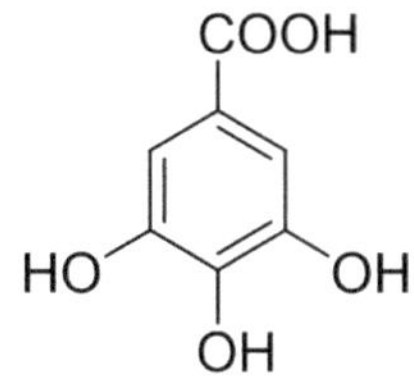

Figure 13.
Gallic acid.

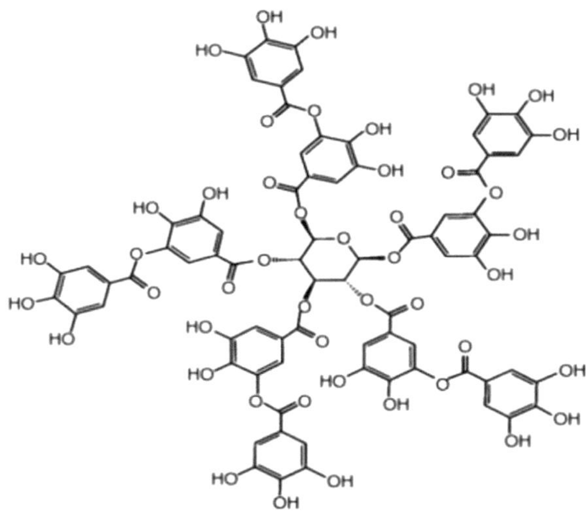

Figure 14.
Tannic acid.

transporters leading to the blockage of a mutagen that was transferred intothe cytosol [40]. One of the mutagenic substances that gallic acid affects is NaN3. It is widely used in agriculture, industry, and medicine, but it is a highly toxicsubstance. If sodium azide is found in the intracellular milieu, azide ions bind Fe3þ in hemoglobin and inhibit the respiratory chain of metabolism [41].

3.2.3 Tannic acid

The anticlastogenic effect of tannic acid (**Figure 14**) was studied *in vivo* in the mouse micronucleus test. Moreover, the antimutagenic effect of tannic acid was investigated *in vivo* in the mouse spot test using male PW and female C57BL/10 mice. The results showed that tannic acid can act as an anticlastogen and antimutagen in vivo [42].

3.2.4 Synthesized β- aminoketones

Theantigenotoxic potential of two newly synthesized β-aminoketones such as2-{(4-bromophenyl)[(4-methylphenyl) amino] methyl} cyclohexanone and 2-{(4-chlorophenyl)[(4-methylphenyl) amino] methyl} cyclohexanone compounds was tested against the mutagenN-methyl-N-nitro-N-nitrosoguanidine (MNNG), acting by DNAmethylation (**Figure 15**) [9]. The antimutagenic potential of these compounds may be related to the inhibition of the production of O6-methylguanine,

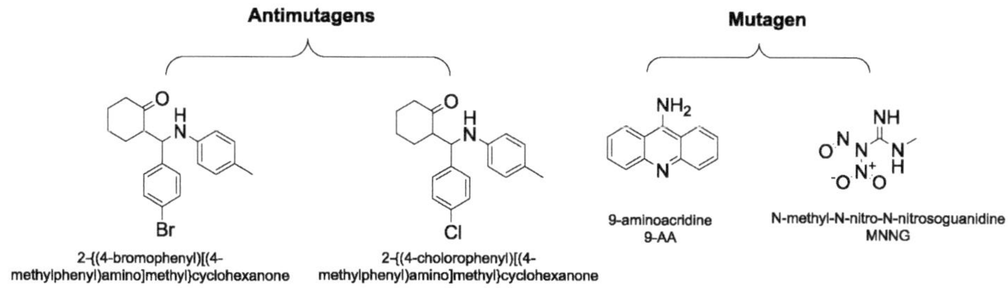

Figure 15.
β-Aminoketones and mutagens.

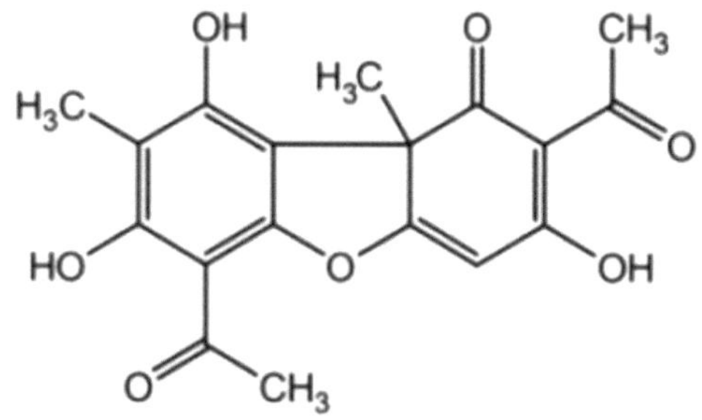

Figure 16.
Usnic acid.

a product of MNNG that is related to its mutagenic effect. Both compounds also abolished mutagenesis induced by 9-AA that binds to DNA noncovalently by intercalation [43].

3.2.5 Phenolic agents

This category of antimutagenics acts against mutagens via either intracellularor extracellular mechanisms [44]. The extracellular mechanism showed interference with the cytochrome P450-mediated metabolismof these mutagens and the interaction with active mutagenicmetabolites [8]. Moreover, the antimutagenic potency of these compounds may be relatedto DNA protection from mutagens presenting electrophilicproperties [8].

Hydroxyphenyliminoligands and their metal complexes [Cu(II), Co(II), Ni(II) and Mn(II) complexes] of usnic acid (**Figure 16**) which is isolated from *Usnea longissima*, were synthesized by Schiff base method with *O-*, *P-*, and *M-*aminophenol compounds to determine their antimutagenic activity against different bacteria species. The results showed that the Co and Mn complexes of the ligands possess potent antimutagenic activity [45].

New polymeric microspheres containing azomethine were designed and synthesized to evaluate their antimutagenic activity against NaN_3, among of them; a new polymeric microspheres containing azomethine (**Figure 17**) which contains R = CH_3 had potent antimutagenic effect against NaN_3 [46].

Chitosan derivatives containing quaternary ammonium groups and di (tertbutyl) phenol (TBPh) (**Figure 18**) in the polymer side chain improved the antimutagenic efficiency of the polymer from 48 to 93% [47].

Hydrazone derivatives were synthesized to study their antioxidant and antimutagenic activity against 4-NPD and NaN3 in *S. typhimurium* TA98 and TA100, respectively, among of them; the hydrazone derivative (**Figure 19**)

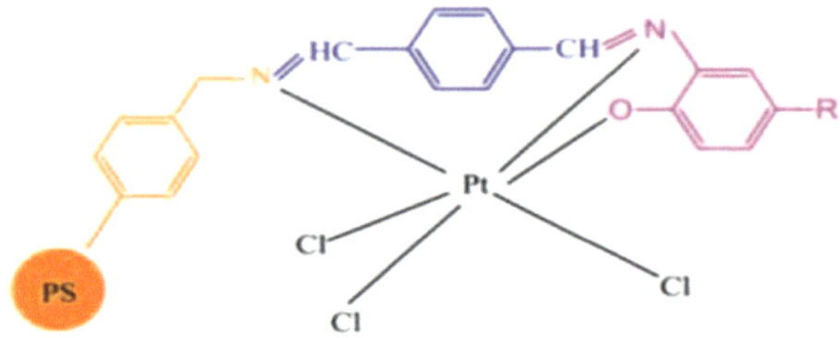

Figure 17.
New polymeric microspheres containing azomethine.

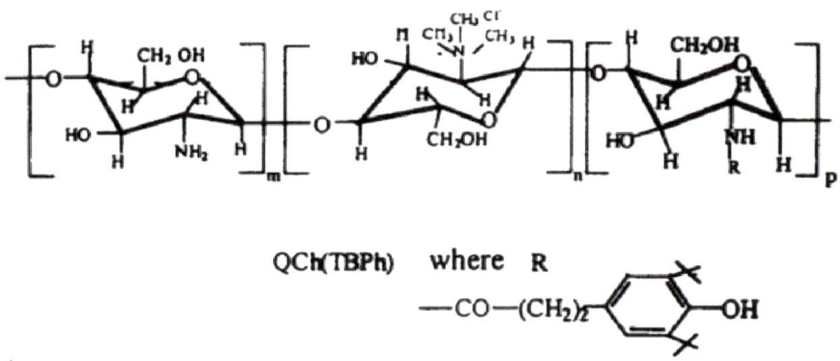

Figure 18.
Chitosan derivatives containing quaternary ammonium groups.

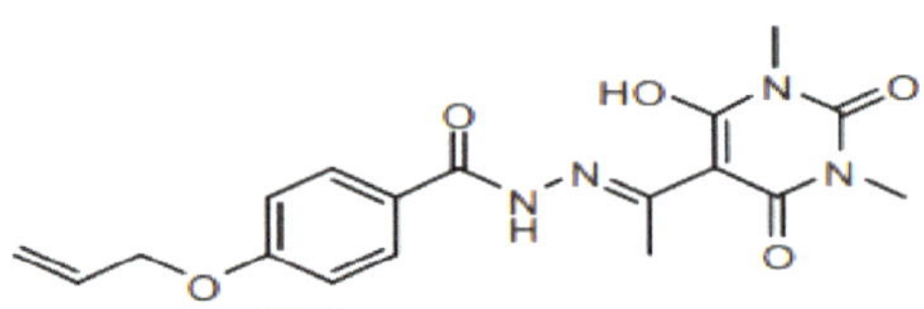
(III)

Figure 19.
Hydrazone derivatives

had high antimutagenic activity. The strongest antimutagenic activity was observed at 5 mg/plate concentration against *S. typhimurium* TA100 strain [48].

3.2.6 Xanthones

The potential antimutagenic of xanthonesis attributed to different mechanisms, such as the rapid elimination of mutagens from bacteria; the interaction between antimutagens and the reactive intermediates of mutagens; and the influence on microsomal enzymes against direct mutagen 4-nitroquinoline-N-oxide (NQNO) (**Figure 20**) [49].

3.2.7 Indols

Novel polymeric-Schiff bases including indol (L1, L2, L3) (**Figure 21**) exhibited the antigenotoxic properties against sodium azide in human lymphocyte cells by micronuclei (MN) and sister chromatid exchange tests [50].

A series of indolizine derivatives have been synthesized to determine their antimutagenic activity, the indolizine derivative (**Figure 22**) had the highest activity [51].

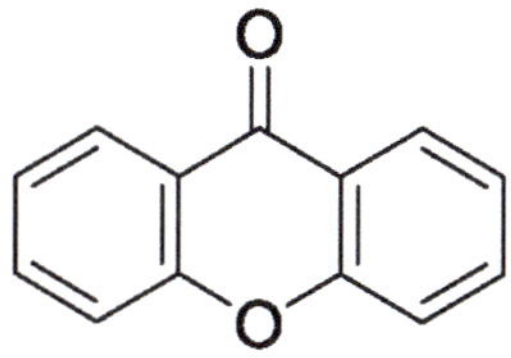

Figure 20.
Xanthone.

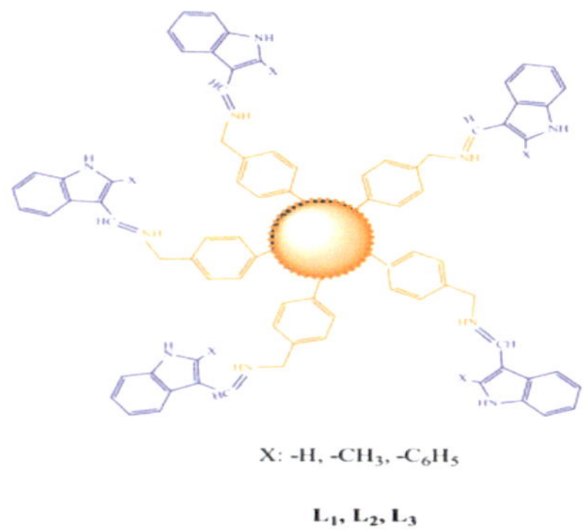

Figure 21.
Novel polymeric-Schiff bases.

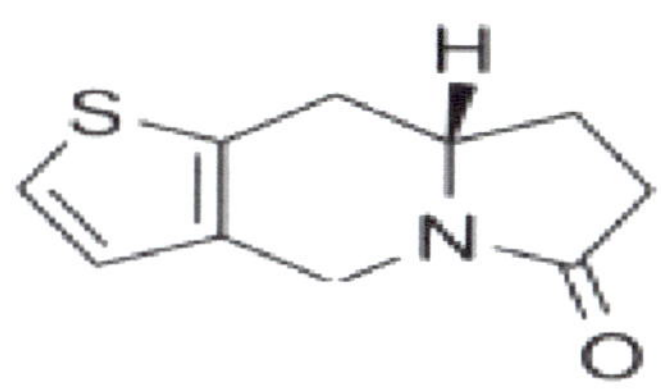

Figure 22.
Indolizine.

3.2.8 Organoselenium

Scientists demonstrated that this series of compounds are protected against genotoxicity and oxidative stress induced by an indirect-acting mutagen CP [52]. This is attributed to effect of CP on DNA through its alkylating properties and free radicals production [53].

3.2.9 Bichalcophenes

The novel bichalcophenes significantly decreased the mutagenicity induced by two mutagens, namely, NaN_3 and BP [54]. It was found that the antimutagenic potential of the compounds could be attributed to their antioxidant activity [55].

3.2.10 Others

New zerumbone-bicarbonyl analogues were synthesized to determine their antimutagenic activity against *Salmonella* tester strains. Zerumbal (**Figure 23**) had significant higher antimutagenic activity than zerumbone [56].

Two newly synthesized oxadiazoles: 1,3-bis(5-benzylthio-1,3,4-oxadiazol-2-yl) benzene (M1) and 1,4-bis(5-benzylthio-1,3,4-oxadiazol-2-yl) benzene (M2) (**Figure 25**) were synthesized and studied in *Salmonella typhimurium* strains TA97, TA100, TA102 and TA1537 in the presence and absence of S9mix. The antimutagenicity of M1 and M2 against H_2O_2, NaN_3, and 4-nitro-o-phenylene diamine (NPD) using the tester strains, was also investigated. The two compounds were found to be nonmutagenic [58].

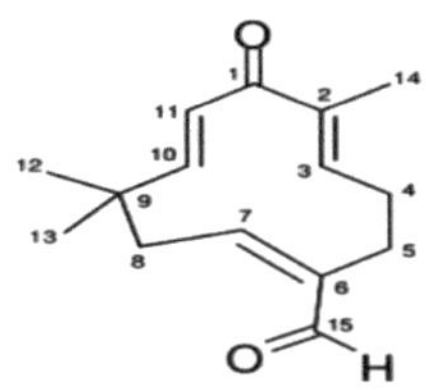

Figure 23.
*1,4-Dihydropyridines (1,4-DHP) (**Figure 24**) possessed antioxidant and antimutagenic activities. The compounds modified the activity of DNA repair enzymes, to protect the DNA in living cells against peroxynitrite-induced damage [57].*

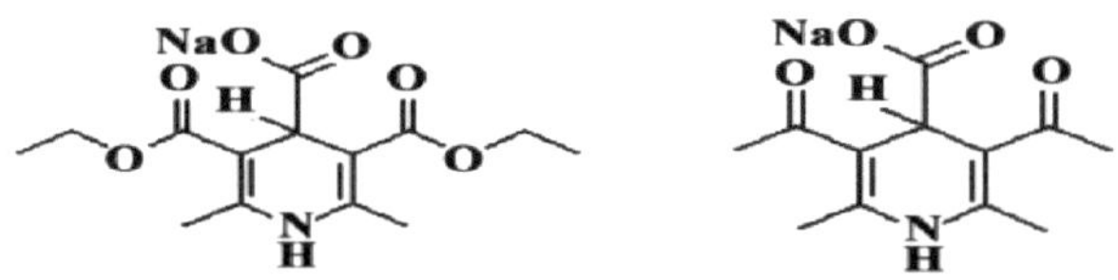

AV-153-Na AV-154-Na

Figure 24.
1,4-Dihydropyridines (1,4-DHP) derivatives.

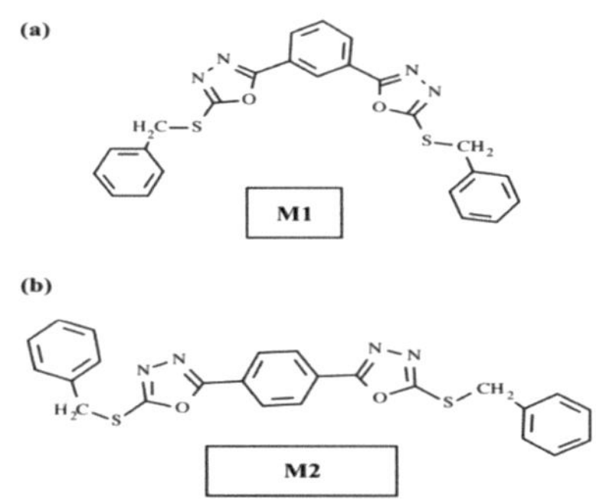

Figure 25.
Oxadiazole derivatives.

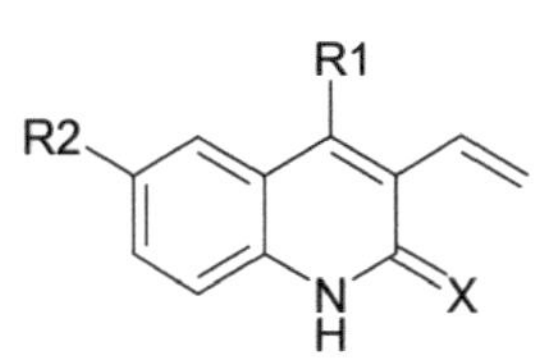

1c R1=C_6H_5 R2=Cl X=O; **1d** R1=C_6H_5 R2=NO_2 X=O

Figure 26.
Dihydrothienoquinoline derivatives.

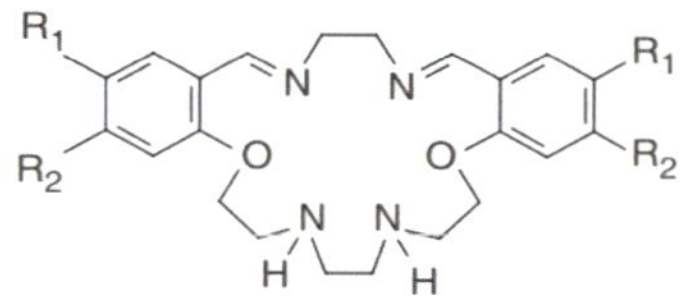

1 $R_1 = R_2 = H$
2 $R_1 = NO_2$, $R_2 = H$
3 $R_1 + R_2 = CH{=}CH{-}CH{=}CH$

Figure 27.
Azacrown ether Schiff bases.

Dihydrothienoquinoline derivatives were designed and synthesized to evaluate their antimutagenicity using Ames test. Several compounds showed good antimutagenicity. The results for compounds (**Figure 26**) were found to be statistically significant (P = 0) [58].

A series of novel azacrown ether Schiff bases have been synthesized, and they were investigated for their antimutagenic activities using the spot test and Ames test using strains TA1535, TA100, and TA97a of *Salmonella typhimurium*. The results showed that compounds 1 and 2 (**Figure 27**) were antimutagenic [59].

Conflict of interest

The authors declare no conflict of interest.

Author details

Adel M. AbdelHakem* and El-Shimaa M.N. Abdelhafez
Faculty of Pharmacy, Department of Medicinal Chemistry, Minia University, Minia, Egypt

*Address all correspondence to: pharmacist_adel2010@yahoo.com

References

[1] Słoczyńska K, Powroźnik B, Pękala E, Waszkielewicz AM. Antimutagenic compounds and their possible mechanisms of action. Journal of Applied Genetics. 2014;**55**(2):273-285

[2] Gautam S, Saxena S, Kumar S. Fruits and vegetables as dietary sources of antimutagens. Journal of Food Chemistry and Nanotechnology. 2016; **2**(3):97-114

[3] Kada T, Inoue T, Namiki M. Environmental Mutagenesis and Plant Biology. In: Environmental desmutagens and antimutagens. New York: Praeger; 1981. pp. 134-151

[4] Bode AM, Dong Z. Cancer prevention research—Then and now. Nature Reviews Cancer. 2009;**9**(7):508

[5] Tian YF, Hsieh CH, Hsieh YJ, Chen YT, Peng YJ, Hsieh PS. α-Lipoic acid prevents mild portal endotoxaemia-induced hepatic inflammation and β cell dysfunction. European Journal of Clinical Investigation. 2012;**42**(6):637-648

[6] Unal F, Taner G, Yuzbasioglu D, Yilmaz S. Antigenotoxic effect of lipoic acid against mitomycin-C in human lymphocyte cultures. Cytotechnology. 2013;**65**(4):553-565

[7] Watanabe M, Kobayashi H, Ohta T. Rapid inactivation of 3-chloro-4-(dichloromethyl)-5-hydroxy-2 (5H)-furanone (MX), a potent mutagen in chlorinated drinking water, by sulfhydryl compounds. Mutation Research/Environmental Mutagenesis and Related Subjects. 1994;**312**(2): 131-138

[8] Marnewick JL, Gelderblom WC, Joubert E. An investigation on the antimutagenic properties of south African herbal teas. Mutation Research, Genetic Toxicology and Environmental Mutagenesis. 2000;**471**(1–2):157-166

[9] Ozturkcan SA, Turhan K, Turgut Z, Karadayi M, Gulluce M. Antigenotoxic properties of two newly synthesized β-aminoketones against N-methyl-N′-nitro-N-nitrosoguanidine and 9-aminoacridine-induced mutagenesis. Journal of Biochemical and Molecular Toxicology. 2012;**26**(7):258-263

[10] Şakiyan İ, Anar M, Öğütcü H, Agar G, Sarı N. Schiff bases attached L-glutamine and L-asparagine: First investigation on antimutagenic and antimicrobial analyses. Artificial cells, Nanomedicine, and Biotechnology. 2014;**42**(3):199-204

[11] Kakinuma K, Koike J, Kotani K, Ikekawa N, Kada T, Nomoto M. Cinnamaldehyde: Identification of an antimutagen from a crude drug, cinnamoni cortex. Agricultural and Biological Chemistry. 1984;**48**(7): 1905-1906

[12] Kakinuma K, Okada Y, Ikekawa N, Kada T, Nomoto M. Antimutagenic diterpenoids from a crude drug isodonis herba (Enmei-so). Agricultural and Biological Chemistry. 1984;**48**(6): 1647-1648

[13] Clarke CH, Shankel DM. Antimutagenesis in microbial systems. Bacteriological Reviews. 1975;**39**(1):33

[14] Zahin M, Ahmad I, Gupta RC, Aqil F. Punicalagin and ellagic acid demonstrate antimutagenic activity and inhibition of benzo [a] pyrene induced DNA adducts. BioMed Research International. 2014;**2014**:1-10

[15] Orhan F, Barış Ö, Yanmış D, Bal T, Güvenalp Z, Güllüce M. Isolation of some luteolin derivatives from *Mentha longifolia* (L.) Hudson subsp. longifolia and determination of their genotoxic potencies. Food Chemistry. 2012;**135**(2): 764-769

[16] Orhan F, Gulluce M, Ozkan H, Alpsoy L. Determination of the antigenotoxic potencies of some luteolin derivatives by using a eukaryotic cell system, *Saccharomyces cerevisiae*. Food Chemistry. 2013;**141**(1):366-372

[17] Vilar JB, Ferreira FL, Ferri PH, Guillo LA, Chen Chen L. Assessment of the mutagenic, antimutagenic and cytotoxic activities of ethanolic extract of araticum (*Annona crassiflora* Mart. 1841) by micronucleus test in mice. Brazilian Journal of Biology. 2008;**68**(1): 141-147

[18] Okuno Y, Marumoto S, Miyazawa M. Antimutagenic activity of flavonoids from Sozuku. Natural Product Research. 2019;**33**(6):862-865

[19] Manon L, Béatrice B, Thierry O, Jocelyne P, Fathi M, Evelyne O, et al. Antimutagenic potential of harpagoside and *Harpagophytum procumbens* against 1-nitropyrene. Pharmacognosy Magazine. 2015;**11**(Suppl 1):S29

[20] Rodríguez-Muñoz E, Herrera-Ruiz G, Pedraza-Aboytes G, Loarca-Piña G. Antioxidant capacity and antimutagenic activity of natural oleoresin from greenhouse grown tomatoes (*Lycopersicon esculentum*). Plant Foods for Human Nutrition. 2009;**64**(1):46-51

[21] Inami K, Mine Y, Tatsuzaki J, Mori C, Mochizuki M. Isolation and characterization of antimutagenic components of *Glycyrrhiza aspera* against N-methyl-N-nitrosourea. Genes and Environment. 2017;**39**(1):5

[22] Verma J, Gautam S. Antimutagenic potential of date palm (phoenix dactylifera) fruit aqueous extract in suppressing induced mutagenesis and purification of its bioactive constituent. MOJ Food Process Technol. 2016;**2**(5): 179-185

[23] Horn RC, Vargas VMF. Antimutagenic activity of extracts of natural substances in the *Salmonella*/ microsome assay. Mutagenesis. 2003; **18**(2):113-118

[24] Mushtaq M, Sultana B, Anwar F, Batool S. Antimutagenic and antioxidant potential of aqueous and acidified methanol extracts from *Citrus limonum* fruit residues. Journal of the Chilean Chemical Society. 2015;**60**(2):2979-2983

[25] Silva VA, Gonçalves GF, Pereira MS, Gomes IF, Freitas AF, Diniz MF, et al. Assessment of mutagenic, antimutagenic and genotoxicity effects of *Mimosa tenuiflora*. Revista Brasileira de Farmacognosia. 2013;**23**(2):329-334

[26] Hong C-E, Cho M-C, Jang H-A, Lyu S-Y. Mutagenicity and anti-mutagenicity of *Acanthopanax divaricatus* var. albeofructus. The Journal of Toxicological Sciences. 2011; **36**(5):661-668

[27] Del-Toro-Sánchez CL, Bautista-Bautista N, Blasco-Cabal JL, Gonzalez-Ávila M, Gutiérrez-Lomelí M, Arriaga-Alba M. Antimutagenicity of methanolic extracts from *Anemopsis californica* in relation to their antioxidant activity. Evidence-based Complementary and Alternative Medicine. 2014;**2014**:1-8

[28] Toscano-Garibay J, Arriaga-Alba M, Sánchez-Navarrete J, Mendoza-García M, Flores-Estrada J, Moreno-Eutimio M, et al. Antimutagenic and antioxidant activity of the essential oils of *Citrus sinensis* and *Citrus latifolia*. Scientific Reports. 2017;**7**(1):1-9

[29] Ruiz-Pérez NJ, Arriaga-Alba M, Sánchez-Navarrete J, Camacho-Carranza R, Hernández-Ojeda S, Espinosa-Aguirre JJ. Mutagenic and antimutagenic effects of *Heterotheca inuloides*. Scientific Reports. 2014;**4**: 6743

[30] Boubaker J, Mansour HB, Ghedira K, Chekir-Ghedira L. Antimutagenic and free radical

scavenger effects of leaf extracts from *Accacia salicina*. Annals of Clinical Microbiology and Antimicrobials. 2011; **10**(1):37

[31] Pesarini J, Zaninetti P, Mauro M, Carreira C, Dichi J, Ribeiro L, et al. Antimutagenic and anticarcinogenic effects of wheat bran in vivo. Genetics and Molecular Research. 2013;**12**: 1646-1659

[32] Satyendra G, Sudhanshu S, Sanjeev K. Fruits and vegetables as dietary sources of antimutagens. Journal of Food Chemistry and Nanotechnology. 2016;**2**(3):97-114

[33] Edenharder R, Kurz P, John K, Burgard S, Seeger K. In vitro effect of vegetable and fruit juices on the mutagenicity of 2-amino-3-methylimidazo [4, 5-f] quinoline, 2-amino-3, 4-dimethylimidazo [4, 5-f] quinoline and 2-amino-3, 8-dimethylimidazo [4, 5-f] quinoxaline. Food and Chemical Toxicology. 1994; **32**(5):443-459

[34] Saxena S, Verma J, Gautam S. Potential prophylactic properties of apple and characterization of potent bioactive from cv."granny smith" displaying strong antimutagenicity in models including human lymphoblast TK6+/− cell line. Journal of Food Science. 2016;**81**(2):H508-H518

[35] Batista ÂG, Ferrari AS, da Cunha DC, da Silva JK, Cazarin CBB, Correa LC, et al. Polyphenols, antioxidants, and antimutagenic effects of *Copaifera langsdorffii* fruit. Food Chemistry. 2016;**197**:1153-1159

[36] Lee H-R, Lim H-B. Antimutagenic and antioxidative effects of polysaccharides isolated from the water extract of *Ganoderma lucidum*. Journal of Applied Pharmaceutical Science. 2019;**9**(04):001-007

[37] Ajith T, Janardhanan K. Antimutagenic effect of Phellinus rimosus (Berk) Pilat against chemical induced mutations of histidine dependent *Salmonella typhimurium* strains. Food and Chemical Toxicology. 2011;**49**(10):2676-2680

[38] Słoczyńska K, Pańczyk K, Waszkielewicz AM, Marona H, Pękala E. In vitro mutagenic, antimutagenic, and antioxidant activities evaluation and biotransformation of some bioactive 4-substituted 1-(2-methoxyphenyl) piperazine derivatives. Journal of Biochemical and Molecular Toxicology. 2016;**30**(12):593-601

[39] Wilpart M, Speder A, Ninane P, Roberfroid M. Antimutagenic effects of natural and synthetic hormonal steroids. Teratogenesis, Carcinogenesis, and Mutagenesis. 1986;**6**(4):265-273

[40] Gao C, Chang P, Yang L, Wang Y, Zhu S, Shan H, et al. Neuroprotective effects of hydrogen sulfide on sodium azide-induced oxidative stress in PC12 cells. International Journal of Molecular Medicine. 2018;**41**(1):242-250

[41] Shan H, Chu Y, Chang P, Yang L, Wang Y, Zhu S, et al. Neuroprotective effects of hydrogen sulfide on sodium azide-induced autophagic cell death in PC12 cells. Molecular Medicine Reports. 2017;**16**(5):5938-5946

[42] Sasaki Y, Matsumoto K, Imanishi H, Watanabe M, Ohta T, Shirasu Y, et al. In vivo anticlastogenic and antimutagenic effects of tannic acid in mice. Mutation Research Letters. 1990;**244**(1):43-47

[43] Gulluce M, Agar G, Baris O, Karadayi M, Orhan F, Sahin F. Mutagenic and antimutagenic effects of hexane extract of some Astragalus species grown in the eastern Anatolia region of Turkey. Phytotherapy Research. 2010;**24**(7):1014-1018

[44] De Flora S, Izzotti A, D'Agostini F, Balansky RM, Noonan D, Albini A.

Multiple points of intervention in the prevention of cancer and other mutation-related diseases. Mutation Research, Fundamental and Molecular Mechanisms of Mutagenesis. 2001;**480**: 9-22

[45] Koçer S, Uruş S, Çakır A, Güllüce M, Dığrak M, Alan Y, et al. The synthesis, characterization, antimicrobial and antimutagenic activities of hydroxyphenylimino ligands and their metal complexes of usnic acid isolated from *Usnea longissima*. Dalton Transactions. 2014; **43**(16):6148-6164

[46] Nartop D, Demirel B, Güleç M, Hasanoğlu Özkan E, Kurnaz Yetim N, Sarı N, et al. Novel polymeric microspheres: Synthesis, enzyme immobilization, antimutagenic activity, and antimicrobial evaluation against pathogenic microorganisms. Journal of Biochemical and Molecular Toxicology. 2019;**34**:e22432

[47] Alexandrova V, Obukhova G, Topchiev D. Synthesis and antimutagenic properties of novel systems based on poly (quaternized ammonium) salts. Journal of Bioactive and Compatible Polymers. 2002;**17**(5): 321-341

[48] Giziroglua E, Sarikurkcub C, Saracc N. Synthesis and characterization of novel Hydrazone based anti-mutagenic and Antioxidative agents. Journal of Applied Pharmaceutical Science. 2015;**5**(3):048-055

[49] De Oliveira APS, De Sousa JF, Da Silva MA, Hilário F, Resende FA, De Camargo MS, et al. Estrogenic and chemopreventive activities of xanthones and flavones of *Syngonanthus* (Eriocaulaceae). Steroids. 2013;**78**(11): 1053-1063

[50] Nartop D, Özkan EH, Gündem M, Çeker S, Ağar G, Öğütcü H, et al. Synthesis, antimicrobial and antimutagenic effects of novel polymeric-Schiff bases including indol. Journal of Molecular Structure. 2019; **1195**:877-882

[51] Olejníková P, Birošová L, Lu Š, Vihonská Z, Fiedlerová M, Marchalín Š, et al. Newly synthesized indolizine derivatives—Antimicrobial and antimutagenic properties. Chemical Papers. 2015;**69**(7):983-992

[52] Roy SS, Chakraborty P, Ghosh P, Ghosh S, Biswas J, Bhattacharya S. Influence of novel naphthalimide-based organoselenium on genotoxicity induced by an alkylating agent: The role of reactive oxygen species and selenoenzymes. Redox Report. 2012; **17**(4):157-166

[53] Zhang J, Tian Q, Yung Chan S, Chuen Li S, Zhou S, Duan W, et al. Metabolism and transport of oxazaphosphorines and the clinical implications. Drug Metabolism Reviews. 2005;**37**(4):611-703

[54] El-Sayed WM, Hussin WA, Al-Faiyz YS, Ismail MA. The position of imidazopyridine and metabolic activation are pivotal factors in the antimutagenic activity of novel imidazo [1, 2-a] pyridine derivatives. European Journal of Pharmacology. 2013;**715**(1–3): 212-218

[55] Collins AR, Azqueta A, Langie SA. Effects of micronutrients on DNA repair. European Journal of Nutrition. 2012;**51**(3):261-279

[56] Kumar SS, Negi P, Manjunatha J, Bettadaiah B. Synthesis, antibacterial and antimutagenic activity of zerumbone-bicarbonyl analogues. Food Chemistry. 2017;**221**:576-581

[57] Leonova E, Rostoka E, Sauvaigo S, Baumane L, Selga T, Sjakste N. Study of interaction of antimutagenic 1, 4-dihydropyridine AV-153-Na with DNA-damaging molecules and its impact on

DNA repair activity. PeerJ. 2018;**6**: e4609

[58] Maslat A, Khalil A, Fares A, Tashtoush H, El-Talib M. A notable antimutagenicity of two nonmutagenic novel oxadiazoles in *Salmonella* mutagenicity assay. Drug and Chemical Toxicology. 2005;**27**(2):157-167

[59] Ashram M, Maslat A, Mizyed S. Synthesis and biological activities of new azacrown ether Schiff bases and spectrophotometric studies of their complexation with [60] fullerene. Toxicological and Environmental Chemistry. 2009;**91**(6):1095-1104

For EU product safety concerns:
IN TECH d.o.o., Prolaz Marije Krucifikse Kozulić 3, 51000 Rijeka, Croatia,
info@intechopen.com or visit our website at intechopen.com.

Meet the editor

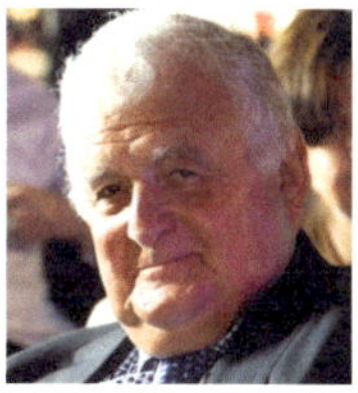

Dr. Jones has been MD of a successful consultancy since 2004. In addition to industrial contacts, he maintains strong academic links with universities in the United Kingdom and internationally and has been appointed external examiner for several Ph.D. and MSc examinations. His extensive list of professional publications includes many technical contributions to the Hydrotransport and Transport and Sedimentation conferences. He takes an active committee role in both organisations. He studied at the University of London. Following an MSc in Thermal Power Engineering and a Ph.D. research degree, Dr. Jones joined the Mining Research and Development Establishment of the National Coal Board. He became a team manager where he led high-value European-funded research projects on the control and management of coal quality, the analysis of coal profiles, and the control of froth-flotation processes. After the closure of British Coal, Dr. Jones became a senior research fellow at the University of Nottingham. He secured research funding for the university with collaborations from Germany, Greece, Belgium, and Holland.

Contents

Preface

Slurries are unusual mixtures. They adopt characteristics quite different from the bulk of solid particles carried with them or the liquids in which they are suspended or partially suspended. They range from mixtures with very fine particles to those with coarse particles such as sand and gravel.

This book is an important collection of technical information on slurry technology. Chapters cover such topics as high-concentration conveying, vertical transport of fine particle slurries, rheology of sludges, pipe wear, and wastewater applications. It begins with an introductory chapter by the editor that summarizes important advances in slurry technology and ends with a chapter on fluidisation.

Slurries are fascinating mixtures that have at least two major manifestations: settling and non-settling. Both types suffer from holdup, a measure of delayed and retained solids in a pipeflow, but the process of modelling it for the two is different. Chapter 2 by the editor models the phenomenon of holdup of settling media in horizontal ducts. It describes the important distinction between in situ concentration and delivered or efflux concentration and its implications. In situ concentration is always greater than efflux concentration because of settling, so there must be a gradation in axial velocity to satisfy the demands of the continuity equation. The two-layer model by Professor K.C. Wilson, invented more than 50 years ago at the time of this writing, simplifies this gradation into two layers: a suspension layer supported by hydrodynamic forces only, and a settling layer gaining additional support from pipe walls and hindered settling.

Vertical ducting is at least as important as horizontal ducting. In Chapter 3, Professor Bartosik presents a study of solid–liquid turbulent pipeflow in a vertical conduit and the mathematical model that it supports. The model centres around an empirical equation for the standard turbulence damping function, which is a factor in the computation of the turbulent viscosity. In its original form, it is a function of turbulent Reynolds number only. The author proposes a modification of the factor to account for variations in particle diameter and volumetric concentration, supported very clearly by experimental evidence. The author is at pains to state that the results apply to specific particle populations and vertical flow but leaves us in no doubt that particle diameter plays an important part in predicting frictional head loss as does solid concentration in a secondary role.

In Chapter 4, Dr. Pullum explains that the upper limit of concentrations for slurries is conventionally limited to 40% (volume/volume) to minimise risks of pipe blockage and restarting difficulties. In pneumatic transport, no such limit applies, and this underlies the motive, perhaps the credo, to extend the concentration range for slurries. The journey is by no means simple because slurries can be very complex mixtures, but the author explains in careful detail how high-concentration hydraulic conveying of coarse particles can be achieved. Inevitable increases in operating costs and specialised equipment to separate coarse and fine are set against lower pumping power requirements and reduced wear.

There is a resonance between Dr. Pullum's chapter and that of Dr. Arno Talmon and his co-author Ebi Meshtaki in Chapter 5 on wall slip in harbour muds. Dr. Talmon covers the very interesting phenomenon of wall slip in rheometry applied to slurries and sludges. Rheometry measures the viscosity of a medium using a variety of techniques. If a vane and cup technique is applied, no wall slip occurs. If a bob-in-cup method is used, shear stress at the wall is sensibly constant for an initial application of shear strain before rising as further strain is applied. The concept has wide implications beyond the laboratory and Dr. Talmon presents results applied to harbour walls and sea defences.

Particle size and the grading of particle sizes are important factors in transporting slurry media. Broadly graded mixtures reduce energy loss due to friction in both horizontal and inclined flows. Ascending and descending flows show predictably different results for hydraulic grading (the rate of pressure loss with downstream distance). Stratification (the selective classification of particles based on size) is an important factor in this difference. In Chapter 6, Professor Matoušek and his co-authors Zdeněk Chára and Jiři Konfršt present a wealth of data on pipe inclination and particle size.

Visualisation of the contents of a slurry duct has informed much of the research into flows of varying concentration distribution. At its simplest level, flow can be passed through transparent sections of pipe and photographed laterally. Penetration of the cross-section can be achieved by a variety of techniques including gamma-ray interrogation, particle image velocimetry, laser Doppler anemometry, and electrical impedance tomography. For some investigations computed tomography, including magnetic resonance tomography, has been borrowed from medical colleagues. A particularly useful technique has been electrical resistance tomography (ERT). Electrodes are positioned around the duct and the resistance experienced by an injected current is used to construct a grid of concentration measurements. ERT can be deployed even when the liquid phase is opaque. In Chapter 7, Dr. Lachlan Graham presents details of the basic theory of ERT and describes the difficult problem of image reconstruction.

Pipe wear is an inevitable consequence of transporting particle-laden liquids. Wear presents a huge cost to industries worldwide and has attracted research to measure, model, and hopefully reduce it. In Chapter 8, Professor Wood and his co-author Alexander Cook explain the research efforts directed at the problem. Computational Fluid Dynamics (CFD) is used to model the flow field with a mesh and to solve the conservation equations (mass, momentum, and energy) at the nodes and spaces. On paper, this technique holds great promise for the future of wear studies, but despite improved particle impact modelling, particle tracking, and dynamically deforming geometry, erosion predictions have so far been disappointing. The Moving Deforming Mesh technique has demonstrated great promise, however. The idea is to update the computational mesh at regular intervals based on local erosion rates and the geometry of the containing walls. In this way, erosive deformations are integrated into the flow field and secondary erosion patterns can be predicted. Pipe layout and internal finish have a great influence on the life of vulnerable components. Professor Wood opines that minor melioration in this area could be influential in increasing component lifetimes.

Sludges and slurries must be dewatered for good practical reasons. In some locations, reclamation of the water they contain is very important to a local community. Municipal sludge must be reduced in volume before transportation and dewatering is a good way to achieve this. The removal of water is also important in improving the calorific value if the waste is to be incinerated. The discharges of wet sludges and slurries can damage the quality of inland waterways. Dewatering can also prevent the release of harmful leachates.

In warm countries, lagoons can be employed to evaporate the water content. If this natural advantage is limited or unavailable, large plate presses can be employed to reduce the moisture content of sludge to cakes of concentrations of about 20% volume/volume. Plate press installations are costly to build and equip, but the running costs are relatively low. An alternative to plate presses are belt filter presses, which are less expensive to install but with relatively high running costs due to the additives that are needed. Professor Fester and her co-author Rössie Werner explain the issues in Chapter 9.

Finally, Chapter 10 covers an important application of slurry flow principles. The use of slurry-bed reactors can be traced back to the Second World War when they were used in the synthesis of oil. Professor Fanhui Meng and his co-author Muhammad Asif Nawaz compare three types of reactors: the mechanically stirred slurry reactor, the bubble column reactor and, the three-phase fluidised bed reactor.

Dr. Trevor Frank Jones
TFJ Consulting Ltd.,
Derby, United Kingdom

Section 1

Introduction

Chapter 1

Introductory Chapter: Slurry Technology – New Advances

Trevor Frank Jones

1. Introduction

Mixtures of particles and liquids are often considered to be *slurries*, but this is not always an accurate description. A gravel extraction might comprise large pebbles in the water, but the solid and liquid components would have distinctly independent behavior (**Figure 1**). A *slurry* has its own character quite different from carrying liquids or entrained bulk solids. The term covers a wide range of mixtures from "non-settling" slurries, usually of very fine particles, to slurry fluidized beds[1].

Before we can study these intriguing mixtures, we must briefly discuss their *settling* propensity. The distinction between *settling* slurries and others is not precise. All particles in a liquid have a gravitational potential however minute that potential might be. A settling rate of 0.6 mm/s has been suggested as the upper limit for a "non-settling slurry", but this is might be considered a little over-prescriptive. If a fine particle slurry can be shown to be effectively a non-settling continuum for a specific application, deposition concerns can be largely ignored and many offline and online measurements carried out. However, many industrial slurries have a settling component, and practitioners are finding new ways to face the challenge of handling them.

When studying the flow of a slurry, frictional headloss and pipe velocity are most important not least because they have a direct bearing on the requirements for a suitable pump. The orientation of the pipe run (horizontal, vertical, or graded) is another major factor. Determination of deposition patterns in horizontal pipelines is a non-trivial task while rising mains have axially symmetric velocity distributions but increased pressure drops. Lastly, the design concentration of the slurry or sludge has a pivotal influence on the choice of pumping system.

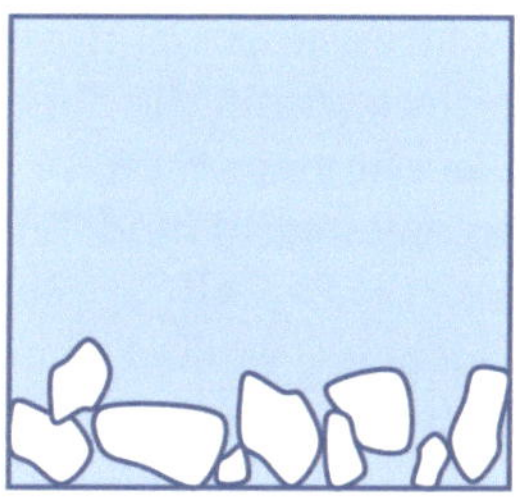

Figure 1.
Solid-liquid mixtures are not always slurries.

[1] Slurry fluidized beds are gas–liquid–solid mixtures often given a category of their own. They have specialized industrial uses, for example in the synthesis of methane.

2. Horizontal slurry ducts

Workers in the 1950s, following an influential study by Durand & Condiolis [1], identified *regimes* for the flow of slurries in horizontal ducts. Categories included a classification by size, but inter-relationships with pipe velocities, particularly those for deposition added a layer of complication in identifying the flow regime. Subsequently four regimes were proposed, based on increasing axial pipe velocity (other factors having been defined):

1. Flow with a stationary bed ($0 < U \leq \boldsymbol{U}_{M1}$).

2. Flow with a moving bed ($\boldsymbol{U}_{M1} < U \leq \boldsymbol{U}_{M2}$).

3. *Heterogeneous* flow with *saltation* heaps. As velocity progresses, these saltation heaps erode and move downstream with a rolling action. At the higher end of this velocity interval, all the solids are in *asymmetric* suspension ($\boldsymbol{U}_{M2} < U \leq \boldsymbol{U}_{M3}$).

4. *Pseudo-homogeneous* mixtures in which all particles are in suspension follow in sequence from the *heterogeneous* pattern ($U > \boldsymbol{U}_{M3}$). Ultimately all the solids are in a *symmetric* suspension and this can be termed a *homogeneous* mixture. Note that many researchers use the terms "pseudo-homogeneous" and "homogeneous" interchangeably.

It is not always straightforward to identify visually the flow regime of a particular slurry against the list of velocity categories alone. An interesting, if rather controversial, approach to this problem was proposed by Turian and Yuen [2] who proposed coefficients based on friction factor, efflux concentration, pipe diameter, and relative density of solid particles in addition to pipe velocity. These coefficients were to be used to choose the regime (0...3). A critical evaluation of the Turian and Yuen method is given by Mediema [3]. The incorporation of slurry flow variables, in addition to pipe velocity, underlines the over-simplification implied by the list, but the convenient four-fold categorization by velocity remains in common use.

Homogeneity in flowing slurries is aided by turbulence. At a small scale, the flow might be extremely complex, but particles are spread by strong mixing actions. At high velocities, concentration profiles across the duct are sensibly uniform. Conversely, non-settling fines in high concentration can be in *laminar flow*. When the mixture is very well mixed prior to transmission, the medium is confined to streamlines and very little mixing takes place within the duct.

When a slurry can be treated as a homogeneous or pseudo-homogeneous liquid, continuum techniques (including rheological modeling) can be applied to the flow as a whole. Strictly, these methods are not really applicable to other regimes, but that does not always prevent them from being applied.

In the discussion above, particle concentration has only briefly been mentioned as an important factor. The transportation of slurry flows in turbulent flow has usually been constrained by a 40% *v/v* limit. The reasons for this limit are in the fear of pipe blockage if greater concentrations are used. Interestingly, much greater concentrations are possible at the cost of improved infrastructure as authors will explore in later pages.

3. Vertical slurry ducts

The flow of slurry in a rising main brings a number of specific challenges. As already mentioned, the most obvious is the increased pressure that the pump must provide in addition to the frictional losses from the pipe wall. The weight in a rising main comes from the density of the slurry being pumped and this changes with elevation. The first task is therefore to establish the density of the slurry in the duct.

The *in situ* concentration, the concentration across a section of duct, yields the density of the slurry at that section. The *in situ* concentration (C_r) should not be confused with the concentration supplied to, or delivered from, the duct (C_v). *Holdup*, the ratio of the relative velocity of the solids to the pipe velocity governs the *in situ* concentration, and this determines the mean density. Holdup is defined here as

$$\mathcal{H} = \frac{U - U_s}{U} = 1 - \frac{C_v}{C_r} \tag{1}$$

where U_s is the velocity of the solids component, and U is the pipe velocity.

Engineers usually have knowledge of the efflux or delivered concentration required (C_v) for an application, but holdup and *in situ* concentrations (C_r) are not generally known at the outset. An *Artificial Neural Network (ANN)* developed by Lahiri and Ghanta [4] is claimed to predict holdup with an absolute average accuracy of 2.5%. The value can be used to determine the mean *in situ* concentration and the appropriate density. Their definition of holdup ($\frac{C_r}{C_v}$) is algebraically linked to the definition given above, but can exaggerate the accuracy obtained, particularly for high values of holdup.

Vertical rising mains are found in many situations. They assume great importance in the mining industry both historically and in present day operations. Interesting, examples of interest to researchers in coarse particle slurry technology are deep-ocean mining and the extraction of coal-water mixtures from depth.

4. Low pipe velocities and non-homogeneous mixtures

At the low to medium pipe velocities found in industrial processes and pipelines, particle concentrations usually vary across a section. We recall the reluctance to pump a slurry of greater efflux concentration than 40% *v/v* for fear of blockages. For horizontal pipe runs, dense regions accumulate at the lower pipe wall as we have already discussed. Despite these difficulties, it is an economic proposition to reduce pipe velocity for at least two reasons:

1. Pumping power is approximately proportional to the cube of pipe velocity. If one can halve pipe velocity, energy consumed in pumping the slurry will be reduced by 87.5% in theory.

2. Pipe wear (per tonne) is approximately proportional to velocity to the power of 2.5. This implies a reduction in wear of approximately 82% for a halving of pipe velocity.

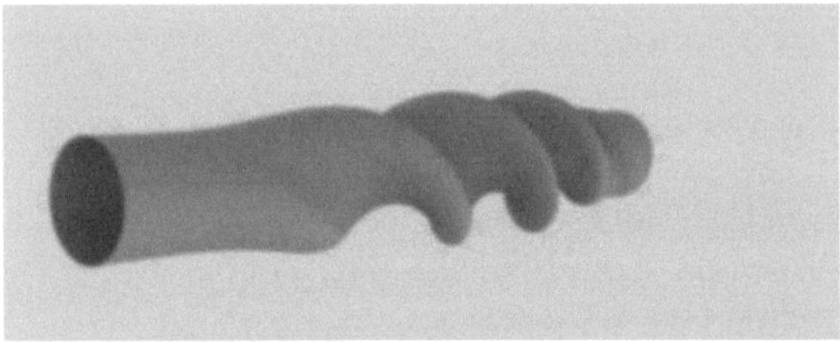

Figure 2.
Swirl-inducing duct. Two-lobe, a low-loss design (illustrated). Four–lobe, for a greater swirl intensity.

These factors have encouraged the development of *swirl-inducing* ducts (**Figure 2**). If sediment from a low to medium-concentration slurry can be swept into suspension at a low velocity, there will be savings in power consumption and pipe wear, not to mention the prevention of pipe blockages. The interested reader is encouraged to visit various contributions to the subject (*e.g.,* Jones [5]).

High-concentration conveying offers an alternative way to exploit the benefits of low pipe velocity as explained in later pages of this volume. An example can be found in the pumping of liquid concrete. This material is a mixture of several particulate elements of widely differing sizes. Utilizing specialized pumping equipment, liquid concrete can be pumped at high concentrations and low velocity. Coarse particles cannot pack at the pipe wall, so a particle-depleted layer exists there. This is sometimes given the rather misleading term: the "lubricating layer" [6].

Broad size distribution in the material to be pumped is an important pre-requisite for pumping at high concentrations in a Newtonian fluid, such as water. There is a very inventive way around this stipulation. Some of the particulate materials can be ground to make a non-settling *visco-plastic* carrier, and the rest of the material can be carried within it. Essentially, at low velocity, the carrier is in *laminar* flow. Machines to create this carrier and to separate coarse particles add to plant costs. Dense-phase horizontal coarse particle transportation for coal slurries became available when a Rotary Ram Slurry Pump (RRSP) was invented [7]. To the incredulity of plant engineers, high-concentration slurries were not required to exceed a minimum velocity and could be stopped and restarted at will.

There are empirical methods to determine headloss in non-homogeneous slurries, but an alternative is a *two-layer model* invented by Wilson [8, 9]. Shook and Roco [10] presented the model "... in a form which should be easier to follow or modify." Over the years, modifications were needed to improve stability and usability of the model, and a completely new interpretation (*2LM*) is now available. The essence of the model is the simplification of the non-homogeneous flow of slurry into two layers. The upper layer represents a component completely supported by hydrodynamic forces, and the lower layer is a component gaining support from pipe walls and hindered settling. This is a severe oversimplification in some eyes, but very good estimates can be obtained.

Designers rely on an estimate of the *critical deposit velocity,* which is the velocity at which a single particle, or perhaps a raft of several particles, will rest immobile at the base of a horizontal pipe. The roughness of the particle surface is greater than that of the pipe alone and this encourages greater accumulations of particles. These particles accumulate into dune-like *saltation heaps*. The curvature of streamlines around the tops of the heaps has an erosive action on the upper particles, which causes a downstream rolling action. This low-velocity downstream motion of dunes characterizes *heterogeneous* flow, but it can be overwhelmed, ultimately causing a pipe blockage. Hence, a fundamental design requirement is to apply a pipe velocity greater than the deposition velocity. The *2LM* model estimates the pipe velocity for a stationary bed. This velocity is not identical to the critical deposit velocity because the stationary bed is not necessarily a single layer of particles but the differences in estimates are relatively unimportant.

5. Instrumentation and measurement of slurry flows

Slurries are fundamental *mixtures,* and this lies at the heart of problems in making useful measurements. Designers have little choice but to use historical empirical evidence often based on examples of differing flow regimes and differing circumstances. It is encouraging to note how successful these designs have been in the hands of experienced practitioners.

Size distributions of industrial slurries can often be broad, non-symmetrical, or perhaps multimodal. Similarly, distracting is the spread of property values in a particle population. This is particularly true of coal slurries in which constituents can have hydrophilic (easily wetted) or hydrophobic (resisting wetting) tendencies and a broad spread of density. The particles themselves can differ markedly in solid geometry from spherical models from which many theoretical predictions have been built.

Setting aside difficulties in accurate prediction, the situation is not entirely bleak. Great progress has been made in online measurements of slurry flows. Radiometric methods have been used to measure the physical properties of a slurry flow. The same methods, at a higher energy level, can indicate the concentration of a flow by interrogating the transmission of the radiometric beam across it. Most interesting of all is visualization technologies which can give us concentration and distribution mapping. These include *Particle Image Velocimetry* (PIV), *Laser Doppler Anemometry* (LDA), and *Tomographic* techniques [11]. Electrical Resistance Tomography stems from early work in the 1930s and 1940s [12], before computational methods opened it up to widespread use. Electrical Capacitance Tomography used to form computed images of pipe contents was investigated from the 1980s [13]. The techniques involve the measurement of electrical properties of the slurry from the pipe periphery. The difficult job has been to reconstruct the interior structure from the measurements obtained—"The Reconstruction Problem."

6. Pipe wear

An unavoidable consequence of flows containing particles is wear. Enormous costs to industry are attributable to wear, but costs can be reduced by careful design. Since 2017, many advances have been made in the study of erosion-corrosion in experimental and *in-situ* monitoring of wear, condition monitoring, the monitoring of wall erosion and computational modeling to name but three.

Designers of slurry systems will often reach for answers from Computational Fluid Dynamics (CFD). There is certainly a promising future for CFD erosion modeling, but that advance is not yet with us. Despite improved particle impact modeling, dynamically deforming geometry and improved particle tracking, the accuracy of erosion predictions is poor. There is hope of improvement from two comparatively new approaches explored by authors in this volume. The Discrete Phase Model (DPM) plots the path of a group of dynamically similar particles through a continuous liquid, while the Discrete Element Model (DEM) tracks individual particles and solves the equations of motion as they interact with each other. In theory, the accuracy of the DPM approach can therefore be improved by a coupling with DEM. A CFD-DPM-DEM combination has been used to model air-particle flows, but no attempt at extending the technique to solid-liquid flows has been reported to date. There is great potential for this combination but a disincentive to its development is the very large computational cost that would be incurred. One of the most significant improvements in the application of CFD is the Moving-Deforming-Mesh (MDM) approach. The computational mesh is updated at regular intervals based on local erosion rate and the geometry of the wall. In this way erosive deformations are integrated into the flow field and secondary erosion patterns can be predicted.

Very little research has been carried out on the influence of pipe layout. on the life of vulnerable components. Pipe geometry upstream of a vulnerable pipe section can have a significant effect on erosion rates. For example, the swirl pipe design described above can show significant wear reductions in adjacent downstream pipe components. Unsurprisingly internal surface finish (particularly in pipe elbows) has a disproportionate effect on the erosion pattern suffered in service. Comparatively minor melioration in this area could be influential in increasing component lifetimes.

7. Sludges, Slurries and Wastewater

The problem of movement, transportation, and *handleability* of slurries and sludges is a major preoccupation for many industries. Their causes are many and various. The character of the particulates, particularly clays, and their size distribution have an important influence. Moisture has a complex relationship with handleability: too much and a slurry must be contained, too little and a sludge can be sticky and difficult to move. The study of flow problems from hoppers has a long history [14] and since the 1950s it has gathered pace as a subject of interest to industry and academia. The Jenike Cell [15–17] was devised to measure the shear forces in particulate materials.

Industrial slurries are generally thickened to a sludge of water content of about 25% *v/v*. The applied stress at which a sludge distorts or moves is termed the *yield stress*. A shear vane tester (**Figure 3**) is a widely-used and readily-available device for measurements of shear stress in cohesive sludges [18]. The vanes are distributed in a cruciform shape around a spindle which can be rotated. Immersed in a sludge the

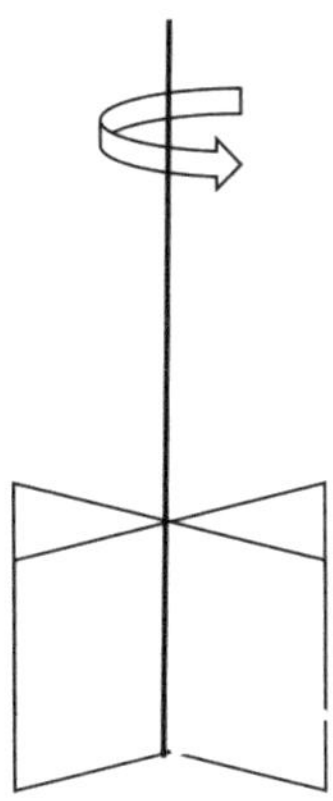

Figure 3.
Vane Tester.

spindle is rotated at between 5 and 12 degrees per minute until the sludge fails and the vane rotates in equilibrium with the RSS or "Residual Shear Stress" [19]. The insertion of the vanes, and the rotation of them, has been suspected of changing the structure of a sludge and causing inaccuracies in measurement [20–22]. The controversy stems from the observation of viscous deformation before the yield point [23, 24]. This "wall slip" phenomenon is fairly important in geo-structures (harbor walls for example) and is not shown by vane tests. Wall slip is explored in later pages of this volume.

Despite controversies over certain critical measurements, the vane tester continues to be the measurement of choice for the shear strength and handleability of sludges.

Dewatering in municipal wastewater treatment is an important field of study. Some reasons for sludge dewatering are as follows.

1. Reclamation of water.

2. The reduction of volume of municipal sludge. The cost of transportation is a large recurring cost for municipal budgets.

3. Reduction of harmful leachate emissions.

4. Creation of a friable product which can be used in agriculture.

5. Production of a calorific product for energy production. Moisture lowers the calorific value of a fuel by virtue of the energy required to evaporate the liquid component.

6. Limiting of damage to the natural environment, including the control of discharges into inland waterways.

Dewatering can be carried out in many ways, for example, in warm countries lagoons can allow the sun to evaporate the water content. Periodically, industrial machines can then be employed to carry off the dried sediment. Large plate presses can be employed to reduce the moisture content of sludge to cakes of concentrations of about 20% *v/v*. Plate press installations are costly to build and equip, but the running costs are relatively low. An alternative to plate presses are belt filter presses which are less expensive to install, but with relatively high running costs due to the additives which are needed [25].

Author details

Trevor Frank Jones
TFJ Consulting Ltd., UK

*Address all correspondence to: info@tfjconsulting.com

References

[1] Durand R, Condiolis E. Experimental Study of the Hydraulic Transport of Coal and Solid materials in Pipes. In: Proceedings of the Colloquium on the Hydraulic Transport of Coal, National Coal Board. UK: Paper IV; 1952. pp. 39-55

[2] Turian RM, Yuen TF. Flow of Slurries in Pipelines. AICHE Journal. 1977;**23**:232-243

[3] Mediema SA. Slurry Transport. TU Delft Open Textbooks, Libre Text Libraries, UC Davis Library, California State University; 2020

[4] Lahiri SK, Ghanta KC. Development of an artificial network correlation for prediction of hold-up of slurry transport in pipelines. Chemical Engineering Science. 2008;**63**(2008):1497-1509

[5] Jones TF. In: Boushaki T, editor. Swirl-inducing Ducts, Swirling Flows and Flames. London, UK, London, UK, Chapter 5: InTechOpen; 2019. pp. 77-95

[6] Chen L, Liu G, Cheng W, Gang P. Pipe flow of pumping wet shotcrete based on lubrication layer. Springerplus. 2016;**5**:945

[7] Boyle BA. Rotating barrel pump. US Patent 3999895. Alexandria, Virginia, USA: United States Patent and Trademark Office (USPTO); 1975

[8] Wilson KC. Slip point of beds in solid-liquid pipeline flow. Proceedings ASCE Journal of Hydraulics Division. 1970;**96**:1-12

[9] Wilson KC. A unified physically-based analysis of solid-liquid pipeline flow. In: Proc Hydrotransport 4 Conference BHRA, Cranfield, UK, Paper A1. 1976. pp. 1-12

[10] Shook CA, Roco MC. Slurry Flow – Principles and Practice. Butterworth Heinnemann; 1991. pp. 119-133 and Appendix 4. pp. 285-290

[11] Beck MS, Williams RA. Process Tomography – Principles, Techniques and Applications. Oxford: Butterworth Heinnemann; 2012

[12] Tikhonov AN. О единственности решения задачи электроразведки. Doklady Akademii Nauk SSSR (in Russian) [About the uniqueness of solving the problem of electrical exploration.]. 1949;**69**(6):797-800

[13] Beck MS, Byars M, Dyakowski T, Waterfall R, He R, Wang SJ, et al. Principles and industrial applications of electrical capacitance tomography. Measurement and Control. 1997;**30**(7):197-200

[14] Jansson JA. Versuche über Getreidedruck in Silozellen. [Tests on grain pressure in silo cells.]. Zeitschrift des Vereines Deutscher Ingenieure. 1895;**35**:1045-1049

[15] Jenike AW. Gravity Flow of bulk solids. In: Engineering Experiment Station. USA: University of Utah; 1961. Bulletin 108

[16] Jenike AW. Storage and Flow of Bulk Solids. In: Engineering Experiment Station. USA: University of Utah; 1964. Bulletin 123

[17] Jenike AW. New developments in the theory of particulate solids flow, Proceedings: reliable flow of particulate solids. European Federation of Chemical Engineers. 1985;**49**:122-131

[18] Cadling L, Odenstad S. The Vane Borer, an apparatus for determining the shear strength of clay soils directly in

the ground. In: Proceedings of the Royal Swedish Geotechnical Institute. Vol. 2. Stockholm. 1950

[19] Meshtaki E, Talmon A, Luger D, Bezujen A. Rheology of Clay-Rich Soft Sediments: From Fluid to Geo-Mechanics, Central Dredging Association, CEDA Dredging Days 2021. Delft, The Netherlands: CEDA Secretariat, Radex Innovation Center; 2021

[20] Cerato AB, Lutenegger AJ. Disturbance effects of field vane tests in a varved clay. Geotechnical and Geophysical Site Characterizationzation. 2004. Vol. 1 and 2. p. 613. https://scholarworks.umass.edu/cee_faculty_pubs/613

[21] Sharifounnasab M, Ullrich CR. Rate of shear effects on vane shear strength. Journal of Geotechnical Engineering. 1985;**111**(1):135-139

[22] Skempton AW. Vane tests in the alluvial plain of the River Forth near Grangemouth. Geotechnique. 1948, 1948;**1**(2):111-124

[23] Barnes HA. A review of the slip (wall depletion) of polymer solutions, emulsions, and particle suspensions: its cause, character and cure. Journal of Non-Newtonian Fluid Mechanics. 1995;**56**:221-251

[24] Cloitre M, Bonnecaze RA. A review on wall slip in high dispersions. Rheologica Acta, Springer Verlag. 2017;**56**(3):283-305

[25] Brown DW. Personal Communication. 2022

Section 2

Process Modelling of Slurry Systems

Chapter 2

Solid-Liquid Pipeflows – Holdup and the Two-Layer Model

Trevor Frank Jones

Abstract

The relative delay of the flow of solids in a pipe, *holdup*, is shown to be an important factor in the evaluation of the flow of settling particle-bearing liquids. Holdup can be determined using a new, modified interpretation of the *two-layer model*, originally published in the 1970s. In the original model, particles in the upper layer of the flow are supported by hydrodynamic forces only, while those in the lower layer are also supported by hindered settling and wall reactions. This concept has been retained in the new model. An initial approximated value of holdup can be refined to allow an increasingly accurate value to be calculated. Innovative coding of the new model overcomes instability and interface positioning problems. Applications for determinations of holdup and the model are examined. Pressure loss, flow rate and the prediction of the pipe velocity to avoid a stationary bed are established. The model allows a locus of stationary bed conditions to be plotted for a family of holdup values. A method to obtain the *centre of concentration* in the cross section is demonstrated. The *locus of centre of concentration (LCC)* gives an indication of the position and size of the particle burden as conditions change.

Keywords: solid-liquid pipe flow, two-layer model, holdup, stationary bed locus, center of concentration

1. Introduction

R.A. Bagnold [1] identified two distinct mechanisms of particle support: fluid suspension and intergranular contact, in his studies of desert sand in Egypt. It was Professor K.C. Wilson [2, 3] who proposed the application to particle-bearing liquids in pipes, i.e., an upper fluid suspension and a lower layer taking support from hindered settling and the pipe walls: the *Two-Layer Model*. This is a gross simplification in some eyes, but a great help in identifying the velocity and magnitude of the stratified burden. **Figure 1** shows a typical concentration map for a liquid with settling particles obtained by *electrical resistance tomography* (*ERT*) for low-velocity pipe flow (0.75 m/s). Interestingly, the supernatant phase (in pale blue) has not stacked itself in height order but has spread around the boundaries of the other pipe contents—actually emphasising the interface between two layers. The two-layer model was later modified for computer modelling by Professor C.A. Shook [4]. Shook proposed a *contact load* within an all-pervading suspension fraction.

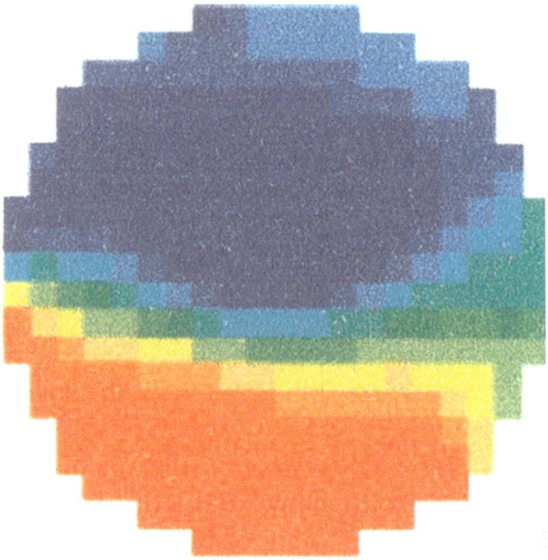

Figure 1.
Concentration map (~5.5% v/v) for 2 mm beads (relative density 1.4) in water, obtained by ERT. High concentration red and low concentration blue.

2. Computer models of slurry pipe flow

The model of two parts, settling and suspended, is not the only classification, which has been applied to component parts of a settling slurry flow. Shook and Roco [4] postulated a notional third layer without lift forces underneath the settling layer, and a three-layer model was proposed by Doron and Barnea [5] to overcome perceived "limitations" of the two-layer representation. The new model provides a way to identify the relative delay of the solids fraction in a duct or holdup, which none of the other classifications achieve, at least not in a direct way. A more recent *four component model* pioneered by Wilson and Sellgren [6] and revised by Visintainer et al. [7] produces useful pump derating calculations but is based on uniform particle distribution.

Since its invention by K.C. Wilson [2, 3, 8, 9], there have been several references to the two-layer model. At the time of writing a new reference volume, Visintainer et al. [10] contain detailed discussion of it. The author's current version (*2LM*) described in the following pages has completely new coding to overcome instability and interface positioning difficulties of the original in obtaining estimates of the downstream velocity of the settling layer and holdup.

The *limit of stationary deposition velocity* over ranges of particle size, pipe diameters and relative density of grains was published by Wilson [3] in the form of an elegant nomogram constructed using techniques originated by Wood [11] (see Annexe C). The original nomogram did not account for volumetric concentrations, but in later work, Wilson et al. [8] modified the nomogram for a range of concentrations. The results are comparable with those obtained later in this chapter (**Figure 2**).

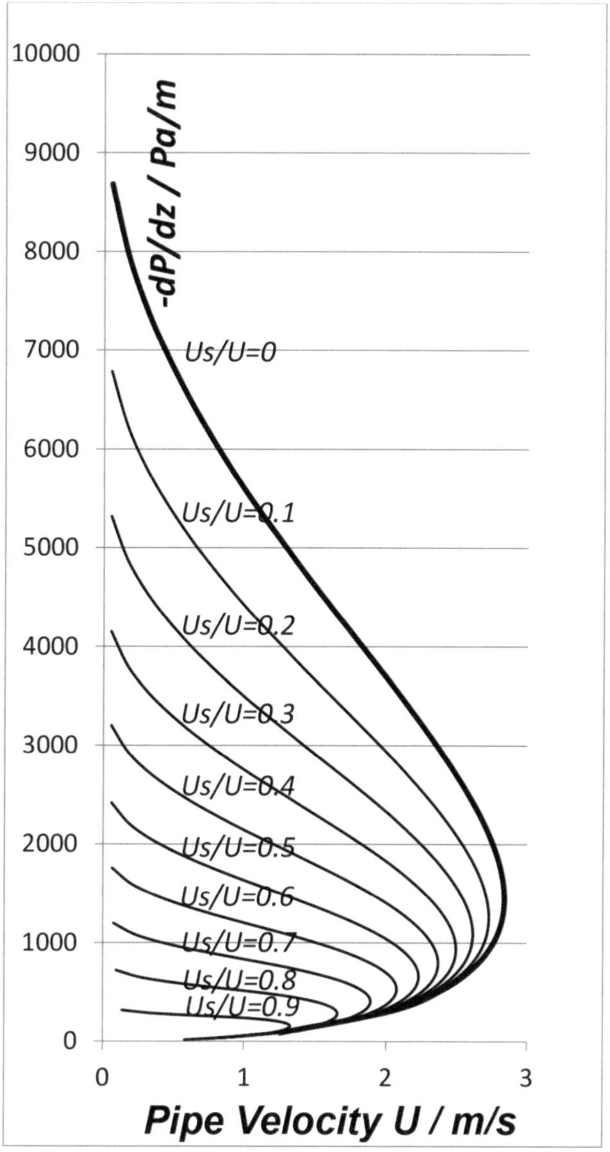

Figure 2.
Stationary bed loci for horizontal flow of sand in water. The concentration is 0.2 v/v, particle size is 2 mm, pipe diameter is 250 mm. U is the axial pipe velocity, Us is the velocity of the solids and dP/dz is the downstream pressure gradient. Note the classification of each locus by the relative velocity of solids, n.b $\mathcal{H}_{SBL} = 1 - \frac{U_s}{U}$.

Among other advantages, the simple geometry of the model provides an accessible alternative to an experimental image of a particle distribution, initially at least. For example, the first moment yields the *centre of concentration* of the particle burden about the centre of the duct. This is an indicator of its position and possibly its wear propensity. The second moment can indicate the energy required to achieve optimal particle suspension by swirling action. If available, experimental images of particle distribution can be obtained using, for example, *electrical resistance tomography (ERT)* or *particle image velocimetry (PIV)*.

3. Inputs and outputs

Inevitably, one must gather the parameters of the slurry flow problem ahead of any model calculation. For example, the pipe bore, the particle diameter, the v/v concentration, *etc.* are all highly influential in the results obtained. **Table 1** gives a list of the initial requirements for the model and suggestions for starting values if they are not known.

4. Flags

The solution can hit obstacles, but these are almost always the result of unachievable entry data (**Table 1**). Convergence of the model is assessed by the convergence of actual efflux concentration with that desired. If this cannot be achieved a flag is raised. The axial pipe velocity for a stationary bed is the solution of a quadratic equation (see Eqs. (37)–(40)). If an imaginary solution is obtained, a discriminant flag is set. The *SB* flag is not really an obstacle, but an indication that the

Parameter	Symbol	Unit		Typical Value
Pipe Bore	D	m		
Particle diameter	d	m		
Mean pipe velocity	U	m/s		
Concentration of solids by volume [0,1]	C_V		The required or delivered concentration of particles (*v/v*)	
Internal roughness height	ε	m	Commercial steel pipe [12] Cast iron [12] Concrete, upper value [12] Concrete, lower value [12] Drawn Tubing [12]	4.5×10^{-5} 2.6×10^{-4} 3.0×10^{-3} 3.0×10^{-4} 1.5×10^{-6}
Coefficient of friction	η	—	For the friction of settled particles with the duct walls. Starting estimate	0.6
Viscosity of liquid vehicle	μ	Pas	At 293°K Water [13] Glycerol [13] Olive oil [13] Paraffin oil [13]	0.001 0.0015 0.08 ~1.0
Density of solid particles	ρ_S	kg/m^3		
Density of Liquid vehicle	ρ_L	kg/m^3		
Limiting concentration of lower layer	C_{LIM}	—	Loosely-packed concentration of particles v/v. Starting estimate *NB* dense particle packing will require a higher value.	0.6
Angle of inclination	θ	°		

Table 1.
Preparatory data gathering.

value obtained for the velocity of the lower layer (U_2) is zero or less than zero. If U_2 is calculated to a value less than zero, this does not generally indicate a reverse flow direction, but an established stationary bed. The model sets it to zero, and the *SB* flag is raised.

The outputs from the model are shown in **Table 2**.

$\mathcal{H}$	Holdup ratio: the relative delay to the solids fraction
$\mathcal{H}_{SBL}$	Holdup if pipe velocity, *U*, were to be reduced to form a stationary bed
C_r	*In-situ* concentration *v/v*
β	Subtending angle for the interface chord
U_1	Pipe velocity, upper layer
U_2	Pipe velocity, lower layer
U_{SBL}	Pipe velocity for stationary bed locus
dP/dz *or* i	Pressure gradient
ρ_1	Density, upper layer
ρ_2	Density, lower layer
ρ_M	Density, mixture
y	Distance of the notional interface chord from the centre line
$\bar{y}$	Centre of Concentration, vertical distance from centre line
$\bar{\bar{y}}$	Radius of gyration of the cross section including the settling bed
C_v	Efflux concentration *v/v*
C_v convergence flag	YES if C_v has converged satisfactorily to the value specified (**Table 1**)
Discriminant flag	YES if discriminant is positive
SB flag	YES for stationary bed. NB if $U_2 \le U_{SBL}$ U_2 is always set to zero and the flag is raised

Table 2.
2LM outputs.

5. Solution of the equations: iteration and approximation strategy

A guiding principle in the development of this version of the model has been to keep trial-correction iterations to a minimum. However, a small number of trial-correction cycles are needed for the solution because many of the variables are only known in an experimental or empirical sense. The first phase, usually six iterations, is concerned with estimating the concentrations in the cross section. These values are established using the best estimate of the vital holdup ratio, the relative delay to the solids fraction. The holdup ratio can be estimated using an empirical correlation and is generally within ±3% of its experimentally determined value. The second, and last, phase of the solution (usually a further six iterations) is concerned with refining the holdup ratio, the velocity in the lower layer, the pressure gradient, the velocity for a stationary bed and, importantly, the convergence of the solids concentration to the specified value.

2LM requires a representative particle diameter, so care should be taken when there is a broad distribution of particle sizes. Wilson [2] suggests that distributions be partitioned into a small series of percentiles, *for example,* d_{02}, d_{25}, d_{50} d_{75}, and d_{98}, so that the model can be run with the fines fraction, the coarse fraction and prominent intermediate size ranges. Individual researchers will approach the results in different ways, perhaps simply taking a weighted mean of a key outcome and applying a tolerance band. Inevitably, such a procedure ignores the packing propensity of small particles to occupy voids between larger particles and the segregation of larger particles when pipe velocities are low. In **Table 1**, a value of limiting concentration, C_{LIM} of *0.6,* is advised as a starting estimate. Published datasets [14] give values between *0.58* and *0.78*, depending on the packing propensity of slurries with broad-size distributions.

A flowchart summarising the stages in the calculation is presented in Annexe A.

6. Concentrations

Figure 3 shows the basis of the idealised concentration distribution. The barchart illustrates the principle used by Shook and Roco [4] to express the concentration of the settling layer, C_2, as an addition to a pervading medium composed of the suspended fraction (a "carrier" medium [6, 7]). This is particularly relevant when the suspended fraction is composed of finely divided solids or particles of a completely different character to the settling medium. When referred to the whole cross section, C_2 is termed the *Contact Load* (C_c), i.e.

$$C_c = C_2 \times \frac{A_2}{A} \tag{1}$$

In this form, it can be added to the concentration in layer 1 to form the *in situ* concentration.

$$C_r = C_1 + C_c \tag{2}$$

The *in situ,* concentration takes no account of the differing rates of flow of the upper and lower layers. The *efflux* or *delivered* concentration (C_v) will be lower than the *in situ* value (C_r) because of the delay or holdup of the lower layer. It can be obtained by expressing the total flow rate as the combination of the two constituent

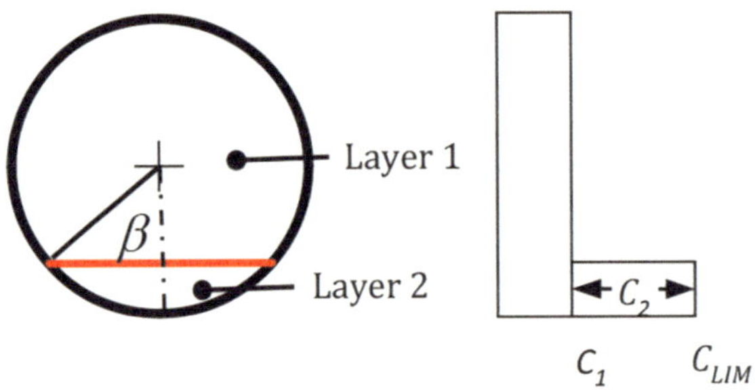

Figure 3.
The two-layer model. After shook [4].

flows, remembering that C_2 represents only the concentration in the lower part of the section.

$$C_v AU = C_1 AU + C_2 A_2 U_2 \tag{3}$$

substituting from Eqs. (1) and (2)

$$C_c = \frac{C_2 A_2}{A} = \frac{U(C_v - C_1)}{U_2} \tag{4}$$

Holdup ($\mathcal{H}$) is the key variable in this version of the model. It is quite difficult to determine with accuracy from experiments, and one must expect some scatter in experimental results. It can be defined in one of two possible ways. Some authors define it as the ratio of the *in situ* concentration to the delivered concentration ($\frac{C_r}{C_v}$). A better definition is given by the ratio of the velocity reduction of the solids to the free stream velocity, and this is the form used here.

$$\mathcal{H} = \frac{U - U_s}{U} \tag{5}$$

where U_s is the axial velocity of the solids at any section. Fortunately, the two definitions of holdup are algebraically linked as shown below.

The delivery flow rate of solids (Q_s) can be calculated using the mean mixture velocity in the duct or the *in situ* velocity of the solids (U_s) at the delivery section. These two expressions must be equal, i.e.

$$Q_s = C_v\left(U\frac{\pi D^2}{4}\right) = U_s\left(C_r\frac{\pi D^2}{4}\right)$$

From which

$$C_v = \frac{U_s}{U} C_r \tag{6}$$

Using Eq. (6), we obtain the influential relationship, which relates holdup ($\mathcal{H}$) to *in situ concentration* (C_r).

$$\mathcal{H} = 1 - \frac{C_v}{C_r} \tag{7}$$

In Eq. (4)

$$C_c = \frac{UC_v}{(U - U_2)} \frac{\mathcal{H}}{(1 - \mathcal{H})} \tag{8}$$

Eq. (8) yields the contact load C_c after the results of the first pass of the calculation have provided U_2 and $\mathcal{H}$. But one-off estimates of C_c and $\mathcal{H}$ are needed at the start of the calculation to make a first estimate of U_2. They are strongly related for a given slurry, but no direct analytical relationship solely between the two is available. A trial-correction strategy for two variables simultaneously is fraught with difficulties, so a good solution procedure is to fix one of them as accurately as possible in the initial stages. Unsurprisingly, the holdup ratio is highly influential in the two-layer model (Jones [14, 15]), so this would be a good choice for a variable to be determined as accurately as possible at outset. Later, the value of the holdup ratio can be refined by a second set of iterations. So, the first task was to search for a strong correlation for holdup in terms of the input variables.

Lahiri and Ghanta [16] have a neural network design, which they claim predicts holdup ratio with an absolute average accuracy of 2.5%. Seshadri et al. [17] demonstrate a strong relationship between holdup and hindered settling velocity using equations from Richardson and Zaki [18]. They suggest a relationship with a dimensionless parameter W/U_*, where W is the hindered settling velocity and U_* is the shear velocity. This cannot be used directly because the shear velocity U_* is not available at this stage of the calculation. However, a simpler direct correlation with holdup emerges when the hindered settling velocity is expressed as a non-dimensional ratio with pipe velocity (W/U). **Figure 4** shows a good general relationship when applied to data collected by Lahiri and Ghanta [16] (predominantly from publications by Hsu [19]), but scatter and uncertainty, particularly at low values of holdup ratio, must be considered. A second set of iterations to refine the estimate of holdup is a necessary precaution with this important variable.

Hence, an initial estimate of the holdup ratio can be obtained from

$$\mathcal{H}^{(0)} \sim 3.1179\left(\frac{W}{U}\right) \tag{9}$$

Richardson and Zaki [8] provide

$$W = v_0(1 - C_v)^Z \tag{10}$$

in which v_0 is the *un*hindered settling velocity. The defining equations are

$$v_0 = \left(\frac{g}{18\mu}\right)(\rho_s - \rho_L)d^2 \quad Re < 1 \text{ (Stokes Law)} \tag{11}$$

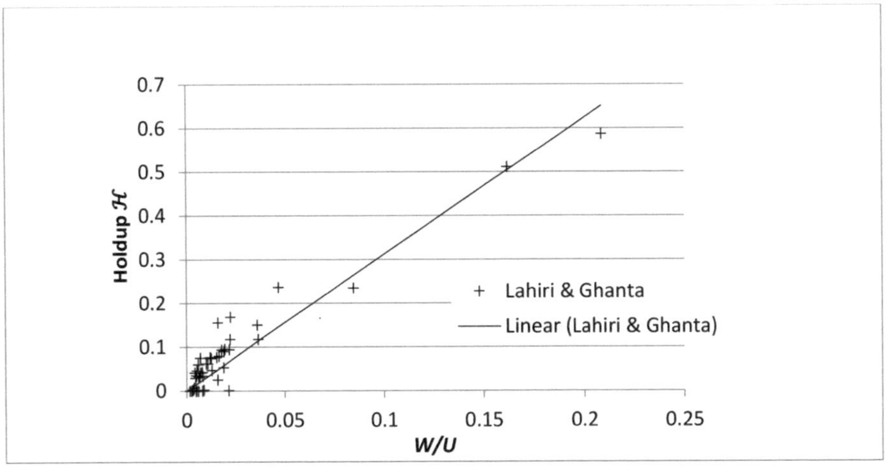

Figure 4.
Holdup vs. W/U ratio from data collected by Lahiri and Ghanta [16]. Linear regression gives $\mathcal{H} = 3.1179 \times \left(\frac{W}{U}\right)$ *with* $r^2 = 0.89$.

$$v_0 = \frac{0.2d^{1.18}\left(\frac{\rho_s-\rho_L}{\rho_L}\right)^{0.72}}{\left(\mu/\rho_L\right)^{0.45}} \quad 1< Re <800 \text{ (Allen's Law)} \tag{12}$$

$$v_0 = 1.74\sqrt{gd\left(\frac{\rho_s-\rho_L}{\rho_L}\right)} \quad Re >1000 \text{ (Newton's Law)} \tag{13}$$

$$Z = 4.65 + 1.95\left(\frac{d}{D}\right) \quad 0.002< Re \le 0.2 \tag{14}$$

$$Z = \left(4.35 + 17.5\left(\frac{d}{D}\right)\right) Re^{-0.03} \quad 0.2< Re \le 1.0 \tag{15}$$

$$Z = \left(4.45 + 18\left(\frac{d}{D}\right)\right) Re^{-0.1} \quad 1< Re \tag{16}$$

where Re = Reynolds number.

A later correlation for the exponent Z for power-law liquids is given by Coulson and Richardson [20].

Shook and Roco [4] suggest two empirical correlations for C_c, the first of which is

$$C_c^{(0)} \sim C_r^{(0)} exp\left[-0.124 \times Ar^{-0.061}\left(\frac{U^2}{gd}\right)^{0.028}\left(\frac{d}{D}\right)^{-0.431}(S_s-1)^{-0.272}\right] \tag{17}$$

where Ar = Archimedes Number defined $\frac{4gd^3(S_s-1)\rho_L^2}{3\mu_L^2}$

S_s = Relative density of solids

and, from Eq. (7) the *in situ* concentration $C_r^{(0)} = \frac{C_v}{1-\mathcal{H}^{(0)}}$

Note that Eq. (17) is simply a starting estimate from which a short- trial correction sequence can be initiated. Initial estimates of concentrations in hand, the solution of the pressure balance equations can proceed.

7. Pressure balance

In a steady-state situation, the pressure per unit length in the upper and lower component must be equal, i.e.,

$$-\frac{dP}{dz}\bigg|_{Layer\ 2} = -\frac{dP}{dz}\bigg|_{Layer\ 1} \tag{18}$$

$$i.e., \frac{\tau_1 S_1 + \tau_{12} S_{12}}{A_1} + \rho_1 g sin\theta = \frac{\tau_2 S_2 - \tau_{12} S_{12}}{A_2} + \rho_2 g sin\theta \tag{19}$$

where τ_{12} and S_{12} are shear stress and surface area at the interface between layers. The essential strategy now is to populate each of the terms in Eq. (19) as a means to provide a solution.

In most cases, the interfacial shear stress is an artefact of the model since there is generally no sharp discontinuity here unless U_2 approaches zero. Shook and Roco [4] put

$$\tau_{12} = \frac{1}{2} f_{12} (U_1 - U_2)^2 \rho_1 \tag{20}$$

where f_{12} is the friction factor at the notional interface. Nikuradse's sand-roughened pipe tests [21] can be characterised as follows:

$$\frac{1}{\sqrt{f}} = 1.14 - 0.86 \, ln\left(\frac{\varepsilon}{D}\right) \tag{21}$$

Putting roughness height, ε, to half the screen size of the sediment and changing the base of the logarithm yields.

$$f_{12} = \frac{1}{\left(1.736 - 1.98 \, log_{10}\left(\frac{d}{D}\right)\right)^2} \tag{22}$$

Colebrook [22] used Nikuradse's results to develop an empirical transition function for the region between laminar flow and fully developed turbulence, which was the basis of the well known Moody diagram [12, 23].

Eq. (21) can be used again to determine pipe friction factor (f), but it has been claimed that a later correlation from a short paper by Churchill [24] delivers better accuracy over a wide range of fluid regimes.

$$f = 2\left[\left(\frac{8}{Re}\right)^{12} + \frac{1}{(A+B)^{1.5}}\right]^{\frac{1}{12}} \tag{23}$$

in which:

$$A = \left\{-2.457 \, ln\left[\left(\frac{7}{Re}\right)^{0.9} + \frac{0.27\varepsilon}{D}\right]\right\}^{16} \tag{24}$$

$$B = \left(\frac{37430}{Re}\right)^{16} \tag{25}$$

There is a trap for the unwary here. Churchill's correlation is for the *Fanning* friction factor, one quarter of the value usually found on Moody charts. Churchill's formula for f is implied in subsequent calculations.

In the upper layer,

$$\tau_1 = \frac{1}{2} f U_1^2 \rho_1 \tag{26}$$

In the lower layer, we must take account of the Coulombic friction of the particle burden and the effect of pipe inclination, *i.e.*,

$$\tau_2 S_2 = \tau_{2m} S_2 + \tau_{2s} S_2 cos\theta \tag{27}$$

The first part of the Eq. (27) uses the density and friction factor of the invested medium.

$$\tau_{2m} = \frac{1}{2} f U_2^2 \rho_1 \tag{28}$$

The second part of the Eq. (27) requires analysis of the weight of the particle burden on the wall of the duct and the application of the coefficient of friction [15].

$$\tau_{2s}S_2 = \eta_s C_2 \frac{D^2}{2} \frac{(1 - C_{LIM})}{(1 - C_2)} (\rho_s - \rho_L) g(sin\beta - \beta cos\beta) \tag{29}$$

Surface peripheral areas S_1, S_2 *and* S_{12} (per downstream length) are functions of the subtending angle β (**Figure 3**) and will be derived below.

8. Subtending angle 2β

The area of the segment at the base of the circular cross section can be expressed as a non-dimensional function of the subtending angle β (**Figure 3** shows this angle).

$$F(\beta) = \frac{4A_2}{D^2} = \beta - \frac{1}{2} sin\, 2\beta \tag{30}$$

The inverse function $\beta(F)$ is difficult to obtain analytically, especially for small values ($F(\beta)$ has an infinite gradient as $\beta \to 0$). However, the sine expansion for the second part of the Eq. (30) gives

$$sin\, 2\beta = 2\beta - \frac{(2\beta)^3}{3!} + O(\beta^5) \tag{31}$$

In Eq. (30), when β is small, $F(\beta) \approx \frac{2\beta^3}{3}$
i.e., for small values of segmental area A_2

$$\beta(F) \approx \sqrt[3]{\frac{3F}{2}} \tag{32}$$

For $F(\beta) \leq 0.00032$ (approximately $\beta \leq 4.5°$) Eq. (32) applies. Above that, given a value of $F(\beta)$, the Taylor series gives us a simple interpolation.

$$\beta_{i+1}(F) = \beta_i + \beta'_i \times (F_{i+1} - F_i) + \beta''_i \times \frac{(F_{i+1} - F_i)^2}{2!} + \dots \tag{33}$$

A look-up table for $F(\beta)$ and the first three derivatives of β is given at Annexe B. The first lookup and interpolation should be enough for most purposes, but an iterative procedure can be applied by substituting $\beta_{i+1}(F)$ into Eq. (30) until $F(\beta_i) \to \frac{4A_2}{D^2}$ to any prescribed accuracy.

9. Contact lengths

With a value of the subtending angle β, we are now in a position to define accurate lengths of contact between layers and the pipe wall. Referring to **Figure 3**, the length of the arc of contact with layer 2 is given by

$$S_2 = R \times 2\beta \tag{34}$$

The length of the arc of contact with layer 1 is given by

$$S_1 = 2\pi R - S_2 \tag{35}$$

The length of the interface between the two layers is given by

$$S_{12} = 2Rsin\beta \tag{36}$$

10. Gathering terms

Eq. (19) can now be populated with finished values from the foregoing analyses. By good fortune, it resolves into a quadratic equation in U_2.

$$aU_2^2 + bU_2 + c = 0 \tag{37}$$

where

$$a = 0.5A_2S_1f\rho_1\left(\frac{A_2}{A_1}\right)^2 + 0.5AS_{12}f_{12}\rho_1\left(\frac{A}{A_1}\right)^2 - 0.5A_1S_2f\rho_1 \tag{38}$$

$$b = -A_2S_1f\rho_1\left(\frac{AA_2}{A_1^2}\right) - AS_{12}f_{12}\rho_1\left(\frac{A}{A_1}\right)^2 U \tag{39}$$

$$c = 0.5A_2S_1f\rho_1\left(\frac{AU}{A_1}\right)^2 - A_1\tau_{2s}S_2cos\theta + 0.5AS_{12}f_{12}\rho_1\left(\frac{AU}{A_1}\right)^2 + A_1A_2(\rho_1 - \rho_2)gsin\theta \tag{40}$$

From the final value of the bed velocity U_2, the velocity of the upper layer can be obtained from the principle of conservation of volume.

$$A_2U_2 + A_1U_1 = AU \tag{41}$$

11. The stationary bed

Conditions for a stationary bed can be obtained from Eq. (37), i.e.
if $U_2 \to 0$ then $c \to 0$
i.e.

$$U_{SBL\theta} = \frac{A - A_2}{A}\sqrt{\frac{(A - A_2)\tau_{2s}S_2cos\theta + (A - A_2)A_2(\rho_1 - \rho_2)gsin\theta}{0.5\rho_1(A_2S_1f + AS_{12}f_{12})}} \tag{42}$$

For a horizontal duct, this is mercifully simplified

$$U_{SBL} = \frac{A - A_2}{A}\sqrt{\frac{(A - A_2)\tau_{2s}S_2}{0.5\rho_1(A_2S_1f + AS_{12}f_{12})}} \tag{43}$$

Note that the velocity for a stationary bed, $U_{SBL\theta}$ or U_{SBL}, is not exactly equivalent to the *critical deposition velocity* to indicate the lowest velocity at which a slurry might be pumped to avoid settling. There is a slight difference between the definition of these two velocities. The *critical deposition velocity* can be defined as the velocity at which the first stationary particle layer will form at the bottom of a duct. Clearly, the stationary bed is not usually a single layer of particles, but in many ways, the velocity for a stationary bed is as useful a concept as the *critical deposition velocity*, if not more useful for the designer.

12. The stationary bed locus

Practitioners often make use of a plot of the pressure gradient (*-dP/dz* or i) against pipe velocity (the "*i-v diagram*"). On this useful plot, the stationary bed envelope can be plotted to indicate safety from a settling bed and potential blockage. Pump characteristics can also be superimposed. The locus of points with $U_2 = 0$ is called the *Stationary Bed Locus* or *SBL*. Delineation between the two layers is most obvious when the bed is stationary. Hence, *2LM* is particularly adept at plotting this locus and identifying a predicted operating envelope to be avoided.

The pressure gradient can be computed from the final values of density, layer velocities, bed friction and surface areas. In Eq. (18), the pressure gradients in both layers must be equal so the layer 1 computation can be used.

$$i = -\frac{dP}{dz}\bigg|_{Layer\ 1} = \frac{\frac{1}{2}f_1U_1^2\rho_1S_1 + \frac{1}{2}f_{12}(U_1 - U_2)^2\rho_1S_{12}}{A_1} + \rho_1 g sin\theta$$

For a stationary bed in horizontal flow, $U_2 \rightarrow 0$, $U_1 \rightarrow U_{SBL} \times \frac{A}{A_1}$ and $\theta \rightarrow 0$ so the loci of pressure gradient with the velocity for a stationary bed are described by Eq. (44).

$$i_{SBL} = \frac{\rho_1}{2A_1}\left(U_{SBL}\frac{A}{A_1}\right)^2 (f_1S_1 + f_{12}S_{12}) \tag{44}$$

Figure 2 shows stationary bed loci of pressure gradient with pipe velocity, U. The advantage of this graph is that pump characteristics can be overlaid to investigate the possibility of a stationary bed. If a stationary bed is implicated, a specific holdup ratio ($\mathcal{H}_{SBL}$) can be obtained. This value of $\mathcal{H}_{SBL}$ only applies when there is a stationary bed and should not be confused with the value obtained when both beds are flowing freely.

To interpret **Figure 2**, one must refer to the fundamental definition of holdup given by Eq. (5): $\mathcal{H} = \frac{U-U_s}{U}$. When $\mathcal{H}_{SBL} = 1.0$, $\left(\frac{U_s}{U} = 0\right)$, the solid particles have zero velocity, and a high pipe velocity is needed to prevent a stationary bed. For $\mathcal{H}_{SBL} = 0.1$, $\left(\frac{U_s}{U} = 0.9\right)$ solid particles are relatively mobile, and only a low pipe velocity is required to keep the settling layer in suspension. Note the shallow slope of the loci at low pressures—a very small change in pressure gradient yields a large change in velocity requirement. The safest policy is, of course, to maintain a pipe velocity entirely to the right of the SBL envelope, 2.84 m/s in this case This is the "maximum velocity at the limit of stationary deposition" in Annexe C. The value from Wilson's original nomogram [8, 11] (Annexe C) is approximately 2.70 m/s. The slightly reduced value (approximately −5%) is attributed to the lack of compensation for volumetric concentration. A later version of the nomogram, including allowance for a range of concentrations is available [9].

13. Validating the *2LM* model

2LM works on a significant simplification of particle concentrations in a duct. Shou [25] suggests a three-layer model for large pipes with a low-concentration supernatant layer at the top of the section. There have been other criticisms, and it is important to contrast predictions with experimental data. For example, the model proposes a sharply defined discontinuity or interface between upper and lower layers not strictly observed in practice. It is closest to reality when the lower layer is stationary. Even then, local effects have been observed at the interface such as bouncing, gusting (where groups of particles leave the interface altogether), surface rippling and cycles of deposition and re-entrainment. Lahiri and Ghanta [16] provide a dataset of 43 slurries with values of holdup for each one. These data can be compared with predictions from *2LM*. Pressure differences can be accurately measured in experiments and **Figure 5b** shows this. Note the greater scatter at higher pressures. **Figure 5a** shows a significant agreement between experiment and model determinations of holdup but considerably more scatter than those for pressure gradient data. At high values of holdup, the local effects of bouncing, gusting, *etc.* can be expected to have a strong influence on the experimental accuracy of holdup measurements.

In testing the model, it was important to explore as wide a selection of examples as possible. The work by Shook and Roco [4] was the motivation for this development, and their example was the first example to be tested [15]. Application and modification over several years have resulted in a utility with wide applicability and stability. The model has been tested over many examples of slurry flow, two of which will be shown in the next section.

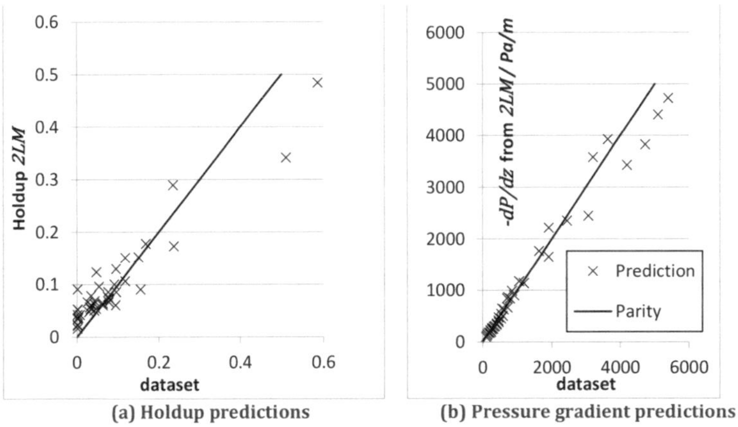

Figure 5.
2LM model validation against experimental results from Lahiri and Ghanta [16].

14. Example calculations from the dataset

Results are presented in two parts. The first part displays iteration progress for a specific example from the dataset. This has a fixed velocity. The second set shows the depth of the settling layer as the velocity is varied.

The corrections shown in **Figure 6** (fine particles in moderately viscous medium) are relatively minor. The algorithm strives to match the given volume concentration, C_v, and achieves this task after the second set of corrections arriving at a value within

DOI: http://dx.doi.org/10.5772/intechopen.112023

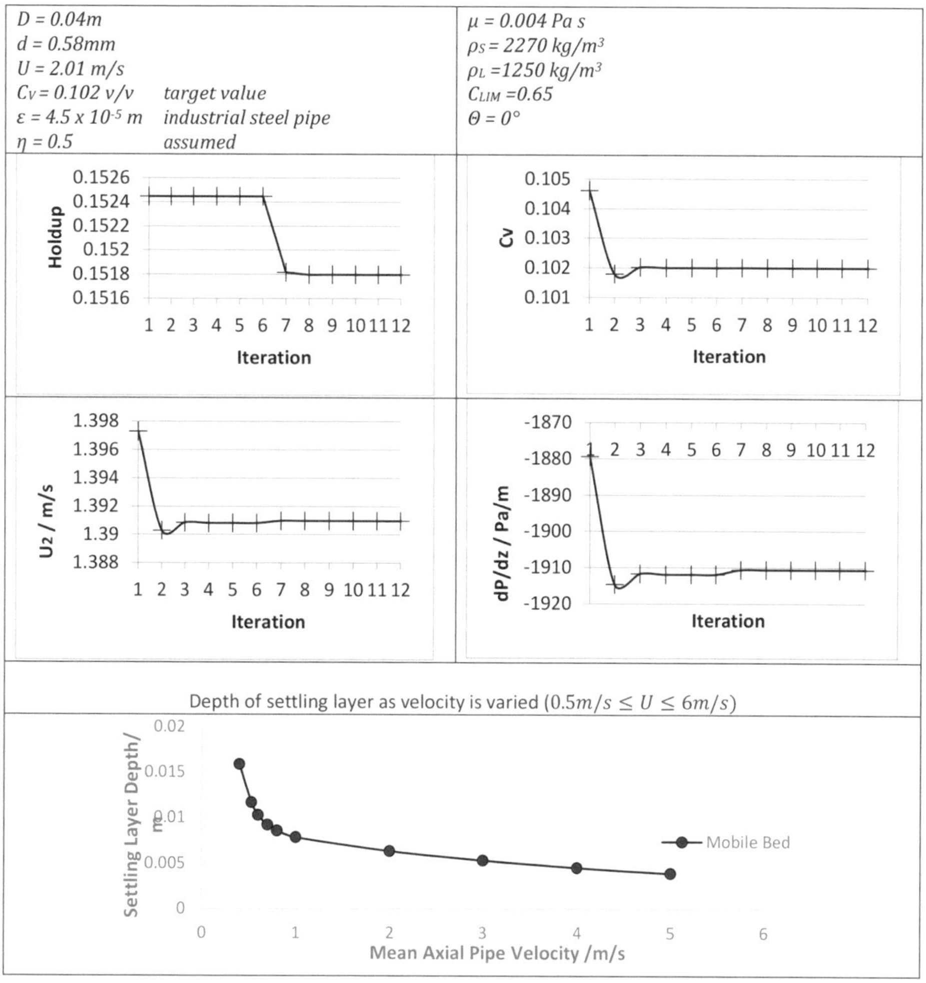

Figure 6.
2LM example — Fine particles in a viscous medium.

approximately 3% on the original estimate. Only 12 corrections are applied in two batches of 6. The depth of the settling layer reduces systematically as the mean pipe velocity is increased.

Corrections required for the second example (very coarse particles in water **Figure 9**) are clearly much greater, but this is to be expected in view of the large particles specified in the case. The second case is the most interesting challenge of the two. Large variations in pressure gradient and volume concentration are becalmed by the second set of iterations. The depth of the settling bed starts from a low value before reducing systematically as in the first example.

15. Centre of concentration

The *centre of concentration* ($G(r,\theta)$ or $G(x,y)$) of particle suspensions can be as important as the *centre of mass* in the mechanics of solids. Uniform suspension is

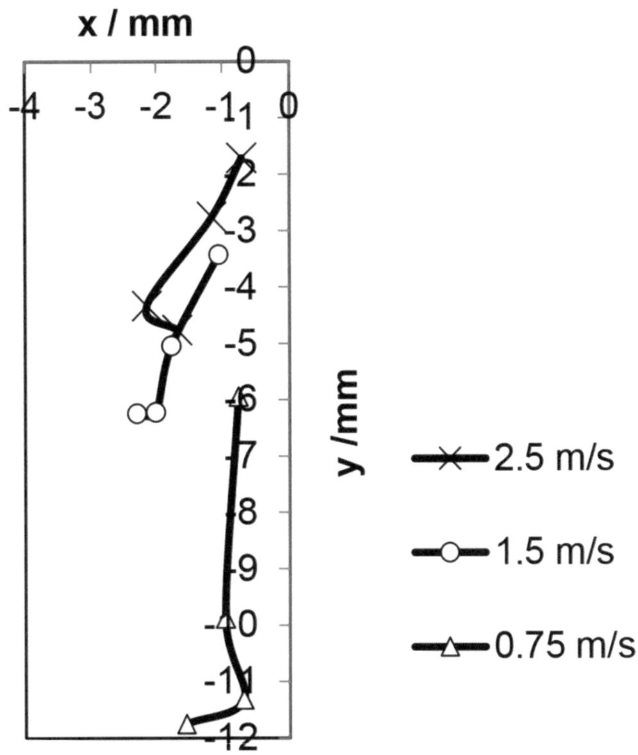

Figure 7.
Locus of Centre of concentration (LCC) from ERT measurements. (2 mm beads of RD 1.4 and concentrations 7.31%, 5.48%, 3.66% and 1.79% v/v in water).

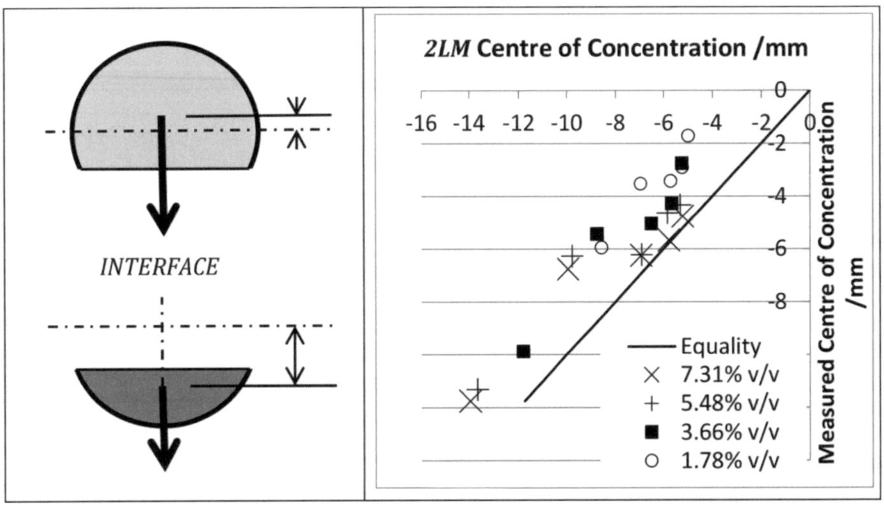

Figure 8.
Centre of concentration calculations using the two-layer model as an approximation to the actual concentration distribution in the cross section.

indicated if G is near the geometrical centre of the duct. If it is near the periphery of the duct, sluggish or static settlement can be inferred.

Figure 7 shows the *locus of centre of concentration (LCC)* for a series of concentrations The origin (0,0) is the centre of the pipe. The position of G for a given pipe velocity changes as concentration increases. This downward trend is a *locus of centre of concentration (LCC)*, which can be used to study the state of suspension of the medium.

The current version of the *2LM* model computes the first moment of the two layers and combines these results to obtain the centre of concentration of the whole. All three results are useful in different ways. The position of the centre of concentration for the upper layer for example may be important when a stationary bed is indicated. The estimates are surprisingly close to those obtained from tomography measurements (see **Figure 8**). The *2LM* estimates are above the parity line because the actual interface between layers is a diffuse boundary rather than a precise chord.

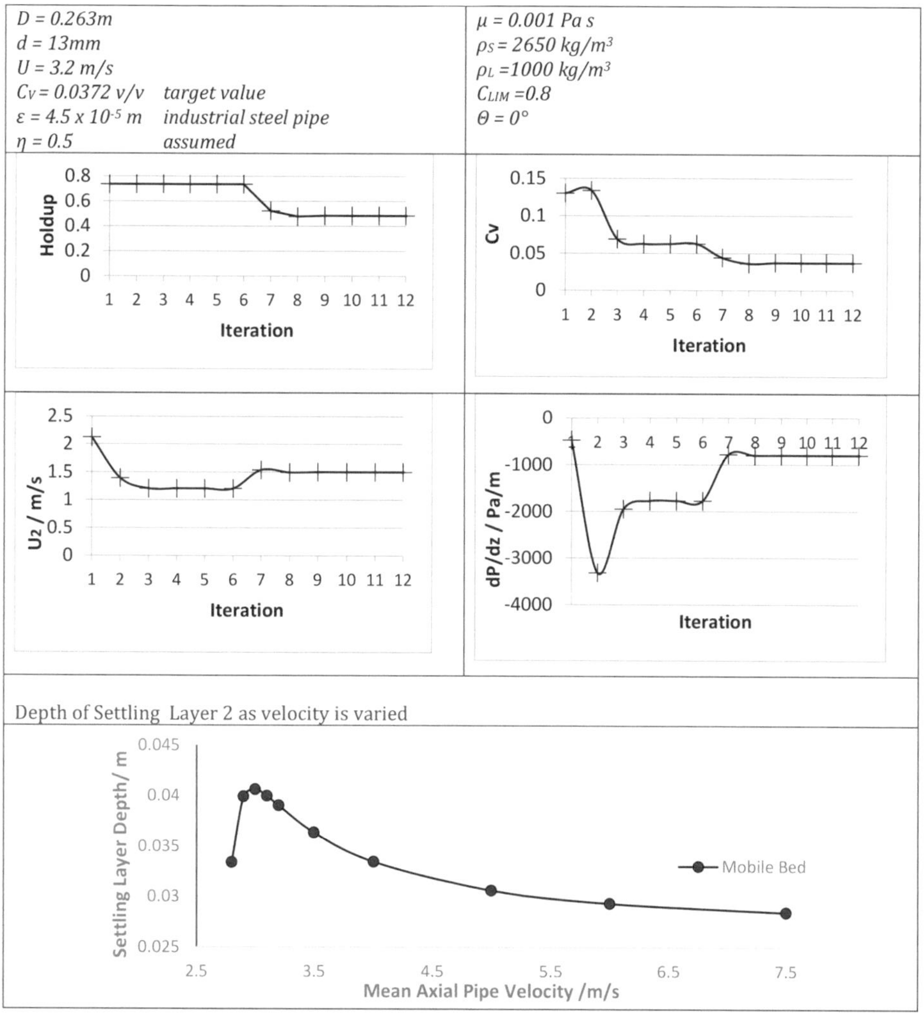

Figure 9.
2LM example — Coarse particles in water.

16. Conclusions

In my conclusions for this chapter, I must first pay tribute to the pioneers of the *Two-Layer Model*: Professors K.C. Wilson and C.A. Shook. They motivated the lengthy process of precise definition of the interface layer, calculation of holdup ratio, accurate estimation of the contact load, estimation of the velocity for a stationary bed, the locus of points for a stationary bed and the calculation of the centre of concentration. The algorithm has a long and useful history, which has been punctuated by a series of incremental modifications. A guiding principle in this model has been to keep trial-correction iterations to a minimum and the two-stage iteration process works extremely well in this endeavour. The first stage — six calculations using an empirical value for the holdup — invites the second stage in which all the variables (including the holdup and contact load) are refined. **Figures 6** and **9** show the progress of the calculations for two widely different examples. They also show how the bed depth reduces as pipe velocity is increased.

Much of the original terminology (from reference (4)) has endured, and the author has been careful to keep to the original symbols where possible. This said much of the *2LM* model described in the foregoing pages is truly new. From a rather unstable computation, a robust and widely applicable system has emerged. In its present form, it has already been used by the author in many calculations for particle-bearing liquids.

Annexe A: flowchart for *2LM* Iterations

Iteration Loops

Repeat $i \leftarrow [1,12]$

Concentrations

Holdup: $i \le 6, \quad \mathcal{H}^{(i)} = \mathcal{H}^{(0)}$

$i > 6, \mathcal{H}^{(i)} = 1 - \frac{C_v}{C_r^{(i-1)}}$

In-situ concentration: $C_r^{(i)} = \frac{C_V}{1-\mathcal{H}^{(i)}}$

Contact Load: $i = 1, \; C_c^{(i)} = C_c^{(0)}$

$i > 1, \; C_c^{(i)} = \frac{UC_v}{\left(U-U_2^{(i-1)}\right)} \frac{\mathcal{H}^{(i)}}{(1-\mathcal{H}^{(i)})}$

Layer concentrations (Upper, Lower) $C_1^{(i)} = C_r^{(i)} - C_c^{(i)}$,

$C_2^{(i)} = C_{LIM}^{(i)} - C_1^{(i)}$

Layer densities (Upper, Lower) $\rho_1^{(i)} = \rho_L\left[1 + C_1^{(i)}(sp-1)\right]$,

$\rho_2^{(i)} = \rho_L\left[1 + C_{LIM}^{(i)}(sp-1)\right]$

Mixture density: $\rho_M^{(i)} = \rho_L\left[1 + C_r^{(i)}(sp-1)\right]$

Pressure Balance

Area of Lower layer $A_2^{(i)} = A\frac{C_c^{(i)}}{C_2^{(i)}}$

Non-dimensional lower layer area function $F^{(i)} = \frac{4A_2^{(i)}}{D^2}$

Subtending angle: $F^{(i)} \le 0.00032\, , \beta^{(i)} \approx \sqrt[3]{\frac{3F^{(i)}}{2}}$

$F^{(i)} > 0.00032 \; interpolate\ for\ \beta^{(i)}$

Contact Areas (Upper, Lower, Interface) : $S_1^{(i)} = D\left(\pi - \beta^{(i)}\right)$

$S_2^{(i)} = D\beta^{(i)}$

$S_{12}^{(i)} = Dsin\beta^{(i)}$

Coulombic wall friction:

$$\tau_{2s}S_2 = \eta_s C_2 \frac{D^2}{2}\frac{(1-C_{LIM})}{(1-C_2)}(\rho_s - \rho_L)g(sin\beta - \beta cos\beta)$$

Lower Layer shear force (including pipe inclination):

$$\tau_2 S_2 = \frac{1}{2} f_1 U_2^2 \rho_1 + \tau_{2s} S_2 cos\theta$$

Velocity of Lower Layer:

Solve $aU_2^2 + bU_2 + c = 0$, for velocity of the bed layer $U_2^{(i)}$, where

$$a = 0.5A_2S_1f\rho_1\left(\frac{A_2}{A_1}\right)^2 + 0.5AS_{12}f_{12}\rho_1\left(\frac{A}{A_1}\right)^2 - 0.5A_1S_2f\rho_1$$

$$b = -A_2S_1f\rho_1\left(\frac{AA_2}{A_1^2}\right) - AS_{12}f_{12}\rho_1\left(\frac{A}{A_1}\right)^2 U$$

$$c = 0.5A_2S_1f\rho_1\left(\frac{AU}{A_1}\right)^2 - A_1\tau_{2s}S_2cos\theta + 0.5AS_{12}f_{12}\rho_1\left(\frac{AU}{A_1}\right)^2 + A_1A_2(\rho_1 - \rho_2)gsin\theta$$

Velocity of the upper layer $U_1^{(i)} = \frac{AU - A_2^{(i)}U_2^{(i)}}{A_1^{(i)}}$

Results:

$$\mathcal{H}, C_r, \beta, U_1, U_2, U_{SBL}, \frac{dP}{dz}, \rho_1, \rho_2, \rho_M, \text{interface height } y, \bar{y}, \bar{\bar{y}},$$

flags: Discriminant Error, Stationary Bed, C_v convergence

Annexe B: look-up Table for β

β	β	$F(\beta)=$	$d\beta/dF$	$d^2\beta/dF^2$	$d^3\beta/dF^3$
degrees	*radians*	$4^*area/D^2$			
0	0	0	1	0	
4	0.06981317	0.00022662	102.7545277	−2938.916414	8053120.117
8	0.13962634	0.001807662	25.81424314	−367.3557681	497829.108
12	0.20943951	0.006071189	11.56677223	−108.8347698	96554.43462
16	0.27925268	0.014293048	6.581029752	−45.90155642	29777.73395
20	0.34906585	0.027672046	4.274316085	−23.48717386	11801.60686
24	0.41887902	0.047306608	3.022340595	−13.57657624	5466.671326
28	0.488692191	0.074173404	2.268566019	−8.5331043	2813.653051
32	0.558505361	0.109108337	1.780535302	−5.698904249	1561.315876
36	0.628318531	0.152790273	1.447213595	−3.983837256	916.1578674
40	0.698131701	0.205727824	1.210138313	−2.884373363	561.0662394
44	0.767944871	0.268249457	1.036161515	−2.145953318	355.3309265
48	0.837758041	0.340497093	0.905363721	−1.630386313	231.1981656
52	0.907571211	0.422423348	0.805203615	−1.258188022	153.8334161
56	0.977384381	0.513792454	0.72748087	−0.981384085	104.3400823
60	1.047197551	0.614184849	0.666666667	−0.769800359	72
64	1.117010721	0.723005344	0.618941539	−0.603755918	50.50151797
68	1.186823891	0.839494706	0.581618596	−0.469978332	36.00772855
72	1.256637061	0.962744435	0.552786405	−0.359222381	26.12198067
76	1.326450232	1.09171445	0.531082227	−0.264827342	19.31211832
80	1.396263402	1.22525333	0.515545602	−0.181809199	14.57906665
84	1.466076572	1.362120726	0.50552345	−0.106265311	11.26033979
88	1.535889742	1.501011505	0.50060973	−0.034963354	8.91045152
92	1.605702912	1.640581149	0.50060973	0.034963354	7.226413536
96	1.675516082	1.779471927	0.50552345	0.106265311	6.00034357
100	1.745329252	1.916339324	0.515545602	0.181809199	5.088747506
104	1.815142422	2.049878203	0.531082227	0.264827342	4.392268907
108	1.884955592	2.178848218	0.552786405	0.359222381	3.84213259
112	1.954768762	2.302097947	0.581618596	0.469978332	3.39094193
116	2.024581932	2.418587309	0.618941539	0.603755918	3.006351647
120	2.094395102	2.527407804	0.666666667	0.769800359	2.666666667
124	2.164208272	2.6278002	0.72748087	0.981384085	2.35774786
128	2.234021443	2.719169306	0.805203615	1.258188022	2.070815141
132	2.303834613	2.80109556	0.905363721	1.630386313	1.800873504
136	2.373647783	2.873343196	1.036161515	2.145953318	1.545575938

β	β	$F(\beta)=$	$d\beta/dF$	$d^2\beta/dF^2$	$d^3\beta/dF^3$
140	2.443460953	2.935864829	1.210138313	2.884373363	1.304395663
144	2.513274123	2.988802381	1.447213595	3.983837256	1.078019326
148	2.583087293	3.032484316	1.780535302	5.698904249	0.867899432
152	2.652900463	3.067419249	2.268566019	8.5331043	0.675922485
156	2.722713633	3.094286046	3.022340595	13.57657624	0.504161945
160	2.792526803	3.113920608	4.274316085	23.48717386	0.354693941
164	2.862339973	3.127299605	6.581029752	45.90155642	0.229459909
168	2.932153143	3.135521465	11.56677223	108.8347698	0.130164791
172	3.001966313	3.139784991	25.81424314	367.3557681	0.058202636
176	3.071779484	3.141366034	102.7545277	2938.916414	0.014603838

Annexe C: nomographic chart for maximum velocity at the limit of stationary deposition

From Wilson [3], with permission

1. Select the pipe diameter/*m* on the left hand axis
2. Place a straight edge to cut the particle diameter/*mm* curve to the middle axis (stationary deposit velocity/ms^{-1} for grains with *RD = 2.65*)
3. Place the straight edge from the value on the middle axis to cut the right-hand function at the correct relative density.

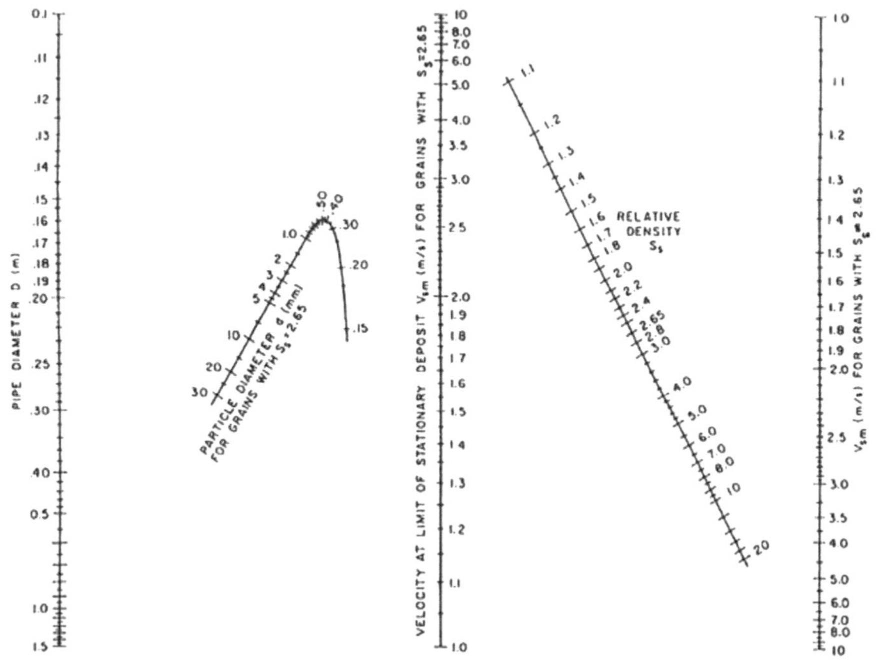

Author details

Trevor Frank Jones
TFJ Consulting Ltd, England

*Address all correspondence to: info@tfjconsulting.com

References

[1] Bagnold RA. The Physics of Blown Sand and Desert Dunes, First edition 1941, reprinted in 1954 by. London: Methuen and Co. Ltd.; 1954

[2] Wilson KC. Slip point of beds in solid-liquid pipeline flow. Proc. ASCE J. Hyd. Div. 1970;**96**:1-12

[3] Wilson KC. A unified physically based analysis of solid-liquid pipeline flow. In: Proc Hydrotransport 4 Conference BHRA. Cranfield, UK: BHRA Group; Paper A1; 1976. pp. 1-12

[4] Shook CA, Roco MC. Slurry Flow – Principles and Practice. MA, USA: Butterworth-Heinnemann; 1991. pp. 119, 285-133 and Appendix 4, 290

[5] Doron P, Barnea D. A three-layer model for solid-liquid flow in horizontal pipes. International Journal of Multiphase Flow. 1993;**19**:1029-1043

[6] Wilson KC, Sellgren A. Hydraulic transport of solids. In: Pump Handbook. 3rd ed. New York, USA: McGraw Hill; 2001. pp. 9.321-9.349

[7] Visintainer R, Sellgren A, Furlan J, McCall G. Centrifugal pump Deratings for a broadly-graded (4-component) slurry. In: 18th International Conference on Transport and Sedimentation of Solid Particles. Poland: Wroclaw University of Environmental and Life Sciences; 2017

[8] Wilson KC. Deposition limit nomograms for particles of various densities in pipeline flow. In: Proc Hydrotransport 6 Conference, BHRA. Cranfield, U.K: BHRA Group; 1979. pp. 1-12

[9] Wilson KC, Addie GR, Sellgren A, Visintainer R. Simplified approach to effect of concentration on deposit limit. In: Proc Transport and Sedimentation of Solid Particles. Poland: Wroclaw University of Environmental and Life Sciences; 2011. pp. 17-25

[10] Visintainer R, Matoušec V, Pullum L, Sellgren A. Slurry Transport Using Centrifugal Pumps. 4th ed. Cham, Switzerland: Springer; 2023

[11] Wood FM. Standard nomographic forms for equations in three variables. Canadian Journal of Research. 1935; **12**(1):14-40

[12] Moody LF. Friction factors for pipe flow. Transactions of the American Society of Mechanical Engineers. 1944; **99**(8):671-684

[13] Tennent RM, editor. Science Data Book. Edinburgh: Oliver and Boyd; 1971. p. 62

[14] Jones TF. Holdup datasets predict critical deposition velocities using a modification of the two-layer model. In: Proc 19th International Conference on Hydrotransport, Golden, Colorado, USA. Cranfield, UK: BHR Group; 2014. pp. 39-46

[15] Jones TF. A spreadsheet version of the two-layer model for solid-liquid pipeflow. In: 15th International Conference on Transport and Sedimentation of Solid Particles, Wroclaw, Poland. Poland: Wroclaw University of Environmental and Life Sciences; 2011. pp. 101-114

[16] Lahiri SK, Ghanta KC. Development of an artificial network correlation for prediction of hold-up of slurry transport in pipelines. Chemical Engineering Science. 2008;**63**(2008):1497-1509

[17] Seshadri V, Singh SN, Fabien C, Mishra R. Hold-up in multi-sized particulate solid-liquid flow through horizontal pipes. Indian Journal of Engineering & Materials Science. 2001; **8**:84-89

[18] Richardson JF, Zaki WM. Sedimentation and fluidization: Part 1. Transactions of the Institution of Chemical Engineers. 1954;**32**:35

[19] Hsu FL, Turian RM, Ma T-W. Flow of non-colloidal slurries in pipelines. American Institute of Chemical Engineers. 1989;**35**(3):429-442

[20] Coulson JM, Richardson JF. Chemical Engineering. 6th ed. Vol. 1. Oxford: Butterworth Heinemann; 1999

[21] Nikuradse J. "Gesetzmäβsigkeiten der turbulenten Strömung in glatten Rohren". [Laws of turbulent flow in Smooth Pipes]. VDI Forsch. 1932;**4**:44

[22] Colebrook C. Turbulent flow in pipes with particular reference to the transition region between smooth and rough pipe Laws. Journal of the Institution of Civil Engineers. 1938;**11**: 133-156

[23] LaViolette, M. (2017), "On the history, science and technology included in the moody diagram", Journal of Fluids Engineering, ASME, Vol 139, pp. 1030801-1 to 1030801-21

[24] Churchill SW. Friction factor equation spans all fluid regimes. Chemical Engineer. 1977;**84**(24):91-92

[25] Shou G. Slurry pipeline blockage, theory and practice. In: 16th International Conference on Hydrotransport, Santiago, Chile. Cranfield: BHR Group Ltd.; 2004, 26-28 April 2004

Chapter 3

Numerical Modelling of Medium Slurry Flow in a Vertical Pipeline

Artur S. Bartosik

Abstract

The study deals with the modelling and experiments of vertical solid-liquid turbulent flow with narrowly sized solid particles of average diameters equal to 0.125 mm, 0.240 mm and 0.470 mm, and solid concentrations by volume from 10% to 40%, called medium slurry. The physical model assumes that the slurry with solid particles surrounded by water is flowing upward through a vertical pipeline with solid concentrations from 10–40% by volume. Experiments with such slurries clearly indicated enhanced damping of the turbulence, which depends on the diameter of the solid particles. The mathematical model constitutes conservative equations based on time averages for mass and momentum. The closure problem was solved by taking into account the Boussinesque hypothesis and a two-equation turbulence model together with an especially designed wall damping function. The wall damping function depends on the average diameter of the solid particles and the bulk concentration. The predictions' results were successfully compared with the measurements. The study demonstrates the importance of solid particle diameter and showed that using a standard wall damping function gives higher friction compared to measurements. The main objective of this study is to present a mathematical model for medium slurry flow in a vertical pipeline, including a specially designed wall damping function, and to demonstrate the influence of solid particle size on frictional head loss. The effect of mean particle diameter and solid concentration on frictional head loss has been discussed and conclusions were formulated.

Keywords: medium slurry flow, experiments on slurry flow, modelling of vertical slurry flow, modelling of slurry turbulence, numerical modelling

1. Introduction

Solid-liquid turbulent flow is an interdisciplinary research area of great technological and commercial importance. It is widely used in mechanical and chemical engineering, power plants, food and mining industries, and in medicine. Solid-liquid flow appears mainly in pump transport in various pipeline systems [1–3]. Such transportation faces problems such as abrasion of the pump's elements, especially between the rotating impeller and the stationary throat bush, the rotating shaft sleeve, and the stationary packing inlet and outlet ducts. Due to the abrasive characteristics of the solid particles, the pumps and pipelines suffer during the work under these conditions. Power, capacity, wear and breakdown resistance, and robustness are the essential keys for efficient pump dredging. The characteristics of dredging pumps and pipelines require a long working life in abrasive conditions, a limited influence of wear on pump performance and a low net positive suction head requirement. Abrasion in a pump or pipeline can be defined by the loss of weight per unit area or the loss of thickness under the dynamic action of solid particles that act on the solid wall [4–6]. In this process, the 'particle-wall' interaction, especially at the high particle size and density, high flow rate, and high solid concentration, plays a crucial role, and research on the determination of the 'particle wall' stress is much desired [7, 8]. Another particular application of solid-liquid flow is related to the drug delivery system in which magnetic targeting offers the ability to target a specific site, such as a tumour [9]. Solid-liquid flow can also exist with extremely high velocity to cut concrete, rock, glass, steel, ceramics, composites and plastics. The finished edge obtained by such a process often eliminates the need for post-machining to improve surface finish [10].

Solid-liquid flow could be classified as stationary bed, moving bed, heterogeneous and pseudo-homogeneous, or as settling or non-settling types [11]. Settling slurry is formed mainly by coarse particles. When predicting frictional head loss in slurry flow with coarse or medium particles, it is reasonable to assume the Newtonian model, as now one can measure the rheology of such slurries [5]. In coarse dispersive slurry flow, one should mention the basic research of Bagnold [7] and mathematical models, such as, for instance, [12, 13], which include solid-liquid and/or solid-solid interactions.

Non-settling slurries usually contain fine particles with an average diameter below 0.040 mm and can form a stable homogeneous mixture exhibiting an increased apparent viscosity. Such slurries usually exhibit yield stress and require a proper rheological model incorporated into the momentum equation. Fine particles demonstrate an increased viscous sublayer, which means that the damping of the turbulence appears in the near-wall region [14]. In this case, the mathematical model includes an apparent viscosity concept, a suitable rheological model [15] and a properly defined wall damping function [16].

Slurries with medium solid particles of average diameter between 0.10 mm and 0.50 mm are usually assumed to be a Newtonian solid-liquid mixture or as a mixture of two separated phases. If the bulk velocity of the slurry is sufficiently high, such slurry can exhibit a non-settling type. If the slurry flow occurs in a vertical pipeline, this flow can be treated as axially symmetric. It is important to emphasise that slurries with medium solid particles exhibit enhanced damping of turbulence because frictional head loss is relatively low compared with carrier liquid flow [17].

Mathematical modelling of solid-liquid flow usually requires reliable experimental data to validate the model. The most desirable measurements are those close to the wall of the pipe. Measurements at high concentrations of the dispersed phase are very difficult. As a result of these difficulties, most measurements regard gas-solid or gas-liquid flow. Mathematical modelling of solid-liquid flow is far away from the knowledge gathered for Newtonian flows, and turbulent flow is still the main challenge of CFD. Analysing the predictions of turbulent solid-liquid flow, the mixture theory models are the most general and are based on rigorous fluid mechanics frameworks [18]. Researchers around the world have been working to develop accurate models for frictional head loss and velocity distribution in slurry flows. Frictional head loss is one of the most important technical parameters to be evaluated by the designers for designing a pipeline slurry transportation system, and the parameter that dictates the selection of pump capacity. Determining the most efficient and economical way to pump any solids into a carrier liquid requires careful consideration and analysis of numerous factors, some of which can have a significant impact on performance and cost. Among them, there are an averaged solid particle diameter, solid concentration, particle density, deposition velocity, carrier liquid properties and properly matched characteristics of a pipeline with the characteristics of a pump.

The main objective of this study is to present a mathematical model for medium slurry flow in a vertical pipeline, including a specially designed wall damping function, and to demonstrate the influence of solid particle size on frictional head loss.

2. Literature review

Analysing measurements with respect to the behaviour of particles suspended in a surrounding fluid, we recognise several techniques. For example, Roberts and Kennedy [19] used pulsed injections of salt water and tagged radioactive particles. Kowalewski [20] used the ultrasound technique, while Altobelli et al. [21] used nuclear magnetic resonance (NMR). Yianneskis and Whitelaw [22], Nouri et al. [23], Nouri and Whitelaw [24], Wildmanet et al. [25] and Chen and Kadambi [26, 27] used Laser-Doppler anemometer (LDA). The necessary condition for the measurement of LDA is that the dispersed phase consists of transparent solid particles, whose refractive index is close to the carrier phase [22–27]. In addition to the above techniques, it is worth mentioning the technique applied by Shook's research team. The authors used the original method to measure the lateral variation of solids concentration in vertical pipelines [28–30].

Yianneskis and Whitelaw [22] measured the local solid and liquid phase velocities in a fully developed pipe flow using the LDA technique. The dispersed phase in the carrier liquid consisted of transparent solid particles with a diameter of 0.270 mm. The most important conclusion from their research was the fact that the slip velocity between the solid and liquid phases clearly decreases with increasing concentration of the solid phase. Sumner et al. [17, 31] and Nasr-El-Din et al. [32] measured the solid concentration distribution in slurry with medium and coarse particles. They concluded that the averaged particle diameter has a crucial influence on friction losses and the profile of solid concentration across a pipe. If the solid particles are coarser, the solid concentration distribution decreases within the near wall region.

The turbulence of the solid particles in the region near a pipe wall was examined by several researchers, such as Nouri and Whitelaw [24], Chen and Kadambi [27], Kuboi et al. [33], Schreck and Kleis [34], and Gai et al. [35]. Researchers observed that the ejection-sweep cycle is affected strongly by particles. They concluded that the slip velocity decreases as the solid concentration increases. The authors emphasised that the presence of solid particles can induce attenuation or amplification of the turbulence. Modification of turbulence depends on the physical properties of the solid and liquid phase. Modulation of turbulence by a dispersed solid particle was also emphasised by Gore and Crowe [36], Sundaresan et al. [37], Jianren et al. [38], Eaton et al. [39], Fessler, J.R.; Eaton [40], and Li et al. [41].

Sundaresan et al. [37] outlined a number of scientific challenges that represent building blocks for a comprehensive understanding of disperse flows encountered in a variety of technologies and in nature. Researchers concluded that new experiments and/or analyses are needed to cast light on the important phenomena that cause turbulence damping or generation. The authors suggested that the experiments should be conducted in simple turbulent flows, such as grid turbulence, fully developed pipe or channel flow, or simple axisymmetric flows. Regardless of geometry, experiments must include a wide range of particle parameters in a single fixed facility. Their conclusions are still outstanding in the mathematical modelling of slurry flow and especially for medium and coarse particles.

In conclusion, one can say that experiments on the influence of solid particles on turbulence are extremely difficult. Measurements at high solid concentrations of the dispersed phase are avoided because of the risk of damage or contamination of intrusive hot film or hot wire probes. With optical methods, the beam is attenuated by particles. As a result of these difficulties, most of the measurements in the literature refer to gas-liquid or gas-solid flows. Other methods of measurement, such as NMR, face problems with resolution, which is fundamental if velocity fluctuations are needed, especially at the pipe wall.

On the basis of the gathered knowledge, we can say that the averaged solid particle diameter has a significant influence on the frictional losses. We know that the difference between the solid and liquid phases is important; however, its importance decreases as the solid concentration increases. Small and medium solid particles can suppress, while large particles can enhance frictional losses. Of course, the phenomenon is more complex as the properties of the solid and liquid phase, and flow conditions, such as the velocity and geometry effect on the level of turbulence.

3. Physical and mathematical model

The physical model assumes that the slurry comprises glass spheres with the cane shape, called Canasphere medium solid particles with average diameters equal to dp = (0.125 and 0.240) mm, and sand particles equal to dp = 0.471 mm, and water as carrier liquid.

All solid particles used in the experiments are rounded and narrowly sized. The solid particle density is 2440 kg/m^3 for Canasphere and 2650 kg/m^3 for Sand. Volume solid concentrations are equal to C_V = (10%, 30%, 40%).

The slurry flow occurs in a vertical pipe with sufficiently high bulk velocity, so the flow can be treated as non-settling and homogeneous. The slurry flow is stationary, turbulent and fully developed. As the vertical flow is considered, it is assumed that the flow is axially symmetric, which means that the velocity components V and W are equal to zero. It is assumed that the viscosity of the slurry is equal to the viscosity of the carrier liquid, while the density of the slurry depends on the solid concentration and is calculated as follows:

$$\rho_m = \rho_L(1 - C_V) + \rho_P C_V \tag{1}$$

The starting point for building the mathematical model is the continuity and the Navier-Stokes equations. Taking into account the physical model, the time-averaged form of the continuity and the Navier-Stokes equations, written in cylindrical coordinates (x, r, φ), can be described as follows:

$$\bar{\rho}_m \frac{\partial \bar{U}}{\partial x} = 0 \tag{2}$$

$$\frac{1}{r}\frac{\partial}{\partial r}\left[r\left(\mu\frac{\partial\bar{U}}{\partial r}-\bar{\rho}_m\bar{u'v'}\right)\right]=\frac{\partial\bar{p}}{\partial x}+\bar{\rho}_m g \tag{3}$$

Eq. (2) indicates that the flow is fully developed. This means that the velocity profile U is unchanged in the flow direction '0x'. The component of the turbulent stress tensor in Eq. (3) is designated by the Boussinesque hypothesis as follows:

$$-\bar{\rho}_m\bar{u'v'}=\mu_t\frac{\partial\bar{U}}{\partial r} \tag{4}$$

The turbulent viscosity (μ_t), stated in Eq. (4), is designated with the support of dimensionless analysis, as follows [42]:

$$\mu_t=f_\mu\frac{\bar{\rho}_m k^2}{\varepsilon} \tag{5}$$

The kinetic energy of turbulence (k) and its dissipation rate (ε), which appear in Eq. (5), are obtained from the Navier-Stokes equation. For the aforementioned assumptions, the final form of k and ε the equations developed by the Launder and Sharma turbulence model [42] are the following:

- equation for the kinetic energy of turbulence:

$$\frac{1}{r}\frac{\partial}{\partial r}\left[r\left(\mu+\frac{\mu_t}{\sigma_k}\right)\frac{\partial k}{\partial r}\right]+\mu_t\left(\frac{\partial\bar{U}}{\partial r}\right)^2=\bar{\rho}_m\varepsilon+2\mu\left(\frac{\partial k^{1/2}}{\partial r}\right)^2 \tag{6}$$

- equation for the dissipation rate of the kinetic energy of turbulence:

$$\frac{1}{r}\frac{\partial}{\partial r}\left[r\left(\mu+\frac{\mu_t}{\sigma_\varepsilon}\right)\frac{\partial\varepsilon}{\partial r}\right]+C_1\frac{\varepsilon}{k}\mu_t\left(\frac{\partial\bar{U}}{\partial r}\right)^2=C_2\left[1-0.3\,exp\left(-Re_t^2\right)\right]\frac{\bar{\rho}_m\varepsilon^2}{k}-2\frac{\mu}{\bar{\rho}_m}\mu_t\left(\frac{\partial^2\bar{U}}{\partial r^2}\right)^2 \tag{7}$$

The turbulent Reynolds number in Eq. (7) is defined using dimensionless analysis, as follows [42]:

$$Re_t=\frac{\bar{\rho}_m k^2}{\mu\varepsilon} \tag{8}$$

The crucial point in the turbulence model is the proper determination of the turbulence damping function (f_μ) in the Eq. (5). This function is also known as the wall damping function. This function is an empirical function and takes low values at a pipe wall. Lower values at the pipe wall cause a decrease in turbulent viscosity and, consequently a decrease in the turbulent stress tensor component, described by Eq. (4). As a function described by Eq. (4) is an empirical function, it is possible to adapt the function (f_μ) for certain applications. For example, Ruffin and Lee [43, 44] successfully used the standard k-ε model of Launder and Spalding [45] and a new wall damping function for the unstructured Cartesian grid solver.

Launder and Sharma [42] proposed the following empirical function for a Newtonian flow, called the standard turbulence damping function:

$$f_\mu = 0.09\,exp\left[\frac{-3.4}{\left(1+\frac{Re_t}{50}\right)^2}\right] \tag{9}$$

For medium slurry flow, Bartosik [46] proposed a new turbulence damping function. This turbulence damping function includes the average particle diameter (dp) and the volume solid concentration (C_V). The proposed turbulence damping function developed for medium slurry flow is the following:

$$f_\mu = 0.09\left\{\frac{-3.4\left[1+A_P^3 d_P^2(8-88A_P d_P)C_V^{0.5}\right]}{\left(1+\frac{Re_t}{50}\right)^2}\right\} \tag{10}$$

where A_P is an empirical constant (A_P = 100).

Eq. (10), which describes the turbulence damping function dedicated for medium slurry, demonstrates that the average diameter of the solid particles plays a primary role, while the solid concentration plays a secondary role. The turbulence damping function (10) was developed based on the comparison between numerical predictions and global measured parameters, such as dp/dx = f(U_b) and velocity profiles for slurry flow in a horizontal pipe in the comprehensive range of mean diameters of solid particle diameters dp = (0.125; 0.240, 0.470) mm and for solid concentrations C_V = (10–40)%. The empirical function (10) approaches the standard turbulence damping function, described in (9), if the solid concentration or the average diameter of the particles is zero.

Figure 1 presents the influence of the average diameter of the solid particles (d) and the turbulent Reynolds number (Ret) on the turbulence damping function, described by Eq. (10). If 'y' goes to zero, the turbulent Reynolds number also goes to zero, as 'k' is approaching zero on the pipe wall. When the averaged solid particle diameter decreases, the turbulence damping function tends to the standard damping function described by Eq. (9) (**Figure 1**). If the diameter of the solid particle increases from dp = 0.125 mm to 0.47 mm, then the turbulence damping function decreases, which is seen in **Figure 1** for Reynolds numbers up to 100. For a turbulent Reynolds

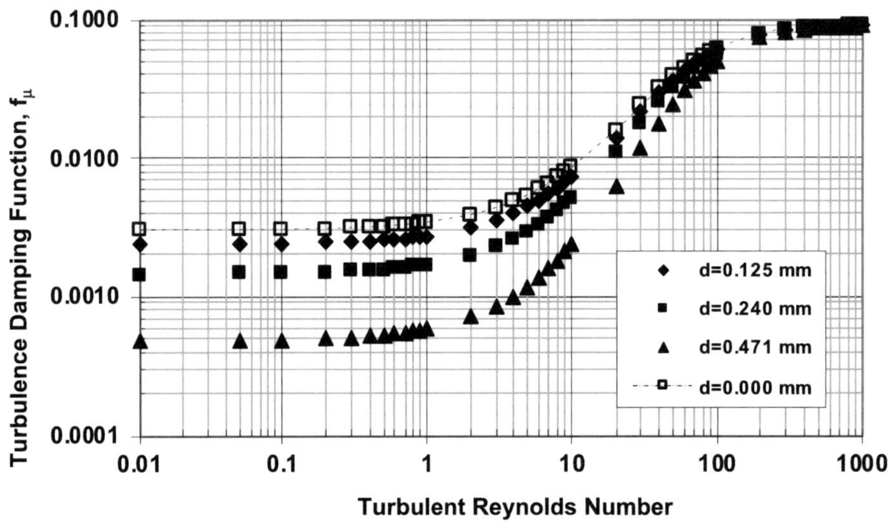

Figure 1.
Dependence of the average diameter of the solid particles and the turbulent Reynolds number on the turbulence damping function at constant solid concentration C_V = 40%.

number greater than 100, the turbulence damping function (10) gives results similar to the function defined by Eq. (9). In **Figure 1** it is seen that the turbulence damping function (10) reaches the minimum value if the average diameter of the solid particles is equal to 0.47 mm. This is in agreement with the Sumner measurements [17].

The turbulence damping function (10), compared to the standard function (9), demonstrates an increase in turbulence damping. It should be emphasised that the lack of measurement of slurry velocity fluctuation components near a solid wall is a limiting factor in the development of new turbulence models suitable for predicting turbulent slurry flow. However, it is possible to suggest a modification of standard turbulence models on the basis of a comparison between predictions and measurements of global parameters, which is demonstrated in this study. The mathematical model of the flow with medium solid particles, which includes the turbulence damping function (10), was developed on the basis of the comparison between prediction and measurements of global parameters. It must be noted, however, that the weakest point of the new turbulence damping function is its dimension.

Finally, the mathematical model of slurry flow with medium solid particles of an average particle diameter between 0.1 mm and 0.5 mm comprises three partial differential equations, namely, (3), (6) and (7), together with the complementary Eqs. (1), (4), (5), (8), and (10). The constants in the turbulence model are the same as those in the Launder and Sharma turbulence model for Newtonian flow [42]: $C_1 = 1.44$; $C_2 = 1.92$; $\sigma_k = 1.0$; $\sigma_\varepsilon = 1.3$. The coefficient A_p in the turbulence damping function was found to be $A_P = 100$. The mathematical model assumes a nonslip velocity at the pipe wall, that is U = 0, and k = 0, and ε = 0. Axially symmetrical conditions were applied at the pipe centre, therefore dU/dr = 0, dk/dr = 0, and dε/dr = 0.

The set of partial differential equations, named (3), (6), and (7), were solved by the TDMA method with an iteration procedure using the control volume method [47] and the author's own computer code.

The criterion of convergence is described as follows:

$$\sum_j \left| \frac{\phi_j^n - \phi_j^{n-1}}{\phi_j^n} \right| \leq 510^{-4} \tag{11}$$

where $\varnothing_j^n$ is a general dependent variable $\varnothing$= U, T, k, ε; the jth is the nodal point after the nth iteration cycle and the $\varnothing_j^{n-1}$ is the (n − 1) iteration cycle.

Numerical calculations were performed for known dp/dx and were performed for 80 nodal points of the differential grid. Nodal points are non-uniformly distributed in the radius of the pipe. Most of the nodal points are located in the vicinity of the pipe wall according to the expansion coefficient. The number of grid points was set experimentally to provide nodally independent computations.

The mathematical model is able to predict the frictional head loss and velocity distribution in a fully developed axially symmetrical pipe flow of medium slurry in a comprehensive range of solid concentrations, that is up to 40% by volume. It is possible to extend the model to the non-isothermal flow if a proper energy equation will be used.

4. Numerical predictions and measurements

To predict the frictional head loss for medium slurry in a turbulent flow, the mathematical model, which includes the new turbulence damping function, is described by Eq. (10), is used. Predictions were made for upward vertical slurry flow containing Canasphere and Sand solid particles in the smooth pipe with an inner diameter equal to D = 0.026 m and for solid concentrations equal C_V = 10%, 30% and 40%. The results of the predictions are compared with the measurements of Shook and Bartosik [8] for the Canasphere particles (t = 27°C) and Sumner [17] for the Sand particles (t = 20°C). Both experiments were performed in a closed vertical loop for fully developed medium slurry flow. The physical properties of the solid particles and slurry, and the carrier liquid, which have been used in experiments and predictions, are collected in **Table 1**.

To demonstrate the importance of the turbulence damping function used in the prediction of frictional head loss, numerical computations were also performed for C_V = 40% using the standard damping function, described by Eq. (9). Such predictions are named 'no damping'.

Figure 2a–c demonstrate a comparison of predictions with measurements [8] of friction head loss in upward vertical slurry flow with average diameter of solid particles dp = 0.125 mm and for solid concentrations C_V = 10%, 30%, and 40%.

Analysing **Figure 2a–c**, it is seen that an increase in solid concentration results in an increase in frictional head loss (dp/dx). Predictions are well-matched measurements for all applied solid concentrations. **Figure 2c** shows that there is no significant difference between the results of the predictions using different wall damping functions. **Figure 2a–c** shows that the frictional head loss of the slurry differs significantly compared to the flow of the water. It looks like it is the effect of different densities between the slurry and water. For example, considering the data presented in **Figure 2c** and choosing a bulk velocity equal to U_b = 5 m/s, we can estimate that the measured dp/dx is equal to ab. 26,500 Pa/m, while for water flow it is 17,500 Pa/m. It means that dp/dx for slurry flow is ab. 1.51 higher compared to water. However, the density of the slurry is equal to that of ab. 1574 kg/m^3, which means that in accordance with the Darcy-Weisbach equation, we expect that dp/dx for the slurry flow should be ab. 1.58 (ρ_m/ρ_L = 1.58) is higher compared to water, while it is 1.51. In such a case, we can say that the results of the predictions are about our expectation, since the difference is rather small.

If the particle diameter increases from dp = 0.125 mm to dp = 0.240 mm, the measurements demonstrate a decrease in frictional head loss for the same solid concentration, which is seen by comparing the measurements presented in **Figure 2a** vs. **Figure 3a**, **Figure 2b** vs. **Figure 3b** and **Figure 2c** vs. **Figure 3c**. On the basis of this, it can be expected that the damping process of turbulence is higher for the slurry with

Solid particles	d_P (mm)	ρ_P, (kg/m^3)	C_V (%)	ρ_m (kg/m^3)
Canasphere	0.125	2440	10	1140.57
	0.240		20	1429.33
			30	1573.71
Sand	0.470	2650	10	1163.38
			30	1493.74
			40	1658.92

Table 1.
Properties of solid particles, slurry and carrier liquid.

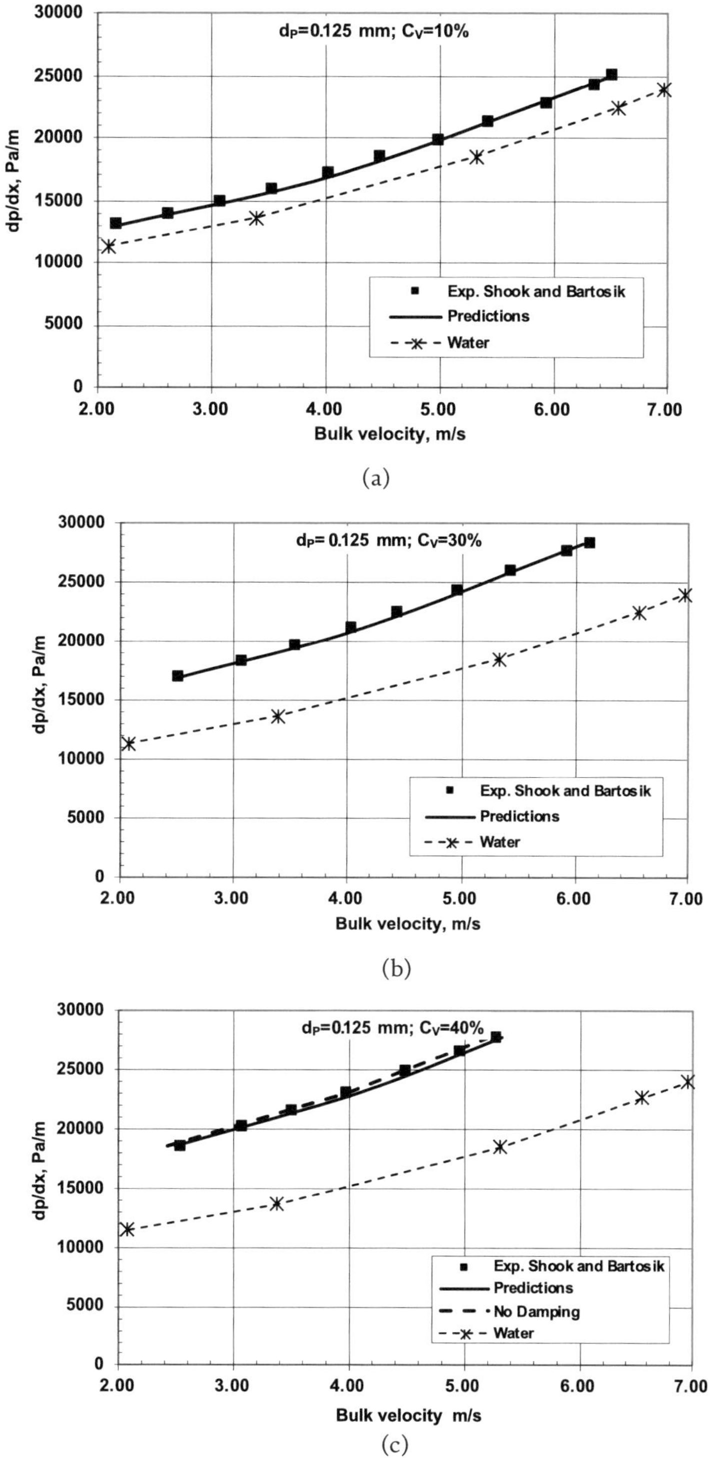

Figure 2.

Predictions and measurements of frictional head loss in upward vertical flow of Canasphere slurry and water in pipe D = 0.026 m: (a) dp = 0.125 mm, C_V = 10%; (b) dp = 0.125 mm, 11C_V = 30%; and (c) dp = 0.125 mm, C_V = 40%.

dp = 0.240 mm than for the slurry with dp = 0.125 mm. To better illustrate this, let us consider the measurements presented in **Figure 3c** for a bulk velocity equal to 5 m/s, which corresponds to dp/dx = 25,000 Pa/m. For the same bulk velocity, the dp/dx for water is 17,500 Pa/m. This means that for slurry flow, the frictional head loss is ab. 1.43 higher compared to water. However, the density of the slurry is equal to that of ab. 1574 kg/m^3, so we expect that dp/dx for the slurry flow should be ab. 1.58 higher compared to water, while it is 1.43. In such a case, we can talk about some damping of the turbulence.

The results or predictions presented in **Figure 3a–c** are in good agreement with the measurements. However, if the standard turbulence damping function is used, Eq. (9), the discrepancy between the predicted and measured frictional head loss is evident; see **Figure 3c**.

If the particle diameter increases from dp = 0.240 mm to dp = 0.470 mm, the measurements demonstrate that for the same solid concentration, frictional head loss continues to decrease, which is seen by comparing the measurements presented in **Figure 3a** vs. **Figure 4a**, **Figure 3b** vs. **Figure 4b** and **Figure 3c** vs. **Figure 4c**.

It is interesting to analyse the data presented in **Figure 4b**, which present frictional head loss for sand slurry with dp = 0.47 mm and C_V = 30%. Bartosik [46, 48] presented such data after subtracting the gravitational term and demonstrated that the frictional head loss is close to the water flow, although the solid concentration is high and equal ρ_m = 1494 kg/m^3.

Trying again to illustrate the damping process of turbulence, let us consider the measurements presented in **Figure 4b** for a bulk velocity equal to 5 m/s, which corresponds to dp/dx = 22,000 Pa/m. For the same bulk velocity of water, dp/dx = 17,500 Pa/m. This means that in the slurry flow, the frictional head loss is ab. 1.26 higher compared to water. However, we took into account the density of the slurry, which is ab. 1494 kg/m^3, and water density, which is 998.20 kg/m^3, we expect dp/dx for the slurry flow to be ab. 1.50 higher compared to water, while it is 1.26. In such a case, we can talk about the damping of the turbulence, which is higher for the slurry with dp = 0.470 mm than for the slurry with dp = 0.240 mm. Experiments presented in **Figure 4a–c** clearly indicate that turbulence damping exists.

Figure 4a–c present the predictions of frictional head loss, with the turbulence damping function depending on particle diameter and solid concentration matching measurements. However, the prediction of slurry frictional head loss using the standard turbulence damping function, described in (9), gives high friction compared to the Sumner measurements [17], which is seen in **Figure 4c**. In this particular case, the predicted frictional head loss using the standard turbulence model is about 22% higher compared to the measurements.

The predictions presented in **Figures 2–4** confirm that the mathematical model, which includes the turbulence damping function depending on (dp) and (C_V), is dedicated to predict the frictional head loss of slurry flow with medium solid particle diameters in the range from 0.125 mm to 0.470 mm.

Comparison of the slurry velocity profile predictions in the vertical upward pipeline with Sumner measurements [17] for dp = 0.47 mm and different solid concentrations and bulk velocities is presented in **Figure 5a** and **b**. Predictions are similar to the measurements; however, in **Figure 5a** the measured velocity profile is slightly steeper compared to the predictions, while in **Figure 5b** it looks opposite; that is, the measured velocity profile is flatter in the core region compared to the prediction.

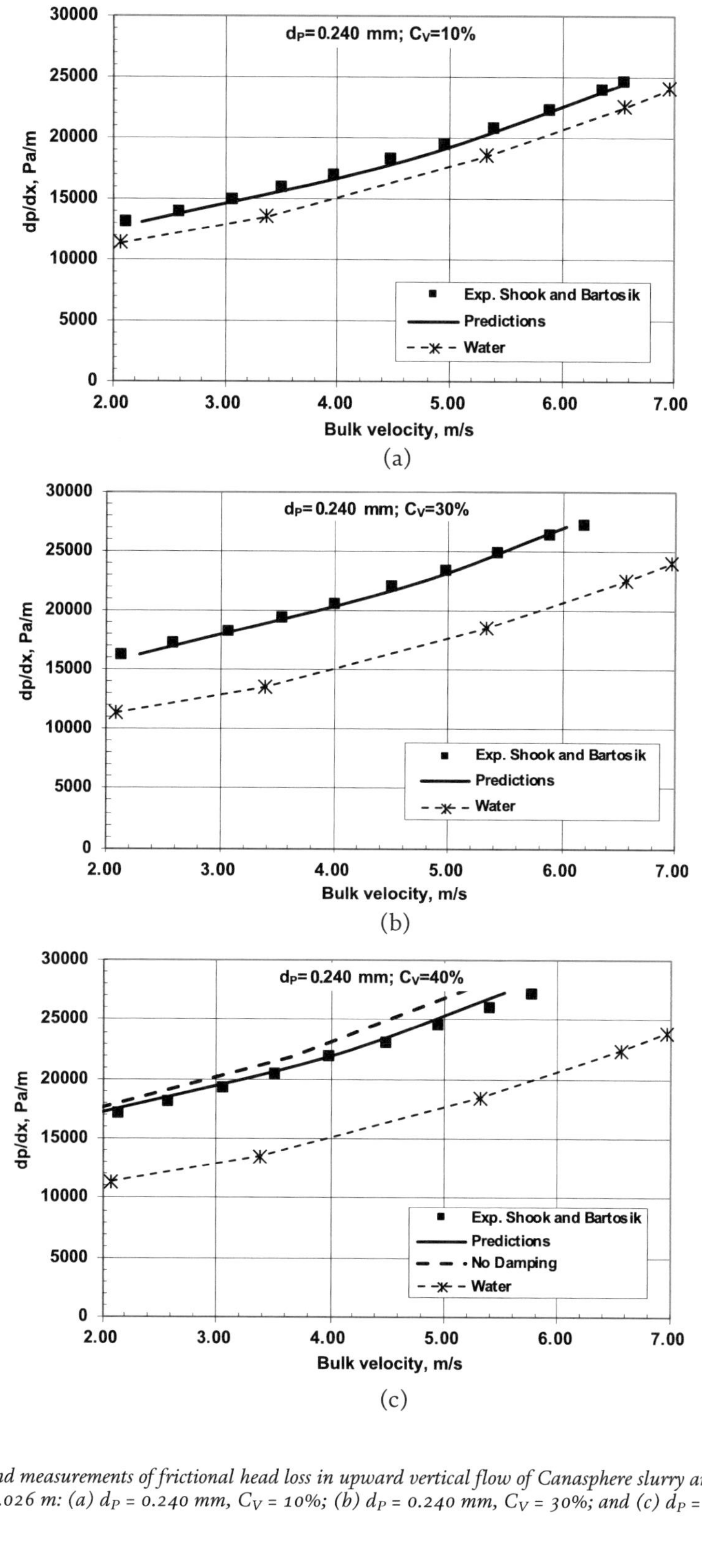

Figure 3.
Predictions and measurements of frictional head loss in upward vertical flow of Canasphere slurry and water in pipe D = 0.026 m: (a) d_P = 0.240 mm, C_V = 10%; (b) d_P = 0.240 mm, C_V = 30%; and (c) d_P = 0.240 mm, C_V = 40%.

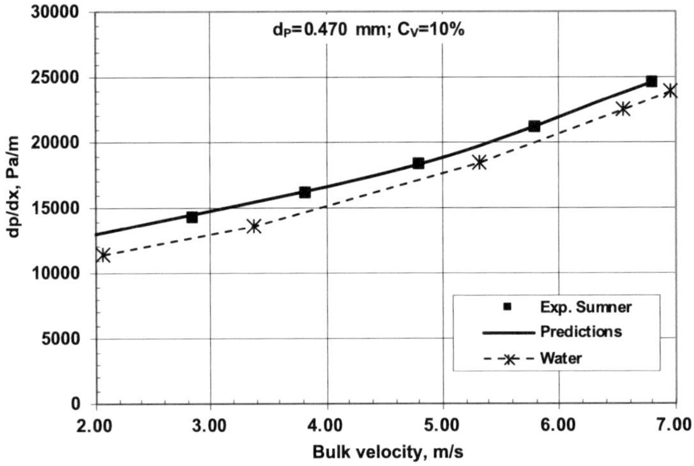

(a)

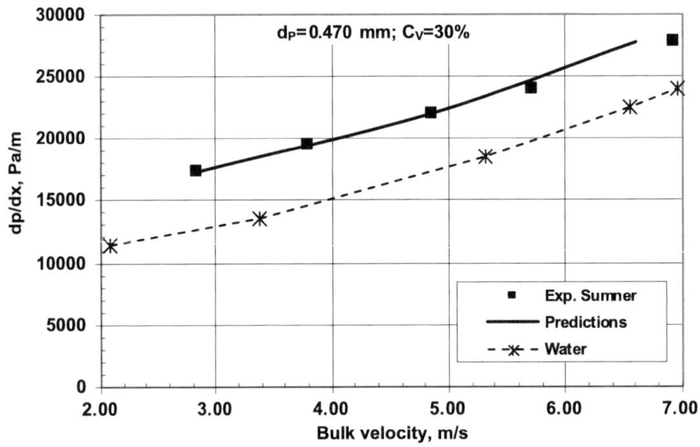

(b)

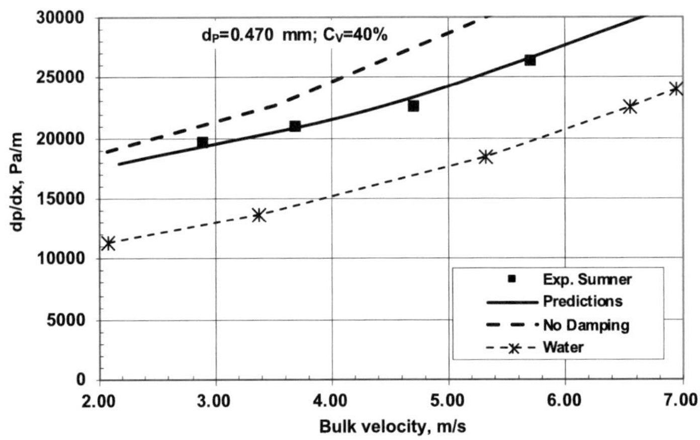

(c)

Figure 4.
Predictions and measurements of frictional head loss in upward vertical flow of sand slurry and water in pipe $D = 0.026$ m: (a) $d_P = 0.470$ mm, $C_V = 10\%$; (b) $d_P = 0.470$ mm, $C_V = 30\%$; and (c) $d_P = 0.470$ mm, $C_V = 40\%$.

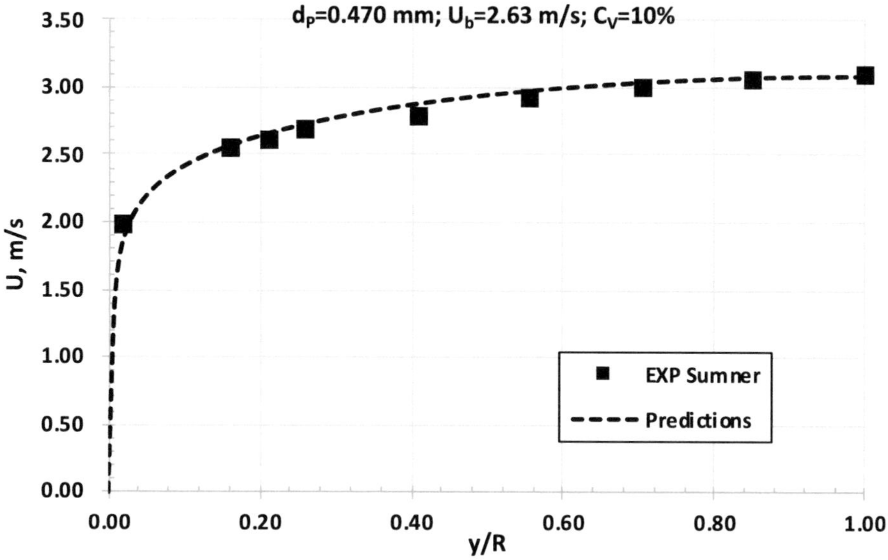

(a)

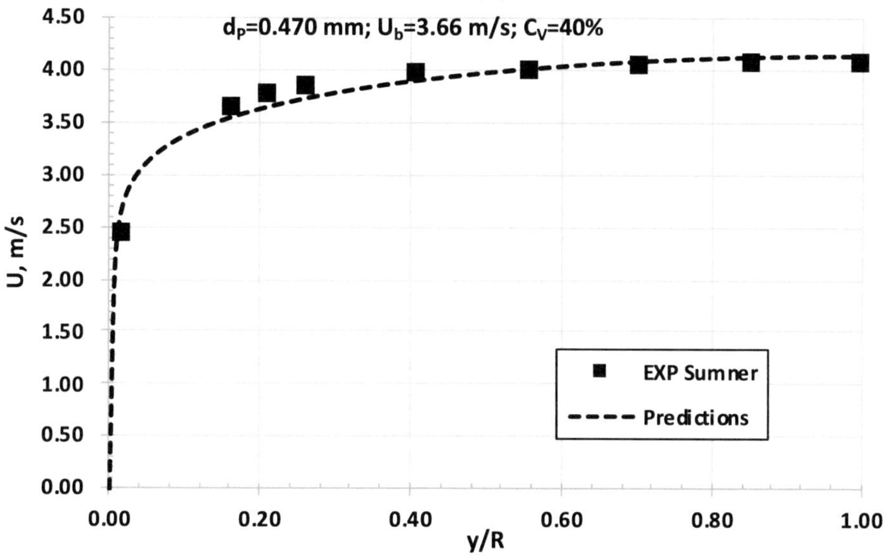

(b)

Figure 5.
Predictions and measurements of the velocity distribution in upward vertical flow of sand slurry in pipe D = 0.026 m: (a) d_P = 0.470 mm, C_V = 10%, U_b = 2.63 m/s; and (b) d_P = 0.470 mm, C_V = 40%, U_b = 3.66 m/s.

In conclusion, experimental data and predictions of medium slurry flow of average diameters equal to 0.125 mm, 0.240 mm and 0.470 demonstrate that the frictional head loss is significantly dependent on particle size and solid concentration. We can say that if the average diameter of the solid particles increases from dp = 0.125 mm to 0.470 mm, the frictional head loss decreases. Such a phenomenon is well predicted if the turbulence damping function, described by Eq. (10), is incorporated into the mathematical model.

5. Discussion and conclusions

If the solid particles are sufficiently fine, the slurry flows usually exhibit non-Newtonian behaviour. This requires the inclusion of a proper rheological model into the mathematical model. Fine solid particles can move freely inside the viscous sublayer, and the friction process proceeds similar to a carrier liquid flow [49]. If the solid particles are coarse or medium, it is impossible to measure the rheology as the sedimentation process occurs. In such a case, it is reasonable to assume that the viscosity is equal to the carrier liquid viscosity and that the density depends on the solid concentration [50]. If a vertical flow is considered, it is reasonable to assume that the flow is axially symmetrical. When the solid density is low or the bulk velocity is sufficiently high, the sedimentation process is limited and, in some cases, we can assume that the flow is pseudo-homogeneous or homogeneous.

When solid particles are larger than the thickness of the viscous sublayer, such as medium and coarse particles, their contact with the pipe wall is limited as a result of the emerging lift forces that push the solid particles away from the wall. Therefore, assuming that there is limited contact of the solid particles with the pipe wall, it can be assumed that the wall shear stress would be similar to the flow of the carrier liquid. Additionally, the presence of solid particles in a carrier liquid can suppress velocity fluctuations. This process is extremely complex, especially in the buffer layer, and is still not well understood. We know from several examples in the literature that in some cases the frictional head loss in turbulent slurry flow in a vertical pipe is similar to the carrier liquid, as presented in this study. This was observed not only by Sumner [17] but also by other researchers who conducted experiments on sand-water mixtures, such as, Talmon [12] for dp = 0.1 to 2.0 mm, Charles and Charles [51] for dp = 0.216 mm, Ghosh and Shook [52] for dp = 0.6 mm, Matousek [53] for dp = 0.37 mm.

This study demonstrates the influence of the average diameter of the solid particles (dp) on the damping of turbulence in the solid-liquid flow with medium solid particles (dp = 0.125–0.470 mm). Damping of turbulence caused by the presence of certain solid particles causes a decrease of the frictional head loss. The other important parameter that affects frictional head loss is solid concentration (C_V).

The study demonstrates that the mathematical model, which uses the standard turbulence damping function, is not suitable to predict slurry flow with medium solid particles. However, it was also demonstrated that using the turbulence damping function in the mathematical model, depending on the averaged solid particle diameter and solid concentration, is the right direction in developing mathematical models to predict the frictional head loss in medium slurry flow. The mathematical model with the turbulence damping function described by Eq. (10) allows predicting the frictional head loss, friction factor and slurry velocity profiles if the slurry flow is fully developed, the stationary, axially symmetrical and averaged solid particle diameters are between 0.1 mm and 0.5 mm. The mathematical model does not include phenomena caused by the slip velocity between the liquid and the solid phase, lift forces acting on solid particles at the pipe wall. However, the model includes the aforementioned phenomena globally through the wall damping function depending on $f_\mu = f(dp, C_V)$.

Considering the upward vertical slurry flow of medium solid particles with average diameters from 0.1 mm to 0.5 mm, one can formulate the following conclusions:

1. The diameter of the solid particles plays an important role in predicting the frictional head loss.

2. In the range of the average diameters of solid particles from 0.125 mm to 0.47 mm, the lowest frictional head loss was achieved for dp = 0.47 mm and C_V = 30%.

3. Experiments and predictions indicate that the process of damping of turbulence occurs and depends mainly on the size of the averaged particle diameter, whereas solid concentration plays a secondary role.

4. It is not recommended to use standard turbulence models for the prediction of medium slurry flow.

5. The wall damping function described by Eq. (10), which depends on the average particle diameter and solid concentration, together with the momentum equation and the Launder and Sharma turbulence model, in which the molecular viscosity of the carrier liquid and the density of the slurry were used, provides reasonable predictions of the frictional head loss and velocity profiles.

The mathematical model requires an additional examination of the predicted velocity profiles, especially in the pipe wall. However, it is difficult to obtain such measurements. To develop new turbulence models dedicated for slurry flow, measurements of fluctuating components of the velocity are needed.

Nomenclature

A_P	constant in the turbulence damping function
C_i	constant in Launder and Sharma turbulence model, i = 1, 2
C_V	solids concentration (volume fraction of solids averaged in cross section), %
d_P	averaged solid particle diameter, μm
D	inner pipe diameter, m
f_μ	turbulence damping function
j	nodal point
k	kinetic energy of turbulence, m^2/s^2
p	static pressure, Pa
Re	Reynolds number
r	cylindrical coordinate, distance from symmetry axis, m
U	velocity component in main flow direction ‘0x’, m/s
V	velocity component in direction ‘0r’, m/s
W	velocity component in direction ‘0φ’, rad/s
u’	fluctuating component of velocity U, m/s
v’	fluctuating component of velocity V, m/s
x	cylindrical coordinate, main flow direction, m
y	radial distance from a pipe wall, m
-	time averaged

Greek symbols

Δx	pipe unit length
ε	rate of dissipation of kinetic energy of turbulence, m^2/s^3

φ	cylindrical coordinate, angle around pipe symmetry axis, deg.
Φ	general dependent variable, Φ = U, k, ε
λ	friction factor
μ	dynamic viscosity coefficient, Pa·s
ν	kinematic viscosity coefficient, m^2/s
ρ	density, kg/m^3
σ_i	diffusion coefficients in k–ε turbulence model, i = k, ε
τ	shear stress, Pa

Subscripts

b	bulk (cross-sectional averaged value)
i	index, i = 1, 2
j	number of nodal points
L	liquid
m	slurry (solid-liquid mixture)
n	number of iterations
P	solid particle/solid phase
t	turbulent
w	solid wall

Author details

Artur S. Bartosik
Kielce University of Technology, Kielce, Poland

*Address all correspondence to: artur.bartosik@tu.kielce.pl

References

[1] Dong H, Abdul Aziz N, Mohd Shafri HZ, Bin Ahmad KA. Numerical study on transportation of cemented paste backfill slurry in bend pipe. PRO. 2022;**10**(1454):1-19

[2] Javed K, Vaezi M, Kurian V, Kumar A. Frictional behaviour of wheat straw-water suspensions in vertical upward flows. Biosystems Engineering. 2021;**212**:30-45

[3] Dai Y, Zhang Y, Li X. Numerical and experimental investigations on pipeline internal solid-liquid mixed fluid for deep ocean mining. Ocean Engineering. 2021; **220**:108411. DOI: doi.org/10.1016/j.oceaneng.2020.108411

[4] Shook CA, Roco MC. Slurry Flow: Principles and Practice. Boston: Butterworth–Heinemann; 1991

[5] Wilson KC, Addie GR, Sellgren A, Clift R. Slurry Transport Using Centrifugal Pumps. 3rd ed. New York: Springer-Verlag; 2006

[6] Chen ZX, Hu HX, Guo XM, Zheng YG. Effect of groove depth on the slurry erosion of V-shaped grooved surfaces. Wear. 2022;**488–489**:204133

[7] Bagnold RA. Experiments on a gravity–free dispersion of large solids spheres in a Newtonian fluid under shear. Proceedings of the Royal Society. 1954;**225**(A):49-63. DOI: 10.1098/rspa.1954.0186

[8] Shook CA, Bartosik AS. The pseudohomogeneous flow approximation for dispersed two-phase systems. Particulate Science and Technology. 1991;**9**:119-134

[9] Wiwatanapataphee B, Chayantrakom K, Wu YH. Mathematical modelling and numerical simulation of fluid-magnetic particle flow in a small vessel. International Journal of Mathematical Models and Methods in Applied Sciences. 2007;**1**(3):209-215

[10] Abdel-Rahman AA. A closed-form expression for an abrasive waterjet cutting model for ceramic materials. International Journal of Mathematical Models and Methods in Applied Sciences. 2011;**5**(4):722-729

[11] Doron P, Granica D, Barnea D. Slurry flow in horizontal pipes experimental and modelling. International Journal of Multiphase Flow. 1987;**13**(4):535-547

[12] Talmon AM. Analytical model for pipe wall friction of pseudo-homogenous sand slurries. Particulate Science and Technology. 2013;**31**(3):264-270

[13] Bartosik A. Influence of coarse-dispersive solid phase on the 'particles–wall' shear stress in turbulent slurry flow with high solid concentration. The Archive of Mechanical Engineering. 2010;**LVII**(1):45-68

[14] Wilson KC, Thomas AD. A new analysis of the turbulent flow of non-Newtonian fluids. Canadian Journal of Chemical Engineering. 1985;**63**:539-546

[15] Lovato S, Keetels GH, Toxopeus SL, Settels JW. An eddy-viscosity model for turbulent flows of Herschel-Bulkley fluids. Journal of Non-Newtonian Fluid Mechanics. 2022;**301**:1-13

[16] Bartosik A. Application of rheological models in prediction of turbulent slurry flow. Flow, Turbulence and Combustion. Springer-Verlag. 2010; **84**(2):277-293

[17] Sumner RJ. Concentration Variations and their Effects in Flowing Slurries and Emulsions. Saskatoon. Canada: University of Saskatchewan; 1992

[18] Soo SL. Multiphase Fluid Dynamics. Beijing: Science Press; 1990

[19] Roberts CPR, Kennedy JF. Particle and fluid velocities of turbulent flows of suspensions of neutrally buoyant particles. In: Zandi I, editor. Advances in Solid-liquid Flow in Pipes and Its Applications. Oxford: Pergamon Press; 1971. pp. 59-72

[20] Kowalewski A. Velocity profiles of suspension flowing through a tube. Archives in Mechanics. 1980;**32**(6): 857-865

[21] Altobelli SA, Givler RC, Fukushima E. Velocity and concentration measurements of suspensions by nuclear magnetic resonance imaging. Journal of Rheology. 1991;**35**(5):721-734

[22] Yianneskis M, Whitelaw JH. Velocity characteristics of pipe and jet flows with high particle concentration. ASME Symposium on Liquid-Solid Flows and Erosion Wear in Industrial Equipment. 1983;**13**:12-15

[23] Nouri JM, Whitelaw JH, Yianneskis M. Particle motion and turbulence in dens two-phase flows. International Journal of Multiphase Flow. 1987;**13**:729-739

[24] Nouri JM, Whitelaw JH. Particle velocity characteristics of dilute to moderately dense suspension flows in stirred reactors. International Journal of Multiphase Flow. 1992;**18**(1):21-33

[25] Wildman DJ, Ekmann JM, Kadambi JR, Chen RC. Study of the flow properties of slurries using the refractive index matching technique and LDV. Powder Technology. 1992;**73**(3):211-218

[26] Chen RC, Kadambi JR. Experimental and numerical studies of solid-liquid pipe flow. ASME Liquid-Solid Flows. 1994;**189**:123-135

[27] Chen RC, Kadambi JR. Discrimination between solid and liquid velocities in slurry flow using doppler velocimeter. ASME Powder Technology. 1995;**85**:127-134

[28] Shook CA. Experiments with concentrated slurries of particles with densities near that of the carrier fluid. Canadian Journal of Chemical Engineering. 1985;**63**:861-869

[29] Sumner RJ, Mckibben M, Shook CA. Concentration measurements in pipelines containing flowing two-phase mixtures. Petroleum Society of CIM. Paper No. PETSOC-SS-89-08. 1989. pp. 1-8

[30] Nasr-El-Din H, Shook CA, Colwell J. A conductivity probe for measuring local concentrations in slurry systems. International Journal of Multiphase Flow. 1987;**13**(3):365-378

[31] Sumner RJ, McKibben M, Shook CA. Concentration and velocity distribution in turbulent vertical slurry flow. Journal of Solid Liquid Flow. 1991;**2**(2):33-42

[32] Nasr-El-Din H, Shook CA, Colwell J. The lateral variation of solids concentration in horizontal slurry pipeline flow. International Journal of Multiphase Flow. 1987;**13**:661-670

[33] Kuboi R, Komasawa I, Otake T. Fluid and particle motion in turbulent dispersion–II—Influence of turbulence of liquid on the motion of suspended particles. Chemical Engineering Science. 1974;**29**:651-657

[34] Schreck S, Kleis SJ. Modification of grid–generated turbulence by solid particles. Journal of Fluid Mechanics. 1993;**249**:665-688

[35] Gai G, Hadjadj A, Kudriakov S, Thomine O. Particles-induced turbulence: A critical review of physical concepts, numerical modeling and experimental investigations. Theoretical & Applied Mechanics Letters. 2020;**10**: 241-248

[36] Gore RA, Crowe CT. Modulation of turbulence by a dispersed phase. Journal of Fluid Engineering. 1991;**113**:304-307

[37] Sundaresan S, Eaton J, Koch DL, Ottino JM. Appendix 2: Report of study group on disperse flow. International Journal of Multiphase Flow. 2003;**29**: 1069-1087

[38] Jianren F, Junmei S, Youqu Z, Kefa C. The effect of particles on fluid turbulence in a turbulent boundary layer over a cylinder. Acta Mechanics Sinica. 1997;**13**:36-43

[39] Eaton JK, Paris AD, Burton TM. Local distortion of turbulence by dispersed particles. AIAA. 2012;**2012**: 3643

[40] Fessler JR, Eaton JK. Turbulence modification by particles in a backward-facing step flow. Journal of Fluid Mechanics. 1999;**394**:97-117

[41] Li D, Luo K, Fan J. Modulation of turbulence by dispersed solid particles in a spatially developing flat-plate boundary layer. Journal of Fluid Mechanics. 2016;**802**:359-394

[42] Launder BE, Sharma BI. Application of the energy-dissipation model of turbulence to the calculation of flow near a spinning disc. Letters in Heat and Mass Transfer. 1974;**1**:131-138

[43] Ruffin SM, Lee JD. Adaptation of a k-epsilon model to a cartesian grid based methodology. International Journal of Mathematical Models and Methods in Applied Sciences. 2011;**3**(3):238-245

[44] Ruffin SM, Lee JD. Flow field prediction accuracy and efficiency using a cartesian grid framework. International Journal of Mathematical Models and Methods in Applied Sciences. 2011;**3**(3): 246-255

[45] Launder BE, Spalding DB. The numerical computation of turbulent flows. Computer Methods in Mechanics and Engineering. 1974;**3**:269-289

[46] Bartosik A. Mathematical modelling of slurry flow with medium solid particles, Monograph: Mathematical Models and Methods in Modern Science, Int. Conf. Mathematical Models for Engineering Science. 2011. Spain

[47] Roache PJ. Computational Fluid Dynamics. Albuquerque: Hermosa Publ; 1982

[48] Bartosik A. Simulation of medium slurry flow with enhanced damping of turbulence. In: Proc. Transport and Sedimentation of Solid Particles. Rostock, Germany; 2013. pp. 215-226

[49] Coulson JM, Richardson JF, Backhurst JR, Hraker JH. Chemical Engineering. Butterworth-Heinemann; 1996

[50] Bartosik A. Validation of friction factor predictions in vertical slurry flows with coarse particles. Journal of Hydrology and Hydromechanics. 2020; **68**(2):119-127

[51] Charles ME, Charles RA. Advances in Solid-liquid Flow and Its Applications. New York: Pergamon Press; 1971

[52] Ghosh T, Shook CA. Freight pipelines. In: Liu H, Round GF, editors. Freight Pipelines. Washington, DC: Hemisphere; 1990. pp. 281-288

[53] Matousek V. Research developments in pipeline transport of settling slurries. Powder Technology. 2005;**156**:43-51

Chapter 4

High Concentration, Coarse Particle, Hydraulic Conveying

Lionel Pullum

Abstract

Conventional coarse particle hydraulic conveying is performed under turbulent flow conditions, usually at concentrations of less than 40% v/v. The last three or four decades have seen the development of much higher concentration conveying, with the successful transport of suspensions of 70% v/v or more. These suspensions can be conveyed at very low velocities and generally exhibit very benign characteristics, having the capability of being stopped and restarted at will. There are generally two methods of pumping coarse materials safely at low velocities. The first method, using a Newtonian such as water, can be applied when the particle size distribution is sufficiently broad to minimize percolation and the concentration sufficiently high to prevent particle restructuring during transport. A second method uses a non-Newtonian, visco-plastic carrier fluid, normally fine particle slurry, to convey the coarser particles. This second method removes the constraints of the first method, allowing a greater range of coarse solid distributions and concentrations to be pumped. In both cases, the conveying characteristics appear similar to laminar flow. Both methods are described and analyzed in this chapter.

Keywords: hydraulic transport, coarse particle, high concentration, no-Newtonian, hybrid suspension

1. Introduction

Except for the transport of pastes and non-Newtonian slurries, most hydraulic transport applications operate under turbulent conditions at low to moderate volumetric concentrations. This contrasts with pneumatic transport systems which operate in both dilute, or lean, phase conveying and dense phase conveying. Dilute phase is analogous to this form of hydraulic conveying, while dense phase conveys solids at much higher solids' concentrations and at lower velocities. Over the last three or four decades, advances have been made in the development of higher concentration hydraulic transport systems, which share many characteristics in common with dense phase pneumatic systems.

Conventional hydraulic transport systems are turbulent, relying on the action of turbulent eddies to suspend and convey the solids in the pipe. At high velocities, the solids' suspension is almost uniform across the pipe, while at lower velocities, a pronounced concentration profile appears, forming sliding and even stationary beds of solids on the bottom of the pipe. Such flows are unstable and solids' transport will stop when the mean velocity falls below a minimum conveying velocity, and may even block the pipe. To minimize this risk of blockage and assist in restarting, a rule of thumb is used whereby the in-line solids' concentration, Cv_i, is generally limited to less than 40% v/v. The minimum conveying velocity is a function of the solids' concentration, size and density, and can typically range from 1 to 2 m/s for fine particles (d < 1 mm say) to 7–10 m/s for coarse particles (d > 5 mm say).

Despite these unstable characteristics, such conveying has many advantages in the main areas where it is practiced, namely inter-process transfer, dredging, tailings disposal and long distant transport of ore or concentrates. It is simple to operate, requiring only that those solids are mixed with water in a suitably agitated vessel of some form, and pumped, normally using centrifugal pumps, through the pipeline to their destination. The low concentration also affords easy separation of the solids from the conveying fluid.

By contrast, outside of the food and some process industries, high concentration conveying is rarely seen, concrete pumping being the most obvious exception. However, high concentration systems have been developed and are finding increasing use in tailings disposal, hoisting and other niche applications. Their attractiveness lies in their benign operation, as they generally do not require a minimum conveying velocity, so lines can be stopped and restarted at will. Their low velocity, typically of order 1–2 m/s, several meters per second lower than their coarse particle low concentration counterparts, results in low particle attrition and pipe wear. This mode of conveying also allows very coarse particles to be conveyed at low particle pipe diameter ratios, e.g., $D/d \leq 5$. The high concentration, $40 < Cv \leq 75\%$ v/v, also produces low specific energy consumption (SEC), producing low operating costs (OPEX) and low greenhouse gas emissions. These advantages, however, are offset against a more complex operating system and the need for more specialized equipment (CAPEX).

Two forms of high concentration conveying have been developed, one using Newtonian fluids, like water, as the carrier fluid to convey the solids, and a second using non-Newtonian carrier fluids. Although sharing many characteristics, these methods will be described separately starting with the Newtonian system.

2. Newtonian high concentration conveying

2.1 Concentration considerations

While weight concentration, *Cw* w/w, or worse weight of solids per volume of liquid, *Cwv* w/v, are common in industry, it is the volumetric concentration, *Cv* v/v, that characterizes and controls the way a suspension of solids behaves. At high concentrations, another more useful way of describing the solids' concentration is the ratio of the volumetric concentration to the maximum packing concentration of the solids, or more usually the maximum dilated or loose poured concentration, i.e., Cv/Cb known as the reduced concentration. The term *Cb* is used here to denote this packing concentration, as this value corresponds to the in-situ concentration of a settled or sliding bed of solids within the pipe. For non-Newtonian systems, described in §3, the bed concentration will be lower than for Newtonian systems, and will be described in greater detail there. This value may be considered to indicate the pipelines obscuration, or particle's mobility.

Cb is a function of the particle's size distribution (PSD) and shape distribution (SSD), from which this value can be calculated (for example [1, 2]), or measured using a procedure outlined by Leuenberger [3], as follows. A tank of initially dry solids is continuously mixed with a pitch-bladed agitator, and the power drawn by the agitator monitored while water is progressively added. An example of such a test is shown in **Figure 1**.

The typical response to the addition of water (**Figure 1b**) is to change the solids from a purely granular flow in air, to one where an increasing number of water bridges are formed. Shearing these as well as the solids requires increasingly more energy. Once all the interstices are filled with water, further addition of water simply separates the particles, reducing the mixer energy requirements. Thus, the value of 1-Cv_{water} corresponding to the peaks in the characteristic curves approximates Cb.

The calculated value of Cb, based on the coal's PSD and SSD, is approximately 89%, whereas the empirical value is around 86%. The discrepancy, although small, is because the empirical value is for a sheared, and hence a dilated bed. It is recommended that the empirical value is used, or that calculated values should be reduced by a couple of percentage points.

2.2 Conveying characteristics

As mentioned in the introduction, both dilute and high concentration conveying is commonplace in pneumatic conveying systems, and the operational or transport characteristics are displayed in what is known as a diagram of state (**Figure 2**).

At moderate to high velocities, the transport characteristics exhibit the familiar hook curves of conventional hydraulic conveying systems, moving from a fully suspended state at high velocities, to sliding beds as the velocity is decreased. After going through a minimum, the pressure gradient rises due to partial obscuration of the pipe and increased particle wall contact. For hydraulic systems, which normally use centrifugal pumps, this is an unstable region, but for pneumatic systems, which use a variety of different feeding systems, e.g., blow vessels, transport can still be obtained down to very low velocities. At these low velocities, the line is filled with solids that

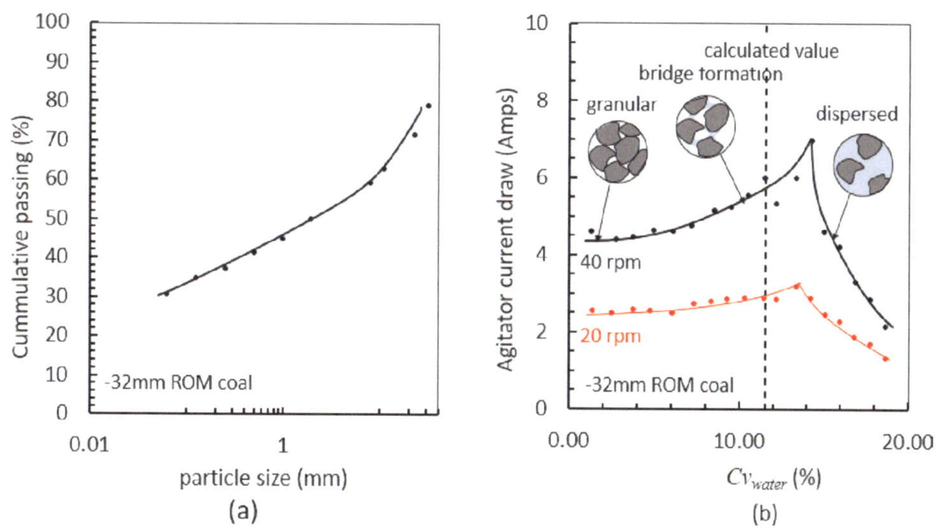

Figure 1.
(a) Broad PSD of typical run of mine (ROM) coal, (b) experimental value for two different agitator speeds and calculated (dashed line) determination of Cb for the same ROM.

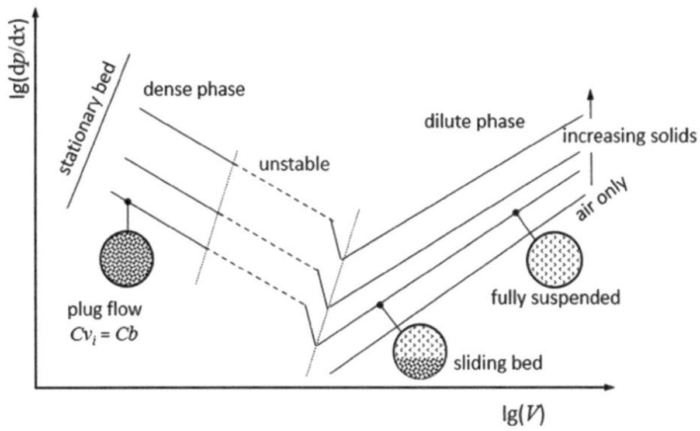

Figure 2.
Diagram of state for coarse particle pneumatic conveying.

move along as a continuous plug, although this plug is often deliberately broken into smaller plugs to reduce the pressure requirements. At intermediary velocities, however, the flow is unstable, exhibiting dune flow that can block the pipe.

Wilson et al. [4] examined the behavior of dense phase hydraulic hoisting, subsequently publishing an analysis of the frictional component of such plug flow [5], and such techniques were employed in the Hansa underground mine to hoist -60 mm coal, 850 m to the surface [6]. To the author's knowledge, though, it was not until the invention of a feeding system called a Rotary Ram Slurry Pump (RRSP), described in §2.7, that dense phase horizontal coarse particle hydraulic conveying was considered at an industrial scale.

The RRSP enabled very high concentrations of coarse particles to be loaded into a pipe using a valving system that opened to the full bore of the conveying pipe. These particles could be conveyed at very low velocities with little, if any, inter-particle movement. This feature was ideal for friable materials such as coal. Transport characteristics for ROM coal conveyed in a 300 mm pipe using this technique are shown in **Figure 3**.

The transport characteristics do not exhibit the typical hooked curves of lower density conveying, although transport below the lowest velocities shown were problematic. Suspensions with concentrations below 65% were also unstable for this particular material. Readings from an isolated electrode probe (see e.g. [7]), inserted into the top of the pipe, registered periodic high activity at these lower concentrations, indicating possible dune formation. A two-layer model, at concentrations close to plug flow, was used to model this flow with satisfactory agreement as shown. However, the adoption of a normal two-layer model is found to substantially overpredict the transport pressure gradients shown, and modification to such a model is needed before the agreement shown here is obtained.

2.3 Two-layer modeling modifications for coarse particles

Only a simple two-layer model (e.g. [8]) will be used in this section for illustrative purposes, and the reader is referred to the chapter on Pipeline Modeling for a more complete description and a more nuanced approach. The early layered models were developed to model the behavior of small sand particle slurries, which become fluidized during transport. This is evident by observing slurry issuing from holes in the upper invert of the conveying pipe, where the slurry behaves as a fluidized jet [9].

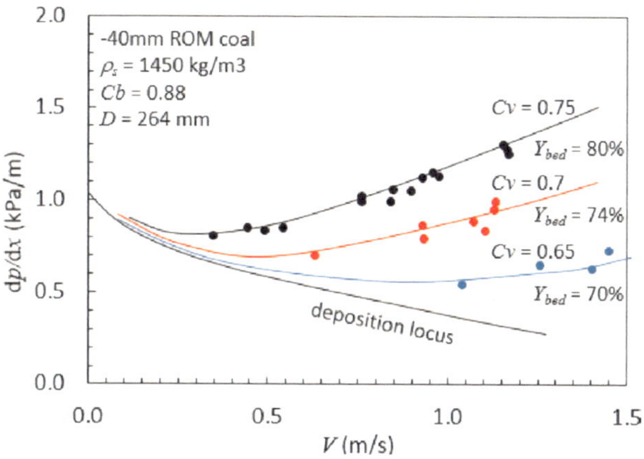

Figure 3.
Typical high concentration, coarse particle, transport characteristics. Computed curves of constant delivered concentrations and partial deposition locus using a two-layer model. The bed depth Y_{bed} *is also shown.*

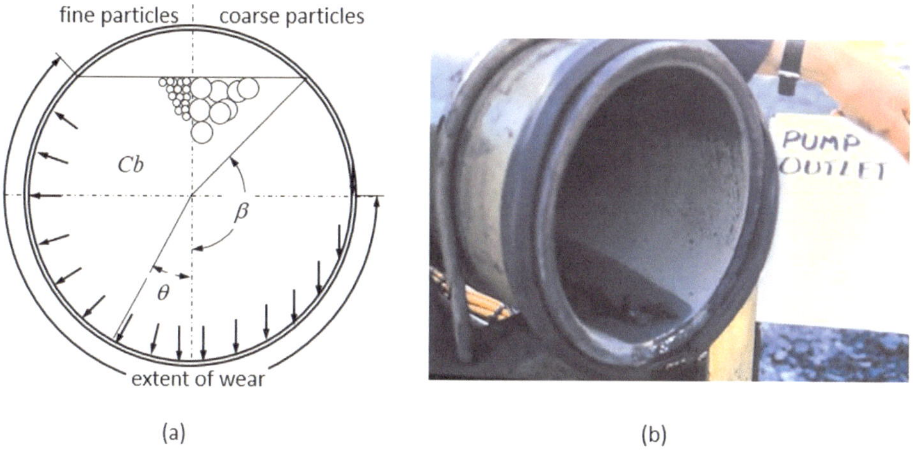

Figure 4.
(a) Schematic of pipe cross section giving the normal force distribution for fine and coarse particles, (b) wear pattern in a 300 mm pipe used for conveying -32 mm solids, showing unworn original oxide coating in pipe upper invert.

Such behavior is not observed in coarse particle flow. This difference has ramifications for the modeling of the resisting force of the bed in a two-layer model. Consider the schematic of the pipe cross section shown in **Figure 4a**.

If the solids are fine and fluidized, the bed presents a hydrostatic pressure at the pipe wall (**Figure 4a**, left hand side), which is normal to the pipe wall. If the density of the fluid and solids are ρ_f and ρ_s, respectively, then the normal force of the bed on the pipe wall is given by

$$N = 2Cb\left(\rho_s - \rho_f\right)gR^2\int_0^{\beta} \cos(\beta) - \cos(\theta)d\theta \tag{1}$$

Where β is the half bed angle shown in **Figure 4a** and which on integrating and rearranging becomes

$$N = 2Cb\left(\rho_s - \rho_f\right)g\frac{D^2}{4}\left(\sin(\beta) - \beta\cos(\beta)\right) \quad (2)$$

Conversely, for unfluidized coarse particles the normal force is simply

$$N = Cb\left(\rho_s - \rho_f\right)g\left(\frac{\pi D^2}{4}\right)(1 - A) \quad (3)$$

where A is the fractional cross-sectional area above the bed and (1-A) is the area of the bed $(1 - A) = (\beta - \sin(\beta)\cos(\beta))/\pi = Cv/Cb$.

The difference between Eqs. (2) and (3) is then a multiplier which accounts for the effect on the resisting force of particle fluidization. Thus, combining Eq. (2), Eq. (3), the bed fractional area and a degree of fluidization $0 < f < 1$, where a value of zero = the unfluidized state, 1 = the fully fluidized state, this multiplier can be written as

$$F = 1 + f\left[2\frac{\sin(\beta) - \beta\cos(\beta)}{\beta - \sin(\beta)\cos(\beta)} - 1\right] \quad (4)$$

and used to describe the bed's normal force for an arbitrarily fluidized bed by

$$N = Cb\left(\rho_s - \rho_f\right)g\left(\frac{\pi D^2}{4}\right)(1 - A)F \quad (5)$$

2.4 Comparison with conventional conveying

Data reported by the Saskatchewan Research Council (SRC) for coarse coal in water [10] show typical results in a similarly sized pipe for -50 mm solids, d_{50} = 3 mm, Cv = 0.457 v/v, D = 234 mm, to be V = 2.5 m/s, dP/dx = 0.64 kPa/m. The conveying velocity is higher than that shown in **Figure 3**, and this, combined with the lower concentration means that particle attrition would be considerable. The pressure gradient, however, is comparable to that of the 70% curve in **Figure 3**. A comparison of the operating costs can be achieved by comparing the *SEC* given by

$$SEC = \frac{\text{suspension pumping power}}{\text{solids mass flow x distance}} = \frac{dp/dx}{3.6Cv\rho_s/\rho_f} \ \text{kWhr}/(\text{tonne km}) \quad (6)$$

where the pressure gradient, dp/dx, is in kPa/m.

Comparing the SRC data with the higher pressure gradient 75% v/v data, the *SEC* for the conventionally conveyed coal is 0.27 kWhr/(tonne km), compared with 0.23 kWhr/(tonne km) for the high concentration conveying. Furthermore, the high concentration system consumes 45% less water. A more detailed comparison of high concentration and non-Newtonian systems, described in §3, with conventional conveying is given in [11].

2.5 Restart capabilities and practical considerations

2.5.1 Restart

As mentioned above, transport at lower concentrations proved problematic through dune formation partially blocking the pipe, resulting in unsteady flow.

Experience gained with the RRSP suggested that an operational concentration range should be limited to $0.75 < Cv/Cb < 0.9$, and that the materials required a broad size distribution such that $Cb > 0.75$ to avoid excessive bed percolation of the low viscosity water carrier.

When operating within these constraints, restart of fully loaded pipelines several kilometers long proved to be immediate once the pumps were activated. The explanation for this is not entirely clear but is expected to relate to the low deposition velocities. The deposition locus for the material in **Figure 5** expressed as a function of Cv/Cb is shown here (**Figure 6**).

At the operational limits for this material the corresponding deposition velocities are approximately 0.6 and 0.2 m/s. Such suspensions started with ease, and it is expected that once the pumps were started, increasing the flow to the normal conveying velocity of a 1 m/s was sufficiently rapid so that reorganization of any particles

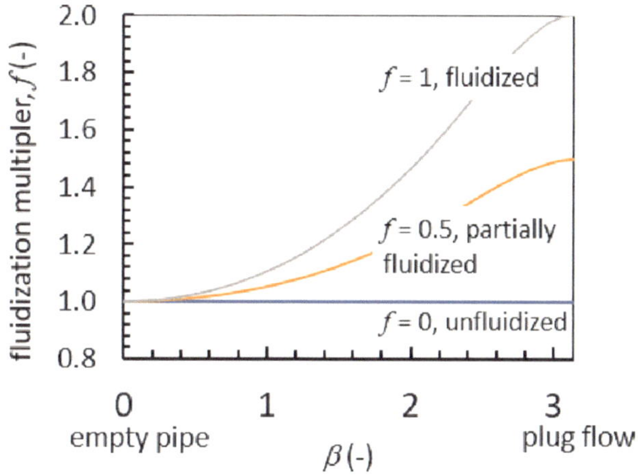

Figure 5.
Normal force fluidization modifier for f = 0, unfluidized coarse particles, f = 0.5, partially fluidized intermediary particles, f = 1 for fully fluidized fine particles.

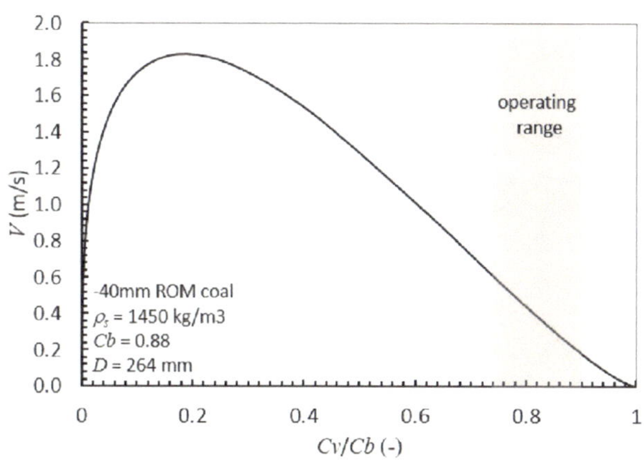

Figure 6.
Deposition locus as a function of Cv/Cb *for the data shown in* ***Figure*** *3. The concentration limits for successful operation are shown shaded.*

above the bed to form a plugging dune did not occur. This is despite the high velocity fluid flowing over the beds, which occupy 75 to 90% of the pipes CSA.

2.5.2 Practical considerations

Production of such suspensions is comparatively easy as the mobility of these suspensions is very high, requiring only gentle agitation in suitable mixing tanks to ensure homogenization. More difficult is maintaining the high concentrations within the required limits, requiring conveyors etc. to be sheltered from rain, and sufficient surge capacity to be installed for constant operation. This last point is less of a problem, as the ability to reduce the transport velocity to very low values or stopping, provides a very large turn down ratio. Maintaining the correct feed to the pump also requires some care, as fluid can be preferentially drawn from the tank diluting the flow into the pump's inlet ducting, producing unstable operation, details of which are described in [12].

2.6 Diagram of state for hydraulic conveying systems

A diagram of state, similar to **Figure 2**, can now be drawn for hydraulic systems, to include high concentration transport, and is shown in **Figure 7**.

The similarities between **Figures 2** and 7 are strong, showing very similar characteristics for dilute or conventional hydraulic conveying, as well as low velocity high concentration flow. In this case, though, rather than the unstable region being simply a function of conveying velocity, it is now a function of solids' concentration being problematic at the intermediary concentrations.

Before leaving this section on Newtonian systems a brief description of the RRSP will be given, although it is noted that other solids feeders can also be successfully employed, e.g. the Kamyr feeder or similar, and various lock hopper systems (e.g. [13]).

2.7 Rotary ram slurry pump

The RRSP was invented by Bede Boyle [14, 15] and further developed by the ASEA Mineral Slurry Transport group [16], who built a 300 mm pipe diameter unit capable of transporting 300 dtph of coarse coal. A schematic illustrating the basic operating principles of this device is shown in **Figure 8**.

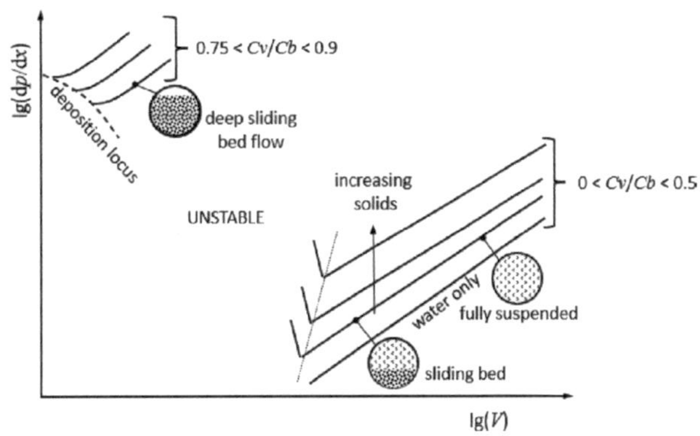

Figure 7.
Diagram of state for water based coarse particle hydraulic conveying.

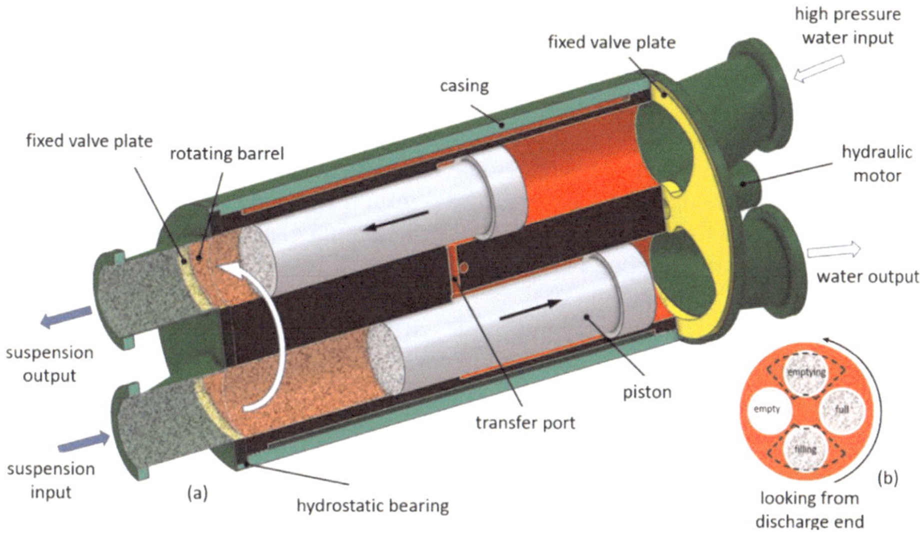

Figure 8.
(a) Partially sectioned schematic of a rotary ram slurry pump, (b) schematic of discharge end of rotating barrel showing the filling and discharging process. Kidney valve locations shown dashed.

The RRSP comprises a barrel, like that in a revolver, containing a multiple number of diametrically opposed paired cylinders and pistons, that rotates on hydro-static bearings inside a casing. The configuration of a four-piston cylinder assembly is shown in **Figure 8a**. Two stationary valve plates each containing a full-bore inlet and full-bore outlet kidney valves are located at either end of the barrel, as shown. Manifolds containing inlet and outlet ducts are attached outboard of these valve plates. The cylinders comprise two bores of different diameters, with the smaller bore at the suspension discharge end of the RRSP. The pistons that run in these cylinders similarly have two diameters to suit the bores in the cylinders. The barrel is rotated by a hydraulic motor, mounted at the water end of the RRSP (right in this Figure), such that the cylinder openings pass the kidney shaped openings in the valve plates, allowing material to periodically enter or exit the cylinders. The upper duct, at the water end, is connected to the output of a multi-stage, high pressure, water pump, and supplies the motive force to drive the suspension. Water is returned via the lower duct to a sump. At the discharge end of the RRSP (left in this figure) the lower duct is connected to a stirred tank containing the suspension to be conveyed, and the upper duct is connected to a matched diameter conveying pipeline. The operation of the RRSP is as follows. While the upper cylinder is exposed through the kidney valve to the high-pressure water supply, the piston is driven forward, discharging the suspension that is in the smaller cylinder into the pipeline. Water contained in the annular volume between the larger upper cylinder and smaller upper piston passes through the transfer port indicated to drive the lower piston backwards. This action induces suspension from the stirred tank through the kidney valve and into the lower smaller cylinder. Since the barrel is continuously rotating, these cylinders move to their horizontal locations, to be replaced by the next pair, indicated in **Figure 8b**, and ultimately to their near vertical location, where the process is repeated. The valving is designed so that contribution from the total of each cylinder pair produces essentially constant continuous flow.

The RRSP's design enables very high concentrations of large particles to be transported, by virtue of the use of the high-pressure centrifugal pumps, rather than by driving the pistons through mechanical means. As the cylinders rotate and the upper suspension cylinder starts to be exposed through the kidney valves to the pipeline, large particles in the cylinder will not be able to pass through the initially small valve opening. The suspension will be compressed, and the piston stopped. As the driving force is supplied by a centrifugal pump, this simply means that the pump's pressure will rise to its shut-off head. The valve opening continues to increase until it is large enough for the trapped particles to pass, and transport continues. This, combined with the full bore opening of the valves, enables very large particles to be conveyed and values of $D/d < 5$ were conveyed as normal practice, compared to the normal upper limit of $D/d > 10$ imposed in conventional conveying.

3. Non-Newtonian high concentration conveying

3.1 A brief history

In the early 70's, tests examining the effect of hydraulic conveying on high concentration coarse coal suspensions [17] showed that as the coal degraded, the transport characteristics changed from the normal turbulent hook curves, to lines that were characteristic of laminar flow, and that the solids could be conveyed at much lower velocities.

These results instigated work into what became known as Stab Flow, whereby research was conducted into the "laminar" behavior of these suspensions, with various researchers (e.g. [18]) reporting linear relationships of the familiar form $\lambda_m = 64/Re_m$, where λ_m and Re_m are the mixture friction factor and mixture pipe Reynolds number. Vertical concentration profiles taken across the horizontal pipes, using traveling densitometers, showed the variation across the pipe to be minimal (e.g. [19]). Such results supported the notion of homogenous behavior for these suspensions. The influence of pH in the data of **Figure 9b** demonstrated that rheology of the underlying

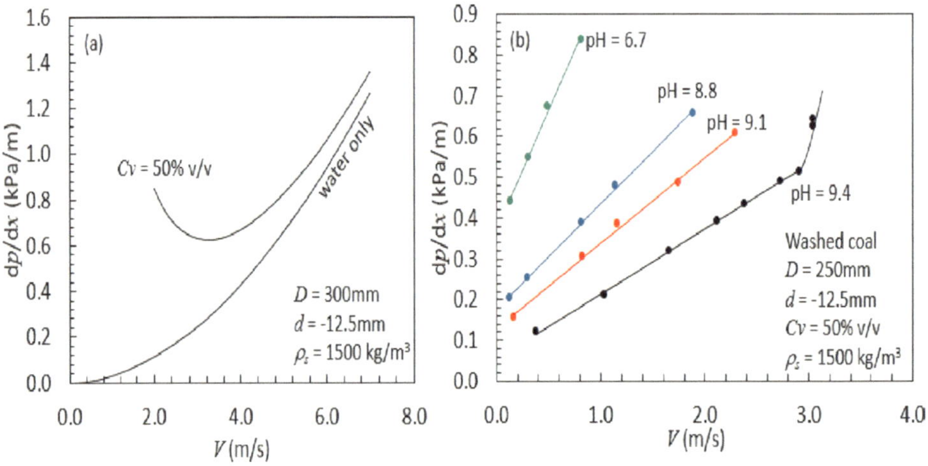

Figure 9.
(a) Typical conventional conveying characteristic for −12.5 mm coal, (b) "laminar" characteristics for degraded −12.5 mm coal, after Elliot & Glidden [17].

carrier slurry, or carrier fluid, was important, but it seemed that the coarse solids, despite their size, could somehow be combined with the properties of the carrier fluid and be modeled using homogeneous non-Newtonian methods.

Figure 10a demonstrates how convincing such an approach can be. Here all suspensions are seen to behave like homogeneous fluids. The originally presented curves were calculated using non-Newtonian laminar relationships and semi-empirical predictions of turbulent flow, using a suspension pseudo-rheology, based on the underlying carrier fluid rheology and coarse particle concentrations, i.e., $\tau_{ym} = f(\tau_{yc}, Cv)$ etc., where subscripts *c* and *m* denote carrier fluid and suspension respectively.

Several groups adopted this pseudo-rheological approach to predict full size data and scale up of test data, but this was found to only be successful for relatively minor increases in scale, and, as demonstrated by the dependence on pH, required that the underlying carrier fluid's rheology would stay constant.

Anecdotal evidence, later confirmed by tomographic studies (described in the chapter on tomography in this text) and flow visualization studies, showed that rather than being homogeneous, such flows were stratified. This allowed mechanistic two-layer models, based on the carrier fluid and particle properties, to be used to predict and scale up the data. Such predictions are shown in **Figure 10b**. Flows such as these are now generally analyzed using layered models, which produce predictions of transport pressure gradients typically within less than 10%.

During this period, the introduction of high rate and deep cone thickeners allowed a new form of tailings disposal to be developed [21], whereby rather than conveying low concentration solids to settle in conventional walled TSFs, high concentration non-Newtonian suspensions were pumped out onto a flat TSF. The discharged suspensions formed cones of solids that were stabilized by the yield stresses in the underlying carrier fluid. Such TSFs had a smaller footprint than their conventional counterparts, did not incur the expense of large bounding walls, were inherently safe, not being susceptible to catastrophic wall breaches, and could be rehabilitated earlier.

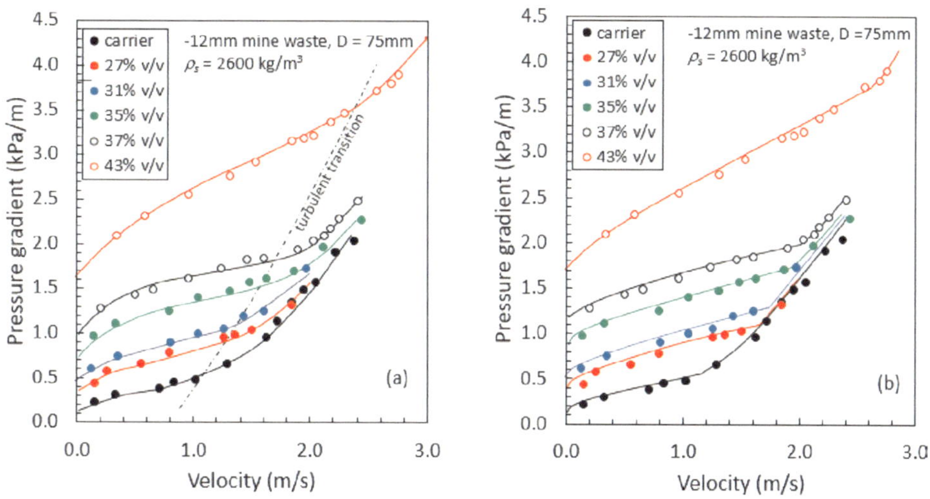

Figure 10.
Coarse mine waste suspensions (after Duckworth et al. [20]). (a) Curves based homogeneous non-Newtonian suspensions with rheology a function of the carrier fluid and coarse concentration, (b) non-Newtonian two-layer model predictions.

Thus, there was a perceived need to adopt this technology to (i) transport coarse materials at low velocities, and (ii) to dispose of large quantities of waste material in a more economic and environmentally safe manner.

3.2 Stratification process

Stratification when the flow is turbulent is performed through a similar process for non-Newtonian based suspensions as it is for Newtonian suspensions. The higher viscosity and differing viscosity distribution means that moderately sized solids are more readily suspended and adopt a more uniform concentration distribution than their Newtonian based counterparts [22].

In laminar flow, there are no turbulent suspending eddies, but if the carrier fluid is a visco-plastic, with a substantial yield stress, this yield stress will be able to support the particle if it exceeds a critical value τ_{yc}, i.e.

$$\tau_{yc} = kgd\left(\rho_s - \rho_f\right) \quad k \approx 0.1 \text{ for irregular particles} \tag{7}$$

However, in sheared visco-plastic flows, the fluid surrounding the suspended solids is subjected to a shear rate equal to the vector total of all applied shear rates, i.e., the local velocity profile, that due to the particles' settling motion and that due to any rotation of the particle. This shear rate is finite, and since visco-plastic flows are very shear thinning, this means that the viscosity of the fluid, local to the particle, will have a high, but finite viscosity, and so the particle will be able to settle through it. It has been shown [22–24] that at particle Reynold's numbers, typical of settling in non-Newtonian pipeline flows, the settling velocity of the particle can be calculated using Stoke's relationship, providing this local viscosity is used.

In visco-plastic pipeline flow, there exists a central core that is unsheared, and thus if the carrier fluid's yield stress exceeds τ_{yc}, any particle that is within this plug will not settle. This argument was used to support the apparent homogenous behavior of Stab Flow, and furthermore it was suggested that Magnus forces, in the sheared annulus, would transfer particles from there into the unsheared plug, such that the flow became a form of lubricated capsule flow, affording very low transport pressure gradients.

Consider the coarse suspension pipeline flow, shown in **Figure 11**, where the carrier fluid has a yield stress greater than that required for static support, i.e., $\tau_y > \tau_{yc}$.,

Suspensions entering the pipe from a well-mixed tank at volumetric concentration Cv_i will be uniformly distributed across the pipe (**Figure 11a**), and once the wall shear stress exceeds the yield stress an annular sheared region ($r > r_p$) will be formed, as shown. Particles within the unsheared core will be statically supported, but those in the annular region will be subjected to shear, and so will settle. Further down the pipe (**Figure 11b**), the particles from the annular region have settled to form a bed (stationary or sliding depending upon the conditions) at concentration C_{vb}. The presence of the bed distorts the flow such that the dynamic center of the flow moves from the pipe axis, to midway between the top of the bed and the upper pipe wall. This distorts the conical stress distribution of the homogenous case, and while it remains linear on the vertical plane of symmetry, it becomes distorted elsewhere. The unsheared plug now adopts an essentially elliptic form, centered on the dynamic center, of major and minor diameters, approximated by

$$p = \frac{\zeta D}{2}; \; q = \frac{\zeta(D - y_b)}{2} \tag{8}$$

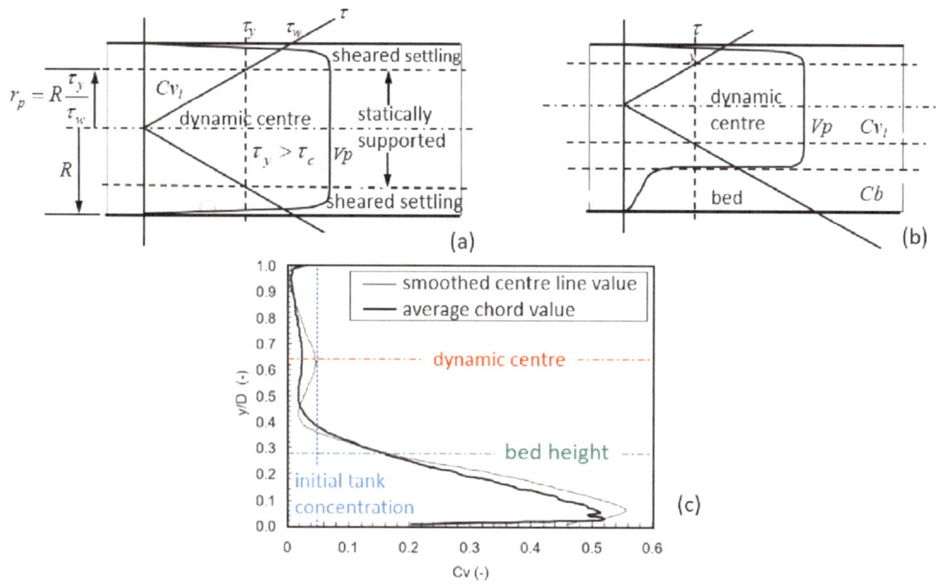

Figure 11.
(a) Initial coarse particle suspension flow as it enters the pipeline, (b) bed development further along the pipe, (c) averaged chord and vertical Centre line concentration profiles, obtained using electrical resistance tomography (ERT) [24].

where $\zeta = \tau_y/\tau_w$ and y_b = the depth of the bed.

The unsheared plug's lower boundary thus recedes upwards, as the bed develops, exposing more particles from the original unsheared plug to shear so that they also settle, and this in turn increases the bed thickness. An example of such behavior is given in **Figure 11c**. Whether a final residual unsheared plug exists or is completely destroyed in the final established flow depends upon the magnitude of ζ.

3.3 Concentration considerations with visco-plastic carrier fluids

The higher viscosity and shear thinning nature of the carrier fluid has an impact on the dilated bed concentration described in §2.1. The packing concentration of the visco-plastic carrier fluids themselves are affected by the applied normal stresses [25], as apparently are beds of coarse particles suspended in such fluids.

Studies in Delft have shown that the coarse particle concentration in the bed adapts itself to the exerted shear stresses [26], where coarse particles, settled from a Couette shear flow, created in an annular flume. Upon increasing the fluid shear stress, the bed compacted more. From considerations of mechanical equilibrium, the shear stresses in the bed are higher than within the flow and the imposed fluid shear stresses are larger than the yield stress, outside of any unsheared plug (which has been shown to exist above the bed). Then, since the strength of the bed increases with solids' concentration, this concentration will increase until bed strength equals the imposed fluid shear stresses [27]. Such analysis has been successfully applied to flow in flumes, tailings deposits, pipelines and computational studies [23, 28–30].

Experimentally obtained values of Cb, or values derived from analysis, are typically 10 to 20% lower than those obtained in §2.1.

3.4 Two-layer considerations for coarse suspensions in non-Newtonian carrier fluids

As before, only a simple two-layer model will be considered in this section and the reader is referred to the chapter on pipeline modeling for more advanced models. Since the behavior, when the flow is turbulent, is similar to Newtonian based systems, varying only in detail concerned with the calculation of wall stresses and the extent of particle suspension, only laminar flow processes will be considered here (see e.g., [31–33]).

The increase in viscosity of the carrier fluid increases the various stresses, and modifies the ways the bed is transported, in particular, it is now possible to convey under conditions where the carrier fluid is in laminar flow.

Changing the rheology of the carrier fluid has profound effects on the bed's behavior as illustrated here.

The example shown in **Figure 12a** is based loosely on data obtained at a diamond mine, where -6 mm grits were conveyed using thickener underflow to the TSF [34] for thickened central disposal. It demonstrates the effect of changing the viscosity of the carrier fluid. In this case the actual carrier fluid was well described by the Bingham plastic model $(\tau = \tau_{yB} + \eta\dot{\gamma})$, where τ_{yB} and η are the Bingham yield stress and plastic viscosity respectively, and τ and $\dot{\gamma}$ the shear stress and shear rate. This model will be used for illustration without any loss of generality. Increasing the viscosity by increasing the yield stress of the carrier, without changing the plastic viscosity, reduces the extent of the deposition locus, such that, for this system, at yield stress values exceeding 55 Pa, the deposition locus has been totally suppressed. Under these circumstances, the coarse solids will move within the pipe as soon as there is any flow. Such a system cannot be blocked. It is worth noting that the disposal system on which this example is based was designed for a carrier yield stress of 50 Pa, very close to this value. It should also be noted that this reduction in the deposition locus is not solely a function of yield stress. Increasing the viscosity through other means, e.g., modifying η, will have similar effects.

3.4.1 Un-blockable systems

The yield stress to ensure that the solids will move as soon as there is flow is obtained by equating the driving and resisting forces on the bed at incipient motion

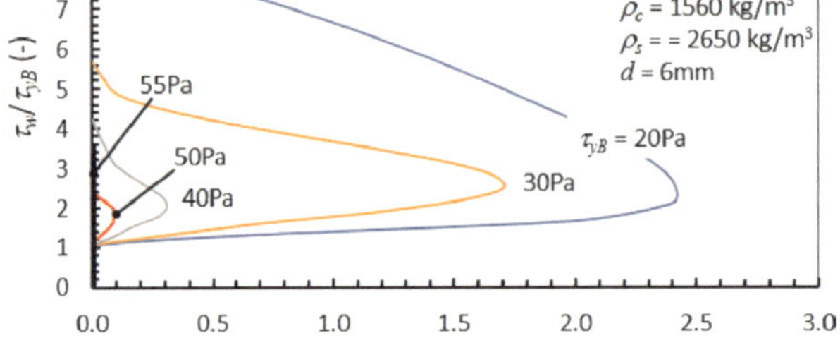

Figure 12.
The effect of yield stress on the deposition locus.

above the bed. At this point on the plane of symmetry, the stress at the pipe wall and the top of the bed will be equal to the yield stress of the fluid, as will the stress under the bed, since it is not moving. Approximating the flow above the bed to that of flow through an equivalent pipe of diameter equal to the hydraulic diameter of the area above the bed [35], it can be shown that the minimum yield stress required to ensure bed motion at all velocities for arbitrary solids' concentration can be written as

$$\tau_{y\,\min} = \frac{\pi D^2 F(\beta, f) C b g \mu_s \left(\rho_s - \rho_f\right)(A-1)}{4\left(\pi\beta + D\sin(\beta) - \frac{\pi D^2 (A-1)}{Dh}\right)} \tag{9}$$

where the area above the bed is $A = 1 - (\beta - \sin(\beta)\cos(\beta))/\pi$ and the hydraulic diameter is given by$Dh = D(\pi - \beta + \sin(\beta)\cos(\beta))/(\pi - \beta + \sin(\beta))$.

Figure 13 demonstrates that for visco-plastic systems, in common with their Newtonian counterparts, the highest deposition velocity occurs at a relatively low concentration (Cv of order 10%), and that this value is a very weak function of yield stress. Substituting this value into Eq. (9) produces a minimum yield stress requirement of 53 Pa, which is consistent with that shown in **Figure 12**. Satisfying though this result is, it is somewhat academic as experience gained in the laboratory and field has shown that restart is not an issue with visco-plastic systems, providing the deposition velocity is within the laminar flow regime. This is probably due to the inability of the laminar flow to resuspend the particles and produce blockages, although reports of viscous resuspension indicate a mechanism that might [36, 37].

3.4.2 Turbulent bed erosion

While this section is primarily concerned with flow that appears to be laminar, there are reports of fine particle beds being resuspended through turbulent action above the bed, before the bed is moved en masse under "laminar" flow and this is now examined.

The velocity displayed in **Figure 12** is the bulk velocity, i.e., $V = 4Q/\left(\pi D^2\right)$, but at deposition, all of fluid flow occurs either above the bed or percolates through the bed.

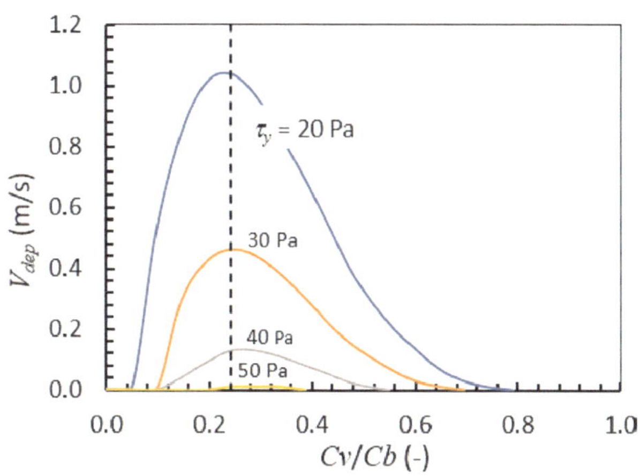

Figure 13.
*Deposition velocities as a function of reduced concentration and carrier fluid yield stress for the system shown in **Figure 12**. Approximate concentration corresponding to the maximum deposition velocities shown dashed.*

Percolation through the bed is very low with these viscous carriers and so may be ignored. Thus, the velocity above the bed is simply

$$V_a = \left(\frac{D}{D_h}\right)^2 V_{dep} \tag{10}$$

Many workers (e.g. [38, 39]) have found that for visco-plastic fluids, in particular those modeled using a Bingham plastic, the transition velocity, V_{tB}, for pipeline flow is insensitive to pipeline diameter and can be approximated by

$$V_{tB} \approx k_t \sqrt{\frac{\tau_{yB}}{\rho_c}} \tag{11}$$

where $22 < k_{tB} < 26$, τ_{yB} is the Bingham yield stress and ρ_c the carrier fluid density.

For small pipes, less than 150 mm, this simple relationship, breaks down. Values for Vt, obtained from the intersection of the appropriate laminar curves and turbulent predictions (e.g. [40]) produce increasingly higher values as the diameter reduces. Nevertheless, the point at which flow above the bed becomes turbulent will be defined here as when V_a, given by Eq. (10) exceeds that produced by Eq. (11), since this produces a more conservative result. Calculations of these velocities for a moderately viscous carrier fluid, transporting 3 mm solids, is shown in **Figure 14**.

The conclusion to be drawn from **Figure 14** is that, even for only moderately viscous carrier fluids, the flow will not become turbulent before the deposition velocity is exceeded, except for large pipes, and then only for low to moderate coarse concentration flows, not for high concentration flows, where the flow will remain laminar.

3.4.3 Testing requirements

At the time of writing, 2-layer model predictions for non-Newtonian carrier-based systems require pipeline or laboratory tests to determine suitable values for Cb and the coefficient of sliding friction. Once obtained however, predictions of industrially sized systems can be made typically to within ±10%.

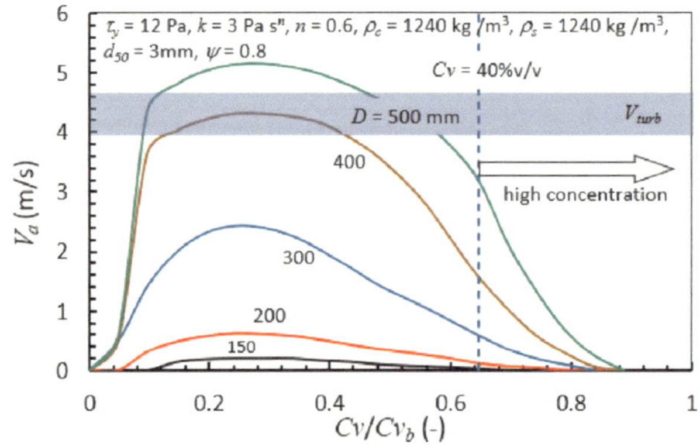

Figure 14.
Variation of the velocity above the bed, Va, for various pipe sizes compared with the transitional velocity range given by Eq. (11) with the limiting values of k_{tB}.

3.5 Comparison with conventional conveying

The thickened tailings of **Figure 12a** will be used as an example, noting that in this case all the solids, both the -6 mm grits and particles that are contained within the thickener underflow are to be disposed. The concentration of the grits was only 10% v/v but when combined with the carrier slurry the total concentration of the solids was 40.5% v/v. While this concentration may be within the range of conventional conveying, it must be remembered that the carrier fluid is a highly thickened slurry, a requirement for the central discharge method employed on the TSF. The transport characteristics for this suspension were very flat, requiring a pressure gradient of 0.97 kPa/m to produce velocities ranging from 0.5 to 3 m/s within the pipe. Using Eq. (6) and based on these values the SEC is found to be 0.4 kWhr/(tonne km).

Using conventional conveying, based on a mean particle size of 3 mm, at this total concentration, would require the solids to be conveyed in excess of 6 m/s and require a transport pressure gradient of around 1.55 kPa/m, giving an SEC of 0.64 kWhr/(tonne km).

By using a non-Newtonian carrier, the solids are transported using only 62% of the energy consumption, which would otherwise be required, and the suspension can be used as a thickened discharge. Conversely, using conventional conveying techniques would produce a very erosive environment, and require construction of a, now deprecated, conventional TSF.

3.6 What constitutes a coarse particle?

Earlier, it was suggested that coarse particles may be those larger than 0.5 mm, but tests conducted with some broad size distribution uranium tailings [41] indicated that it was only particles less than 40 μm that contributed to the carrier fluid's rheology, the rest being coarse and reporting to the sliding bed. Carrier fluid rheology is of course material specific, but it is most likely that similar lower limits exist for other mineral slurries.

4. Discussion and conclusions

Two forms of high concentration conveying have been described, both of which enable very coarse particles to be conveyed at low velocities, and in such a way that stopping and starting the flow is easy. While normally requiring higher transport pressure gradients than those required by fine particle flows, their high solids' concentrations result in low *SECs*. They both have very low minimum conveying velocities, if any at all, allowing solids to be conveyed at low velocities and providing very large turn down ratios. The low velocities also means that pipe wear and particle attrition is similarly low.

The first form, using water, or similar, as the carrier fluid, has the advantage that separation of the solids from the carrier fluid is simple and does not require facilities to manufacture a special non-Newtonian carrier fluid. However, there are considerable restrictions on the solids that can be pumped, requiring both a broad size distribution and a high, but limited, range of solids' concentrations, $0.75 < Cv/Cb < 0.9$. These restrictions are beyond the capabilities of normal centrifugal or positive displacement pumps and require specialized feeding systems.

The second form employs a visco-plastic carrier fluid. This ameliorates or removes the PSD and concentration restrictions of the former method and has the advantage that it can be transported using conventional pumps. However, unless the material to be pumped naturally forms a suitable carrier fluid, e.g., contains a high clay content or has a friable component, equipment and techniques are required to produce the necessary carrier and maintain appropriate rheological characteristics during normal lifetime process variabilities. Separation of the coarse material from the carrier, if required, can be costly and involved, although sheared settling, described above, can be exploited to assist in this. Disposal of the used carrier material may also be problematic. Where separation is not required or desirable, e.g., waste disposal, the presence of a yield stress in the carrier fluid means that deposits are stable. Distribution of these suspensions across a TSF can no longer rely on the simple ring main distributions of conventional TSFs, and requires single or multiple central discharge systems to be employed.

Both means of conveying are successfully characterized and predicted using layered models, which provide a mechanistic means to scale up from test data with confidence.

Acknowledgements

The author would like to thank the CSIRO's Division of Mineral Engineering and Advanced Fluid Dynamic Laboratory, for support in this work, to Dr. Lachlan Graham, in particular, for his imaging of many of these flows, and assistance in developing a deeper understanding their behavior and to Dr. Arno Talmon for his insights into the bed structure when using non-Newtonian carriers.

Author details

Lionel Pullum
Private Consultant, Olinda, Australia

*Address all correspondence to: lpullum@bigpond.net.au

References

[1] Tanaka T, Ouchiyama N. Coordination numbers and porosity of packing calculated from particle size distribution. 4th International Symposium on agglomeration. Royal York Hotel, Toronto, Ontario, Canada: National Research Council of Canada; 1985:9-16

[2] Cross M. Prediction of the Voidage of packed beds. 4th International Symposium on agglomeration. Royal York Hotel, Toronto, Ontario, Canada: National Research Council of Canada; 1985:713-717

[3] Imanidis G, Winzap S, Leuenberger H, editors. Agglomeration kinetics and process monitoring in rapid mixers. In: 4th International Conference on Aglomeration. Toronto: Canada; 1985

[4] Wilson KC, Brown NP, Streat M. Hydraullic hoisting at high concentration: A new study of friction mechanisms. In: 6th International Conference on Hydrotransport of Solids in Pipes: Hydrotransport 6 BHRA Fluid Engineering. Canterbury, UK: BHRA Fluid Engineering; 1979. pp. 269-282

[5] Wilson KC, Brown NP. Analysis of fluid friction in dense-phase pipeline flow. Canadian Journal of Chemical Engineering. 1982;**60**(1):83-86

[6] Jordan D, Dittmann FW. The hydraulic hoisting of coarse coal from a depth of 850 metres. Journal of the Southern African Institute of Mining and Metallurgy. 1980;(May):177-182

[7] Ercolani D, Ferrini F, Arrigoni V. Electric and thermic probes for measuring the limit deposit velocity. 6th International Conference on Hydrotransport of Solids in Pipes: Hydrotransport 6. Canterbury, England: BHRA; 1979. pp. 27-42

[8] Wilson KC. A unified physically-based analysis of solid-liquid pipeline flow. In: 4th International Conference on Hydrotransport of Solids in Pipes: Hydrotransport 4. Banff, Canada: BHRA; 1976. pp. A1-A16

[9] Tan RBH, Davidson JF. Liquid-particle jets from fluidised beds. Chemical Engineering Science. 1989: **44**(12):2899-2907

[10] Gillies RG, Haas DB, Small MH, Husband WHW. Coarse coal in water slurries - full scale pipeline tests. In: SRC laboratories. Saskatoon, Canada: Sakatchewan Research Council; 1982 Report No.: E-725-10-C-82

[11] Pullum L, McCarthy DJ. In: Round GF, editor. Ultra High Concentration and Hybrid Hydraulic Transport Systems. Freight Pipelines: Elsevier Science Publishers; 1993

[12] Pullum L, McCarthy DJ, Longworth NJ. Operating experiences with a rotary ram slurry pump to transport ultra high concentration coarse suspensions. In: Bhr gr Conf Ser Publ. Johannesburg: RSA: BHRA; 1996. pp. 657-671

[13] Geisler P. Three-chamber pipe feeder systems n- further technical development and new fields of application. In: 13th International Conference on Slurry Handling and Pipeline Transport. Johannesburg, South Africa: bHr group; 1996. pp. 347-356

[14] Boyle BA. Slurry Transport (Australian Patent No. AU1981066639), IP Australia. 1981

[15] Stewart DB. High head slurry pump. In: 2nd International Conference on Hydrotransport of Solids in Pipes: Hydrotransport 2. Warwick, England: BHRA; 1972

[16] Bhattacharya A, Imrie I. Development of the Asea mineral slurry transport system for coarse coal. In: 10th International Conference on Hydrotransport of Solids in Pipes: Hydrotransport 10; 29–31 October. Innsbruck, Austria: BHRA; 1986. p. C1

[17] Elliot DE, Gliddon BJ. Hydraullic transport of coal at high concentrations. In: 1st International Conference on Hydrotransport of Solids in Pipes: Hydrotransport 1. Cranfield, UK: BHRA; 1970. p. Paper G2

[18] Lawler HL, Cowper NT, Pertuit P, Tennant JD. Application of stabilised slurry concepts of pipeline transportation of large particle coal. In: 3rd International Technical Conference on Slurry Transportation. Las Vegas: Nevada; 1978

[19] Brookes DA, Snoek PE. Stabflow slurry Development. In: 10th International Conference on Hydrotransport of Solids in Pipes: Hydrotransport 10. Innsbruck, Austria: BHRA; 1986. pp. 89-100

[20] Duckworth RA, Pullum L, Lockyear CF. Pipeline transport of coarse materials in a non-Newtonian carrier fluid. In: 10th International Conference on Hydrotransport of Solids in Pipes: Hydrotransport 10. Innsbruck, Austria: BHRA; 1986

[21] Robinsky EI. Thickened discharge-a new approach to tailings disposal. Canadian Mining and Metallurgical Bulletin. 1975;**68**:47-53

[22] Matousek V, Chryss A, Pullum L. Modelling the vertical concentration distributions of solids suspended in a turbulent visco-plastic fluid. Journal of Hydrology and Hydromechanics. 2021; **69**(3):255-262

[23] Talmon AM, Huisman M. Fall velocity of particles in shear flow of drilling fluids. TUSP. 2005;**20**(2): 193-201

[24] Pullum L, Graham L, Wu J. Bed establishment lengths under laminar flow. In: 18th International Conference on Hydrotransport of Solids in Pipes: Hydrotransport 18; 22–24th September. BHRA: Rio de Janeiro, Brazil; 2010

[25] Wildemuth CR, Williams MC. A new interpretation of viscosity and yield stress in dense slurries: Coal and other irregular particles. Rheologica Acta. 1985;**24**:75-91

[26] Talmon A, Mastbergen D. Solids transport by drilling fluids: Concentrated bentonite-sand-slurries. In: 12th Transport and Sedimentation of Solid Particles. Prague, Czech Republic. Wroclaw, Poland: Wroclaw University of Environmental and Life Sciences; 2004

[27] Talmon AM, van Kesteren W, Sittoni L, Hedblom E. Shear cell tests for quantification of tailings segregation. Canadian Journal of Chemical Engineering. 2012;**92**(2):362-373

[28] Talmon AM, van Kesteren WGM, Mastbergen DR, Pennekamp JGS, Sheets B. Calculation methodology for segregation of solids in non-Newtonian carrier fluids. In: Jewell RJ, Fourie A, Wells PS, Zyl DV, editors. Paste 2014: 17th International Seminar on Paste and Thickened Tailings. Vancouver, Canada: Australian Centre for Geomechanics; 2014. pp. 139-153

[29] Van Rhee C, Dobbe P. CFD simulation of shear settling in non-

Newtonian flow. In: 19th Conference on Transportation and Sedimentation of Solid Particles. Cape Town: RSA; 2019

[30] Van Rhee C, editor Simulation of the settling of solids in non-Newtonian fluid. 18th Conference on Transport and Sedimentation of Solid Particles. Prague, Czech Republic. Wroclaw, Poland: Wroclaw University of Environmental and Life Sciences; 2017

[31] Pullum L, Graham L, Slatter P. A non-Newtonian two layer model and its application to high density hydrotransport. In: 16th International Conference on Hydrotransport of Solids in Pipes: Hydrotransport 16. Santiago, Chile. PRS1: BHR group; 2004

[32] Rojas MR, Saez AE. Two-layer model for horizontal pipe flow of Newtonian and non-Newtonian settling dense slurries. Industrial and Engineering Chemistry Research. 2012;**51**(20):7095-7103

[33] Fraser C, Goosen P. Evaluation of a non-Newtonian two-layer model for high concentration suspensions. In: Paste 2019. Cape Town: RSA; 2019

[34] Houman J. Commissioning and operation of the paste thickening farm at Kimberly combined treatment plant. In: 2003 International Seminar on Paste and Thickened Tailings; 14-16th May, 2003. Melbourne: ACG; 2003. p. Section 11

[35] Sparrow EM, Haji-sheik hA. Flow and heat transfer in ducts arbitary shape with arbtary Lthermal boundary conditions. Journal of Heat Transfer. 1966;351-358

[36] Charru F, Mouilleron-Arnould H. Instability of a bed of particles sheared by a viscous flow. Journal of Fluid Mechanics. 2002;**452**:303-323

[37] Schaflinger U, Acrivos A, Stibi H. An experimental study of viscous resuspension in a pressure-driven plane channel flow. International Journal of Multiphase Flow. 1995;**21**(4):693-704

[38] Slatter PT, Wasp EJ. Transition velocity estimation for visco-plastic fluids. In: 13th International Conference on Transport and Sedimentation. Tiblisi, Georgia. Wroclaw, Poland: Wroclaw University of Environmental and Life Sciences; 2006

[39] Darby R, Mun R, Boger DV. Predicting friction loss in slurry pipes. Chemical Engineer. 1992;**99**:116-119

[40] Wilson KC, Thomas AD. A new analysis of the turbulent-flow of non-Newtonian fluids. Canadian Journal of Chemical Engineering. 1985;**63**(4):539-546

[41] Coghill M, Jarvie N, Pullum L. Characterisation of thickened tailings suspensions using a 100NB and 150NB pilot test facility. In: 19th International Conference on Transport of the Hydraulic Transport of Solids in Pipes. Denver, USA: bHr; 2014

Chapter 5

Rheology, Rheometry and Wall Slip

Arno Talmon and Ebi Meshkati

Abstract

In diverse resource, processing and dredging applications wall slip occurs. In hydraulic transport of highly concentrated particulate mixtures, wall slip can be beneficial as it may substantially reduce hydraulic gradients. In other occasions, for instance in rheometry, wall slip may obscure rheology. Rheometric wall slip is not specific to industrial slurries and appears in natural (fluid) mud as well, mostly found in harbours and estuaries. In natural (fluid) muds, in contrary to industrial muds, coarse solids are absent. However, similarly, (clay) colloids govern their non-Newtonian flow characteristics. It is exciting to see that wall slip does not only occur in the case of dispersed coarse materials but also in the absence of those. In this chapter, we elaborate on wall slip in some existing resource industry rheometry data and compare them with typical recent results of fluid mud rheology. Moreover, measurement of a (stationary) fluid mud's longitudinal profile in a harbour basin is used to examine consequences of utilising slippage data. We finally evaluate measuring element usage and implementation of rheology in calculation methods.

Keywords: Rheometry, wall slip, viscometry, particulate slurries, clay aggregates, non-Newtonian, fluid mud, lutocline

1. Introduction

Rheology is the study of the flow behaviour of materials. Rheometry is the means of quantifying flow (rheological) characteristics of materials. Rheology strongly depends on the fabric of the material and how that changes with time, stress and shear rate. In rheology, the flow behaviour of a given material is visualised by a flow curve in a diagram that depicts the relationship between shear stress and shear rate.

Roto- and capillary-viscometers are standard tools used to carry out rheometry. Often flow (rheological) characteristics of a material are described by a set of parameters, so-called rheological parameters, such as various yield stresses and viscosity. These parameters are important to the characterisation and the modelling of the flow of clay-rich mixtures (consisting of fine and coarse solids) and are often used as a basis in the design and optimisation of soft sediment management plans and processes, amongst many, such as pipe flow, deposition flows, mixing and flocculation processes, emplacements, and the flow in other unit process operations. In these applications, when it comes to initiating flow, the static yield stress (SYS) is a key governing parameter to be determined. Dynamic yield stress (DYS) and viscous properties are, on the other hand, important to the study of fluid flow. The yield points are defined later in this chapter. Rheology and rheometry can also be relevant in the study of stagnant conditions of soft sediments. For instance, static yield stress governs the critical state of stagnant material not only in tailings storage facilities but also in harbour basins.

Ideally, rheometry results should be independent of applied measuring elements. However, in practice, it is often seen that different measurement elements result in different rheological values. The difference may be originated by: i) no or wrong correction factor when it comes to conversion of machine (i.e. rheometer) shear rate to physical shear rate; ii) an ill-defined rheological protocol and iii) occurrence of wall slippage during rheometry. Particularly, wall slip of mixtures in smooth walled measuring geometries can be deceiving. Wall slip occurs when the composition of the mixture at the wall is not exactly the same as in the interior of the mixture [1]. One way to detect the occurrence of wall slip in rheometry is to compare the flow curves of a given material obtained from various geometrical dimensions (pipe/capillary diameter, or sheared gap size). In the presence of wall slip, the rheological results from different geometrical dimensions would differ (shifted flow curves) (Mooney (1931)) [2].

In long-distance pipe flow of highly concentrated mixtures, wall slip may also occur and potentially constitutes a convenient and energy-efficient way of transportation (Goosen and Patterson (2014)) [3, 4]. In the emplacement of industrial tailings, there are many occasions where laminar flow prevails. In the simplest form, lubrication type of shallow flow models (Coussot and Proust (1996)) [5] can be applied for predicting tailings deposition behaviour on beaches in tailings storage facilities [6, 7]. For constant properties, the analytical outcome of such a theory, for a slowly advancing mass or a 1-D deposit on a horizontal base, is a square-root (SQRT) thickness vs. distance longitudinal profile. Assuming critical state conditions of a slowly advancing mass, the shear stress at the bottom equals yield stress [6]. There exist comparable theories for material on mildly sloping inclines, the frontal shape is very similar, but further up the slope, an equilibrium depth is reached. For Newtonian fluid on inclines, see [8]. For stagnant material at a critical state, see [9]. The shape of the frontal profile for other rheological models falls in between. If incorrect yield stresses are applied in such theories, the calculation of deposit depth or flow depth in combination with velocity is strongly affected. In reverse, the desktop Bostwick rheometer, which releases a small mass of material to an inclined channel, uses a similar principle to quantify the strength (i.e. yield stress) of material. For tailings rheology, an upscaled apparatus was developed by [10].

Tailings generally demonstrate time-varying strength properties. This may originate from progressing formation of clay aggregates at constant porewater content known as thixotropy or consolidation (loss of porewater and hence densification-related strength increase). Time/distance varying properties can be included in a numerical version of a lubrication model, but this does not really help to verify the relation between strength (yield stress) and the geometry of an emplacement, which we are pursuing in this chapter.

Rheometry of industrial materials can be difficult because of their inherent time dependency of strength, as well as their dewatering and shear settling of solids. Moreover, materials may have experienced treatment, e.g. by polymers, hence increasing difficulties to properly assess their flow properties. We examined a somewhat simpler material: fluid mud in harbours and estuaries where sand has already settled elsewhere, and the mud predominantly consists of colloidal clays. Rheological properties of fluid mud appear of a comparable magnitude to those of industrial materials where similarly, the colloids are responsible for non-Newtonian rheological properties and where similarly wall slip signatures are observed in rheometry data. In one of the recent fluid mud researches, wall slip is described as two-step yielding (e.g. Shakeel et al. 2020 [11]).

Since rheological characterisation cannot be seen without considering its application, this chapter elaborates on wall slip in pipelines. Some existing industry rheometry data is revisited and recast in formats that allow a more straightforward comparison with the latest measurements that reveal similar slippage. Typical recent results of fluid mud rheology, affected by and checked for wall slip, are presented in the format of flow curves and viscosity curves. Referring to a prototype measurement of a fluid mud's longitudinal profile in a harbour basin, eventually a proxy for emplacements, we examine the consequences of utilising slippage. We finally evaluate measuring element usage and application of rheology in computational fluid dynamics (CFD) and analytical methods.

The present contribution may also connect readers to a number of classical papers/manuscripts, pointing out similarities with recent data and sharing findings.

2. Rheological approach and wall slip experiences

2.1 Rheology in the plastic regime

In rheology, one needs to distinguish between conditions below and above the yield point. Below the yield point materials depict viscoelastic behaviour with no to limited flow (in other words, plastic deformation). In this domain, the viscoelastic behaviour of materials is characterised by shear modulus and loss modulus. For our engineering application, we investigate rheology at and above the yield point where materials experience plastic deformation or, in other words, flow. In this regime, the material's viscosity generally reduces with increasing shear rate and thus are characterised as a yield-shear-thinning material.

The existence, definition and determination of yield points in non-Newtonian materials are debated in the literature [12]. The yield point is defined as the lowest shear stress value above which material will act as a fluid and below which it behaves like a very soft solid matter. This definition is subjective, because the boundary between the fluid-like and solid-like state is not discrete but continuous. Many materials have time- and shear-dependent properties, and under different applied rheometry protocols, they give (somewhat) other yield points. Moreover, transition direction (i.e. from fluid-like to solid-like or vice versa) may occur at different stress levels. This is why in materials with time-dependent strength (thixotropic), at least two different yield points can be distinguished. Engineering applications may require knowledge of various yield points, depending on the application. Principal yield points are as follows:

- The static yield stress (SYS): defined as the minimum stress required for initiating the (shear) flow in a stagnant material under stress.
- The dynamic yield stress (DYS): defined as the minimum stress required for maintaining a given material in flow.

Time-independent materials have unique flow curves. However, the flow behaviour of time-dependent materials may vary depending on their shear and resting history, resulting in different flow curves. Our materials are easily remoulded, and recovery is relatively slow. The section of the flow curve where the shear rate returns to zero after experiencing high shear rates is hence called the remoulded flow curve. Equilibrium conditions may be achieved under continuous shearing at discrete shear rates. By plotting those equilibrium conditions (shear rate-shear stress pairs), an equilibrium flow curve (EFC) is obtained. Remoulded and equilibrium flow curves are amenable for description by mathematical time-independent models such as Bingham, Hershel-Bulkley, Worrall-Tuliani and Oswald-DeWaele power law.

For modelling purposes of flow, segregation and settling, it is preferred to have rheological information of the carrier fluid and rheology of the mixture [13]. The current state of the art stands where we may be satisfied if we can quantify one of these in detail and relate it to the other via single-point tests, for instance, through detailed measurements without coarse to determine the rheology of the carrier fluid as a baseline, supplemented by vane yield stress measurement of mixtures with different ratios of fines and coarse, in case of model materials similar to [14], or vice versa conducting vane-type rheology of mixtures, utilising vane-in-cup method (Barnes and Carnali 1990 [15]) or the vane-in-bucket method (Fisher et al. 2007 [16]) in combination with removal of coarse to determine the colloid's carrier fluid rheology.

2.2 Wall slip

2.2.1 Origin/nature of wall slip

In a non-Newtonian mixture under motion (flow), the velocity appears not always to reduce to zero at the wall because the mixture may have a subtle difference in composition here. Wall slip in a pipe may occur in two different ways, schematised in **Figure 1a,b**:

a. for the same flow rate: the velocity profile flattens, with slippage at the wall.

b. for the same pressure gradient along a pipeline segment: the velocity profile offsets in downflow direction, with slip at the wall.

Both these conditions boil down to the same state where there is a mismatch between flow velocity, pressure drop and rheology of the bulk of the material.

In concentric cylinder rheometry, a proxy for Couette shear flow, wall slip is imagined to occur at the inner cylinder as the shear stresses are highest there. Upon

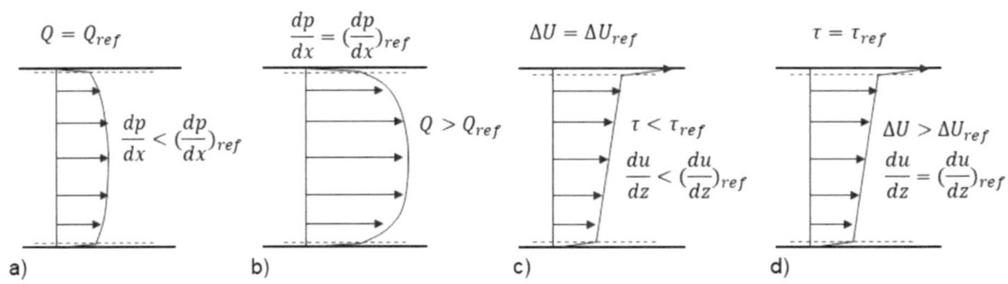

Figure 1.
Wall slip (a, b) in a pipe and (c, d) in Couette shear flow. Wall slip is demarcated by the dotted red line adjacent to solid line representing the wall.

increasing the angular velocity, slippage at both walls (i.e. at the outer surface of the bob and at the inner wall of the cup) may be speculated, as shown in **Figure 1d**.

2.2.2 Industrial flows: bulk slipping of non-Newtonian mixtures

In hydraulic pipe transport of highly concentrated non-Newtonian mixtures, the lower the water content of slurries, the higher their strength, and therefore, higher flow velocities are needed to keep the flow in turbulence to counteract the settling of particles (on this, a practical transition criterion is given by [17]).

Figure 2 depicts measured and calculated deposition velocities in a series of different pipe diameters [3, 4]. Increasing the density, the non-Newtonian properties increase and laminar flow is found for velocities below the red curve. Beyond 1580 kg/m^3, the flow velocity needs to be above the red line for turbulence to keep the material suspended, but beyond 1650 kg/m^3 the material slides as one bulk and laminar flow at low velocities is possible here. If the material would not slide as one bulk, internal shear would lead to settling of the solids [18].

The onset of this wall slipping phenomenon is hard to predict. To achieve sliding flow condition, material needs to be self-supportive. For instance, coarse should not settle in unsheared mixture (a condition referred to as gelled bed by [19]; or freely settling concentration by [3, 4, 20]).

Bulk slipping is also experienced in the transport of cement, shotcrete and fresh grouts [21]. In the construction industry, this allows the pumping of highly concentrated (thick) mixtures over significant distances both horizontally and vertically.

To control thickener operation, it is often not sufficient to rely only on underflow density. Hence, rheological properties of the material are also required. One reason is that the yield stress is found to correlate with the compressive strength of thickened tailings (Green and Boger (1997 [22])), governing the thickening process. As a new advancement, industrial-scale online pipe viscometers are built to measure tailings

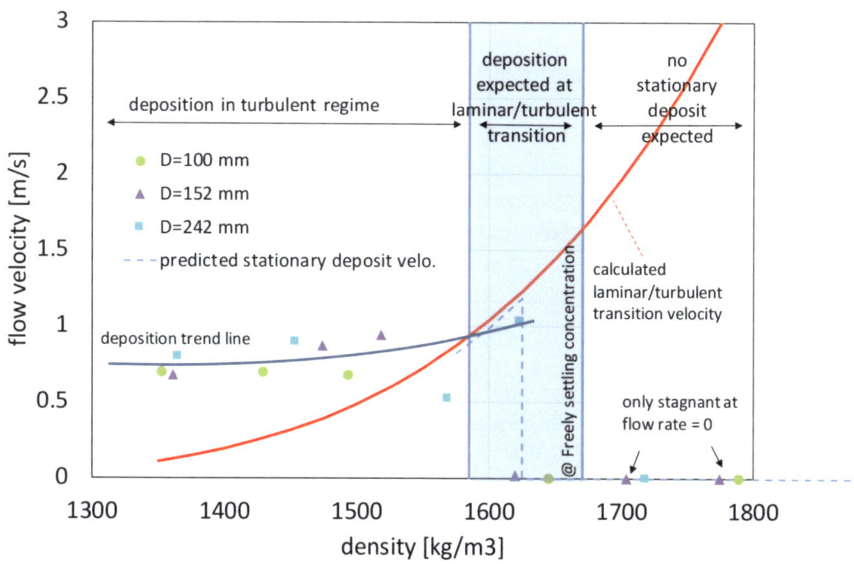

Figure 2.
Observed deposition conditions and stagnant material for different pipe diameters, after [3, 4].

rheology for controlling of thickener's operation, e.g. Chryss et al. 2019 [23] and Boomsma et al. 2022 [24]. These viscometers have multiple measurement units with different tube diameters to enable correction for wall slip.

2.2.3 Industrial flows: wall slip in the presence of water as carrier fluid

In the case of Newtonian carriers, like water, rheometry is difficult because of fast settling solids. In that case, accumulated experience with pipe flow serves as a basis for detecting indirect evidence of wall slip. Two distinct occasions at which wall slip is likely, in the presence of water as the carrier fluid in hydraulic pipeline transport of a mixture, are as follows:

Particles experience off-the-wall forces and therefore tend to move towards the centre of the flow, leaving a fluid-rich layer adjacent to the wall. Bartosik & Shook (1995) [25, 26] experienced such flow conditions in vertical pipe flows.

If solid particles do not fit within the laminar sublayer of turbulent flow, wall friction is found to not obey homogenous mixture theory enabling semi-analytical mathematical modelling of wall slip in these specific conditions [27]. In homogenous mixtures, the components are uniformly distributed throughout the mixture. In other words, only one phase of matter exists in a homogeneous mixture model.

2.2.4 Rheometric wall slip

Checking for wall slip in rheometry data can be conducted by comparing the rheometry data obtained from conducting:

- capillary rheometry using different capillary pipe diameters;
- concentric cylinder bob-cup (BC) rheometry using different annular gap widths;
- parallel plate (PP) rheometry using different gap (standoff) distances;
- rough/grooved/serrated/splined/profiled geometries;
- vane testing (as a radical check for wall slip).

In case of wall slip, the unprocessed flow curves of smaller gaps are expected to be shifted somewhat towards higher shear rates compared to larger gap. In other words, when wall slip occurs, a given shear stress value is achieved at a smaller shear rate with increasing gap size. Mind that, in the case of concentric cylinder rotoviscometry, a Couette-inverse transformation might need to be applied first for larger gap size because of non-uniform shearing across the gap.

An effective way to verify for occurrence of wall slip in rotoviscometry with well-defined shear rates is to additionally conduct tests with a vane (Barnes and Carnali 1990 [15], Boger et al. 2008 [28, 29], Buscall et al. 1993 [30]) and compare the results, as shown in **Figure 3**. Unrealistic steep branches in flow curve plots have been revealed accordingly at low shear rates (**Figure 3a**). We experience that the wall slip affected BC shear stresses can be a factor 5 lower than of those measured by vane (Section 3).

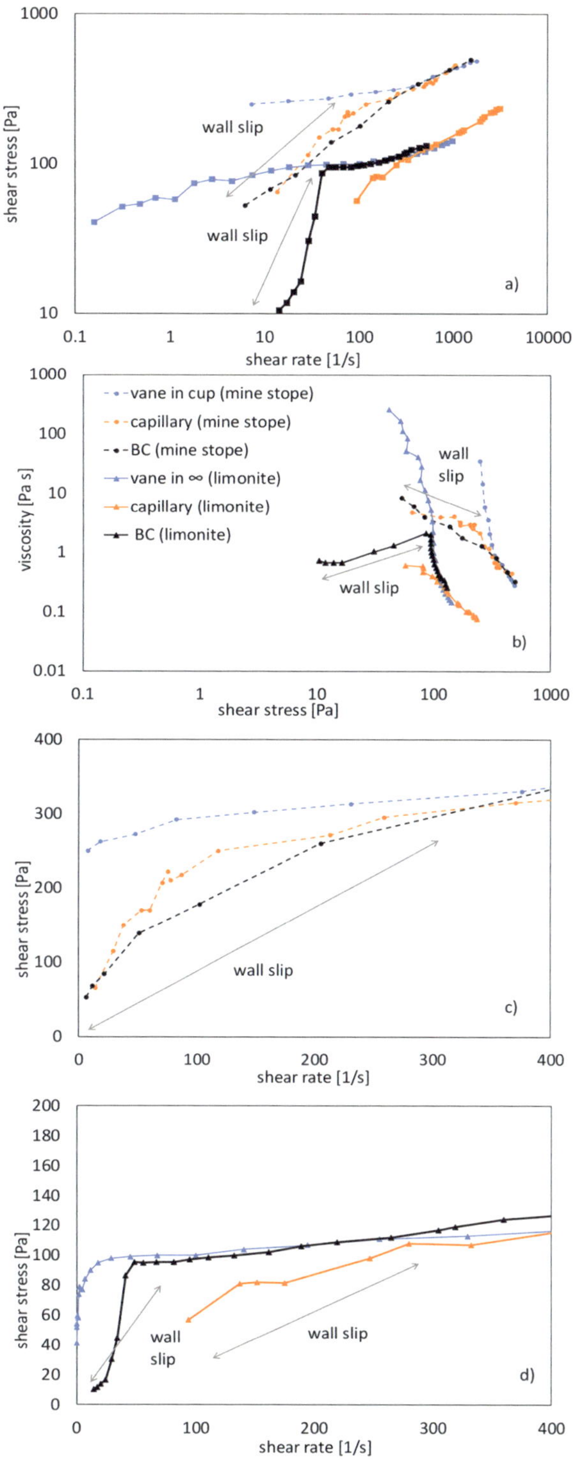

Figure 3.
Vane eradicates wall slip (a,b,c,d). Mine stope fill [28, 29] and nickle limonite [28]. Plotted in original [29] log-log coordinates (a), viscosity plot (b) and lin-lin coordinates (c, d).

2.3 Inverse Couette problem (non-uniform shear rate in gap)

Shear stresses and shear rate that are outputted by a rotoviscometer are derived from measured torque and rotational velocity. When either one, or both, is non-uniform within the mixture in the element, the rotoviscometer's conversion is based on Newtonian fluid conditions. Users may need to apply corrections in post-processing if deemed necessary. A complication with concentric cylinder elements is that the shear stress varies with radial position per conservation of torque with radial position. Hence, a non-ideal Couette flow is tested, and the shear rate across the annular gap is a function of the non-Newtonian properties of the fluid itself. Therefore, it is best to use small gaps. For wider gaps, needed for instance when there are coarse in the mixture, this constitutes the so-called inverse Couette problem: how to calculate the shear rate at measured shear stress [31]?

2.4 Mooney correction for wall slip

In capillary rheometry, it is possible to detect wall slip and to apply a correction to quantify the true rheology of the bulk of the material by applying tubes of different diameter [2]. The method can also be applied to sheared gaps of different sizes. In using a series of different gaps sizes or pipe diameters, it is assumed that the wall slip velocity is identical for the same shear stress. Since the minute thickness of the wall slip layer, consisting of base fluid, is difficult to predict, it remains necessary to rely on rheometry for quantification of wall slip.

2.5 Viscosity regularisation

Yield pseudo-plastic models (e.g. Bingham model) fitted to rheological measurements do not quantify stresses below the yield stress. Fluid flow calculation methods nevertheless need info in this regime: see the central plug in Bingham pipe flow where shear stresses are lower than the yield stress. A CFD model usually solves the flow relying on viscosity. Without intervention, the viscosity would unacceptably rise to infinity at a shear rate of zero. This needs to be limited in the model by providing shear stress values below the yield stress. This is achieved by regularisation of viscosity at low shear rates [32].

3. Detailed rheometry of mixtures without coarse

3.1 Material

Detailed rheology measurements are possible only when the coarse fraction is removed from the mixture. An alternative is to revert to a system where natural segregation has already removed the sand fraction. Natural fluid muds constitute such a system and as mentioned earlier it also appears to display wall slip signature. Results of rheometry [33] conducted on natural fluid mud from Beerkanaal, the port of Rotterdam, The Netherlands, with an initial density of 1263 kg/m^3 will be presented. Earlier measurements of the fluid mud from the port of Hamburg and Emden are also analysed [11, 34–37]. The yield stress of natural fluid muds is considered decisive for navigable depth in ports and waterways.

Fig. ref	Element	CSR [1/s]	CSS [Pa]	Ramp-up [s]	Const [s]	Ramp-down [s]
4	BC	0 to 100	0 to 120	180	60	180
4	VC	0 to 116	0 to 120	180	60	180
5	BC	0 to 100	n.a.	180	60	180
5	gBC	0 to 100	n.a.	240	60	240
5	VC	0 to 580	n.a.	240	90	240
6	PP	n.a.	0 to 50	50	n.a.	n.a.
6	VC	n.a.	0 to 50	50	n.a.	n.a.
6	BC	n.a.	0 to 50	50	n.a	n.a.
9	BC	0.1 to 90	n.a.	n.a.	7*35	n.a.

Table 1.
Applied measuring elements and protocols (B = bob CC25DIN, gBC = grooved bob CC25Din, C = cup CC25 DIN, V = vane FL22, PP = parallel plate P35).

3.2 Configuration and protocol

Configurations with well-defined shear rates such as concentric bob-cup (BC) cylinders are preferred in rheometry. However, as already mentioned, a BC system is prone to slippage: following Boger [29] on usage of vane, slippage appears also to be radically prevented in a vane-cup (VC) configuration, interestingly. The shear rate in a VC, on the other hand, has to be defined.

Two standard rheometry protocols, namely controlled shear rate (CSR) and controlled shear stress (CSS), are applied and compared to investigate the occurrence of wall slip in BC, PP and VC configurations. The vane is applied with 1 mm bottom clearance. **Table 1** provides information on the applied measuring elements and testing protocols. Tests are conducted by Haake Mars 1. The basis protocol consists of a linear ramp-up of either shear rate or shear stress during a certain time, followed by a constant phase and a ramp-down phase.

3.3 Results and discussion

3.3.1 Wall slip signature in bob-cup (BC) configuration

A definite difference is found between tests conducted in BC and VC. **Figure 4a** depicts the result of CSR and CSS tests in a BC configuration. At low shear rates (< 10 [1/s]), the ramp-down part of the curve crosses the ramp-up part in both CSR and CSS tests. This is because the measured shear stresses during the initial part of the ramp-up are underestimated, a typical wall slip signature in a BC configuration, compared with **Figure 3**. **Figure 4b** shows the result of CSR and CSS tests in a VC configuration where no wall slip is observed. The viscometer's outputted rotational velocity has been transformed to an equivalent shear rate at the rim of a virtual cylinder encompassing the vane, similar to the BC configuration, to allow comparisons. The shear stress-shear rate relationships over the ramp-down (remoulded) phase are in excellent agreement.

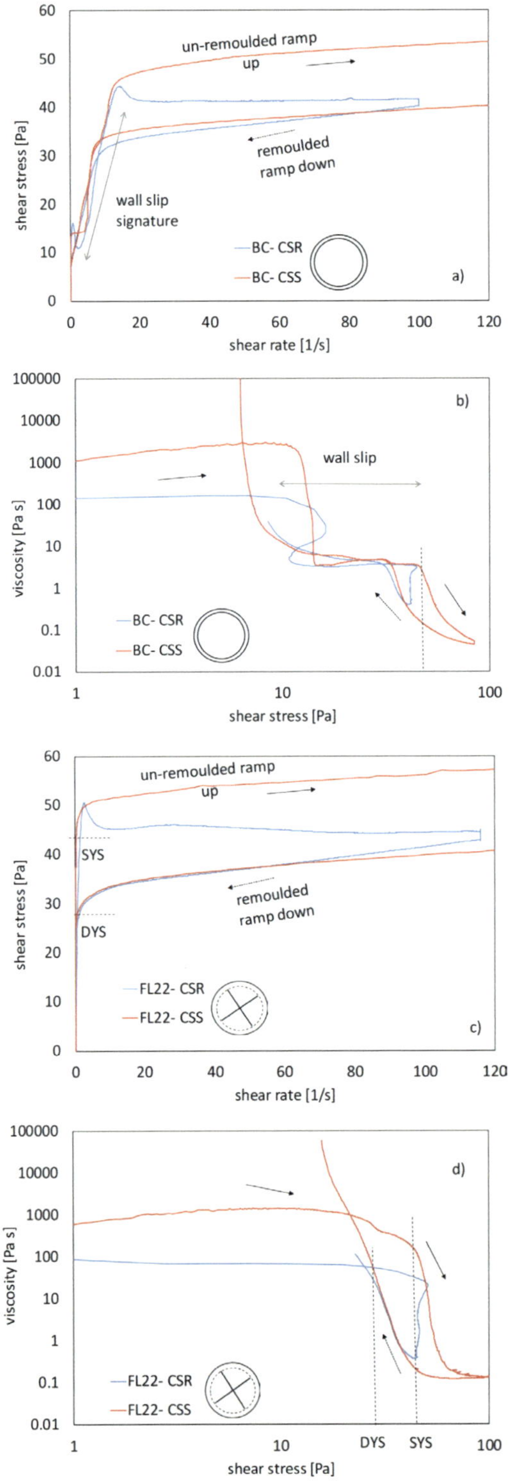

Figure 4.
Example of rheometric results on fluid mud from Beerkanaal, port of Rotterdam, The Netherlands, flow curve (a, c) and viscosity plot (b, d) with different elements and protocols.

3.3.2 Quantification of static and dynamic yield stress

The static yield stress is retrieved from CSS tests in the VC configuration: the shear stress at the point where the linear part of the ramp-up curve leaves the vertical axis and deflects to the non-linear part (at 45 Pa, **Figure 4b**). At this point, the pronounced wall slip also stops (**Figure 4a**): the shear stress has reached the yield stress of the unsheared material in the middle of the gap. The dynamic yield stress can be obtained from both CSR and CSS methods in the VC configuration: the intercept of the ramp-down curve and the vertical axis. In the BC configuration, the dynamic yield stress is underestimated by a factor 3 (comparing **Figure 4a** and **b**) and the static yield stress by a factor 5.

Here, we see that viscosity plots on the log-log scale are magnifying yielding at low shear rates but are also magnifying artefacts when the material transitions from an elastic state to plastic. Other utilised elements such as grooved bob or parallel plate elements may reveal more.

3.3.3 Slippage with rough/profiled elements

Utilising rough measuring elements is a well-known remedy to reduce wall slip, but it may not solve the wall slip problem entirely. We experienced that a rough element may only shift the wall slip problem to lower shear rates, as shown in **Figure 5**. Further roughening measures might be necessary to fully eliminate the wall slip.

Figure 5 shows the rheometry results of three different elements/protocols on the same mud. CSR ramping mode is applied. We see that the BC (blue) starts slipping at about 10 Pa, reaching a maximum shear stress at 40 Pa (end of steep slippage branch), completing a loop and returning finally back to 10 Pa, paralleling with the wall slip of the ramp-up. The vane performs differently; it peaks at 55 Pa and merges

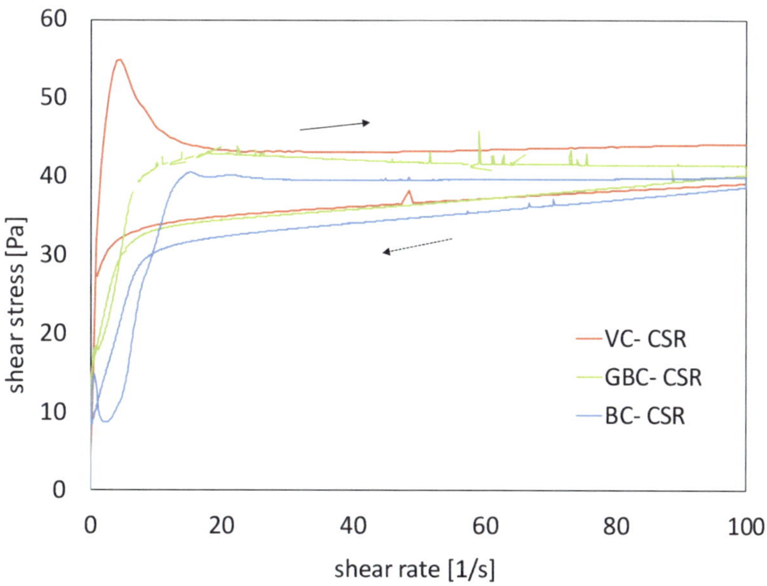

Figure 5.
Grooved bob (GBC) rheometry results compared to smooth bob-cup (BC) and vane-in-cup (VC), fluid mud from Beerkanaal, the port of Rotterdam, The Netherlands.

with the up-ramp of the BC. Upon return, it only bends down a little before cessation of shear. The grooved bob (green) slips at 15 Pa and follows a course between the CSR bob and the CSR vane results. This grooved bob result is positioned similarly with respect to BC in CSS measurements conducted by [11].

3.3.4 Gap variation parallel plate (PP) elements

A way to investigate wall slip and enable correction (e.g. Mooney transformation) is by conducting a rheometry method using a series of different gaps. This is easily done with a parallel plate (PP) measuring element. **Figure 6** includes such exercise.

This figure illustrates a combination of rheometry data of Shakeel et al. [11] that contributed to their rejection of wall slip, while in contrary revealing wall slip upon closer inspection of the data from the PP element. These data are very similar to a PP measurement presented in Ewoldt et al. (2015) [38] on Nivea lotion. When repeated with sandpaper glued to the plates, their result was similar to our vane result for >1 [1/s].

The PP outputs higher shear stress, calculated at the rim of the element utilising Newtonian fluid theory, than the other elements. In reality, with non-Newtonian shear-thinning fluids, a higher torque is measured for the same shear stress at the rim: the stresses in the centre part of the plates are comparably higher; hence, the

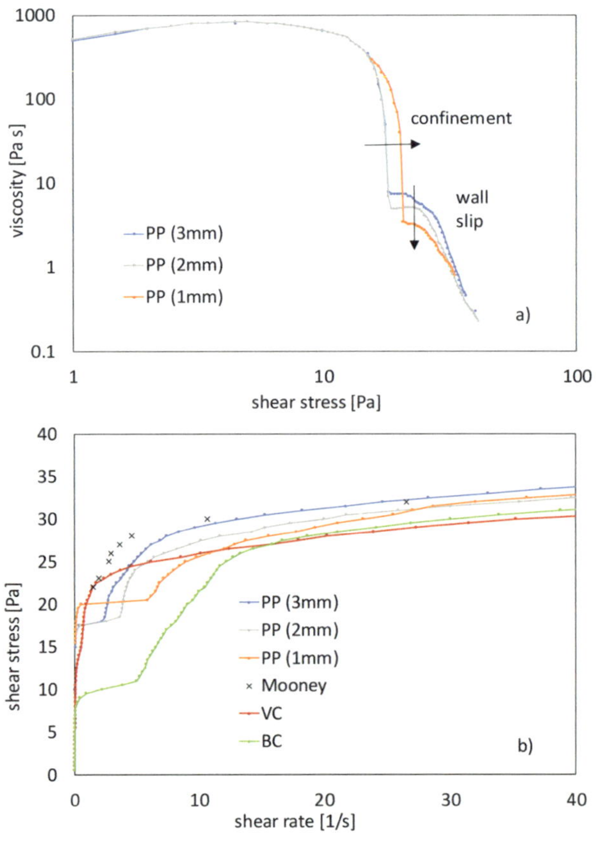

Figure 6.
From viscosity plot to flow curve, fluid mud from the port of Hamburg, Germany: a): Data presentation after [11] and b): Transformed into flow curve, including Mooney wall slip correction and comparison with BC and VC.

outputted calculated shear stress is higher than the true shear stress at the rim, hence a tendency for higher shear stresses.

The shear rate of the vane is calculated as described in Section 3.3.2 and is hence comparable to the BC element: an associated shear rate in a Newtonian fluid. Despite the virtual wider annular gap of the vane, no Couette inverse method has been applied to convert to the actual shear rate in the non-Newtonian fluid. If such correction would have been applied, the steep branch of the vane would have shifted somewhat to the right, in other words to higher shear rates.

Usage of a too small gap size may also play a role, increasing shear stresses because of confinement. Yan et al. (2009) [39] show rheometry results where the yield stress increases for axial gaps smaller than 0.2 mm. It is conjectured that this occurs when the plate distance becomes smaller than the correlation distance of the structure of the fluid. Hence, jamming effects emerge. So, the higher shear stresses for the 1 mm gap, for shear rates <5 [1/s], indicate that the unsheared clay aggregates have a size of 1 to 2 mm.

Figure 6 shows that the commencement of wall slip with a parallel plate system is postponed with respect to a concentric cylinder. This could be due to non-uniform conditions over the plate's surface, and hence total slip commences when yield stresses are exceeded at most of its surface.

Perfect alignment should not be expected. We applied the Mooney wall slip correction procedure to the PP result of [11], despite that shear stress and slippage velocities are not uniform in a PP element, compromising the basic assumption of the Mooney transformation. Also, the bottom clearance of the vane is smaller than its virtual annular gap. Hence, it is conceivable that data for <0.6 [1/s] is influenced by local failure here.

As we see in **Figure 6**, the Mooney wall slip correction procedure projects data back to lower shear rates, close to vane results. This implies that, practically speaking, a vane is a better element to address the internal strength properties of mixtures in rheometry.

4. The pitfall of using wall slip affected rheometry data: a case study example

4.1 Emden outer harbour

Fluid mud, such as at the bottom of harbours and estuaries, constitutes a simplified composition compared to slurries in mineral, resources, and processing industries which often contain a substantial amount of coarse settling solids.

In this subsection, we examine rheological measurements carried out on fluid mud from the Emden Outer Harbour and their importance to the lutocline (= the fluid mud's longitudinal profile) based on mechanical equilibrium.

The ecological-economical and maritime problem of continuous fines settlement in harbour basins is in Emden approached through a sediment managing scheme consisting of recirculation of accumulated fluid mud over a trailing suction hopper dredger (TSHD) to prevent densification into stiff material, through which vessels cannot sail.

As mentioned earlier, thixotropic strength gain during rest increases the static yield stress beyond the dynamic yield stress. After conditioning by the TSHD, or after vessels manoeuvred through the mud, we can assume the strength state of the mud layer to be somewhere between the static and dynamic yield stress and apparently high enough to prevent the mud from flowing to the river Ems fairway.

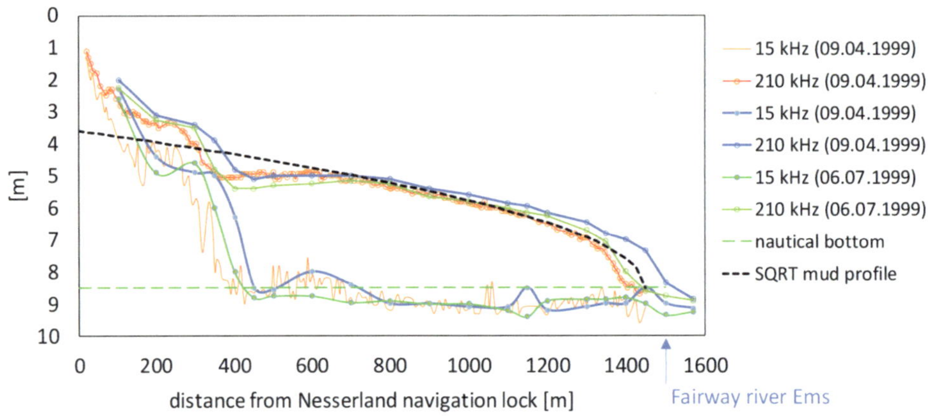

Figure 7.
Fluid mud profile in outer harbour Emden (after [34, 35]) and superimposed calculated lutocline for excess density 123 kg/m³ and 10 Pa yield stress.

Reported rheological measurements on Emden Harbour mud are comparable with the BC data in **Figures 4–6**. In the following, skipping problematic wall slip conditions in the existing data, the yield stress is again estimated by drawing the tangent to the flow curve for >10 [1/s], hence quantifying yielding at the intersection with the vertical axis.

Multibeam echo sounder measurements conducted in the harbour of Emden contain a 15-kHz profile showing a nearly horizontal reflection line indicating a strong transition at the base of the mud, as shown in **Figure 7**.

At a higher frequency, i.e. 210 kHz, a curved profile is found that represents the surface of the fluid mud layer (lutocline): [34, 35]. At about 1 km from the fairway of the river Ems, this layer has grown to a thickness of about 3 m. The 210-kHz profiles show a typical SQRT profile, associated with a stagnant slump or slowly advancing mass of material of uniform density and strength. The SQRT profile can be used as a validation case for yield stress measurement (rheometry data) of the fluid mud of this harbour, which will be discussed further in this section.

4.2 Mechanical equilibrium of longitudinal mud profile

Examples of models for laminar deposition profiles applied in deposition modelling are published by [6, 7]. The essential mechanical equilibrium of such models is repeated here and sketched in **Figure 8**. A density variation with depth can be schematised into a homogenous density. Static vertical pressure profiles are then

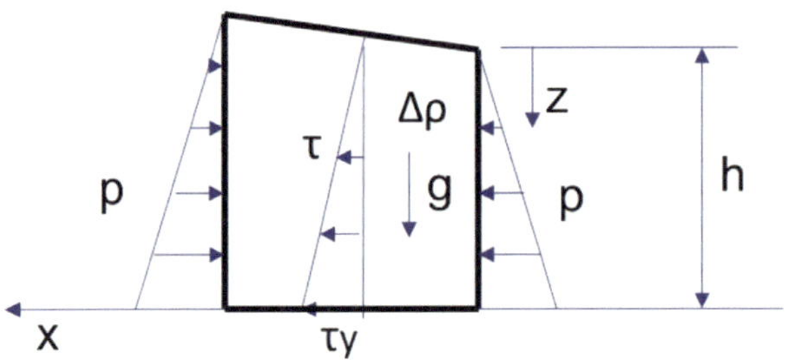

Figure 8.
Definition sketch of mechanical equilibrium of cohesive material on a horizontal base.

linear and equal to $p = \Delta \rho g z$, where z is the vertical distance under the mud surface profile and Δρ is the density difference with supernatant water.

The resulting horizontal driving force follows from the integration of the pressure profiles as: $F_p = \Delta \rho g h \Delta h$. The friction force at the bottom is $F_\tau = \tau_y \Delta x$ Mechanical equilibrium gives $\tau_y = \Delta \rho g h \frac{\mathrm{d}h}{\mathrm{d}x}$. Integration from the toe (x = 0) of the mud profile gives a square-root (sqrt) profile for layer thickness $h = \sqrt{\frac{2\tau_y}{\Delta \rho g} x}$.

4.3 Emden outer harbour mud rheology

4.3.1 Flow curve

Rheology of fluid mud from the Emden Outer Harbour is reported in [35–37]. These measurements are conducted using a smooth BC and applying a shear stress ramp-up (CSS) as well as a controlled shear rates (CSR) protocol. Equilibrium flow curves obtained from the latter protocol are shown in **Figure 9**.

4.3.2 Yield stress

In transitioning from soft soil condition to flow, two yield conditions are distinguished in fluid mud research. One is at the first sign of yielding, when the viscosity strongly declines, and a second condition is originally termed as 'maximum fluidization', Wurpts and Torn (2005) [35]. Similar is applied by [36, 40]. The yield stress at maximum fluidisation is determined by drawing a line through the flow curve beyond 10 [1/s] and extrapolating it towards the vertical axis. Since the data in **Figure 9** represents equilibrium conditions, the intercept of this fitted tangent line with the vertical axis is however close to the static yield stress. A similar yield stress, but probably a bit higher, is found by Shakeel (2022) [41] via viscosity plots of up-ramped CSS and calls it fluidic yield stress (probably very close to 'maximum fluidisation'). Yield stress data of Emden mud, collected from diverse sources, are

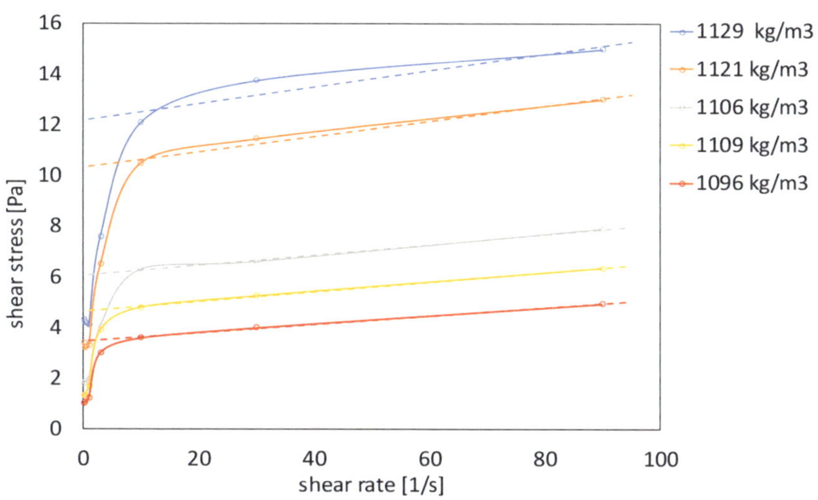

Figure 9.
Equilibrium flow curves of fluid mud from the Emden outer harbour, Germany, after [36]. Dotted lines: Extrapolation to zero shear rate.

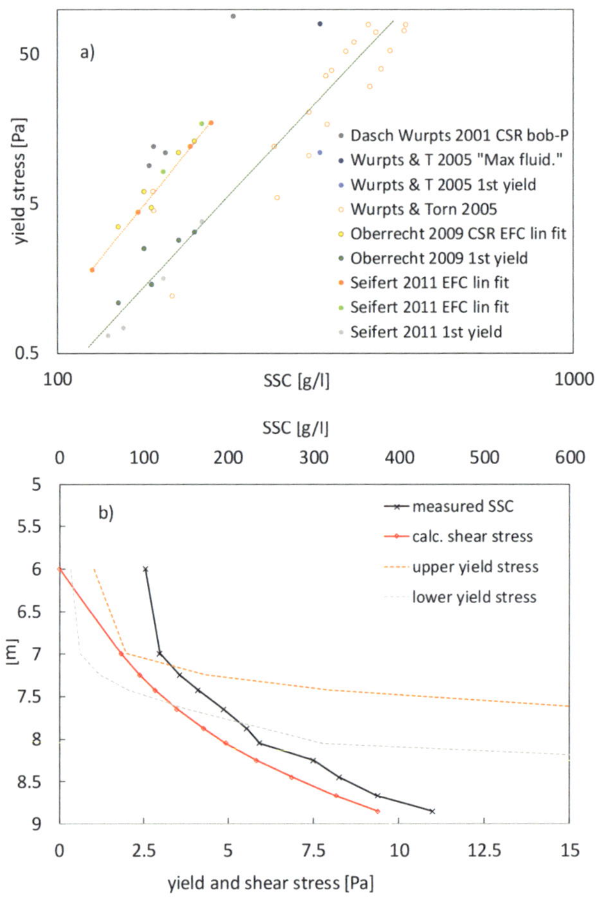

Figure 10.
a) Lower and upper yield stresses of Emden outer harbour samples collected. b) Measured vertical SSC profile and calculated shear and yield stresses.

plotted against their corresponding solid concentrations in **Figure 10a**. As can be seen, the collected data forms two data groups. One group organises itself around a lower diagonal (first sign of yielding, pseudo or slip-yield stress, [1]), and the other groups around an upper nearly parallel line. A factor 4 difference in yield stress is found between these two data groups.

The data of [35] extends to higher solids concentrations. There is also some supportive data in an earlier paper by [34] on maximum fluidisation, where a profiled bob element was used, and the simpler rotoviscometer could only be operated in CSR mode. This data lines up a bit above extrapolated upper yield stress data.

4.4 Application of longitudinal mud profile theory

To ensure mechanical stability, the yield stress of the mud should at least exceed the local shear stress. Suspended solids concentrations (SSCs) in the Emden Outer harbour are in the range of 105 g/l to 400 g/l [37]. Without counter force by the muds' yield stress, the material may flow out of the harbour basin. The mean excess density of the fluid mud is 123 kg/m^3, which is calculated on basis of a measured SSC profile, a water density of 1015 kg/m^3 (=average of low tide and high tide) and a solids density of 2636 kg/m^3 ([42] Dollard mud). Referring to **Figure 7**, a bottom yield stress of 10 Pa suffices to keep the circulated fluid mud at its position respecting the shape of longitudinal profile.

We though also have to evaluate if stability conditions along the entire depth are satisfied. **Figure 10b** shows that the lower yield stress values, which we earlier showed to originate from rheometric wall slip, are not compatible with the muds's conditions in the upper half of the profile. The fluid mud in Emden Outer Harbour would not be able to stay in place and have to run off to the fairway of the river Ems according to wall slip affected rheometry data, which is not the case.

5. Evaluation and takeaways

5.1 Application of rheological characterisation

In using rheology in calculation methods, the entire shear stress-shear rate relation needs to be carefully quantified. Primarily, the remoulded/equilibrium flow curve is needed. Only in exceptional cases where the material is set in motion, un-remoulded conditions, as obtained with CSS ramp-up applied for Hamburg and Emden mud earlier, apply. So, up- and down-ramping (CSS or CSR) is necessary to capture the remoulded/equilibrium conditions. Depending on the application, we need the rheology as a function of fine and coarse constituents.

There exists the risk that wall slip data is mistaken for actual rheology. The rheometric wall slip branch appears akin to viscosity regularisation. Wall slip is, though, situated at relatively higher shear rates, and it does not extend down to a shear stress of zero. In natural fluid muds, this branch appears to be taken for real in some approaches. In CFD modelling of the Elbe-Dollard area [43], the rheological fit (Worrall Tuliani [44]) is laid through this branch, and upon implementation in a CFD code, the viscosity measured at yielding is applied down to zero shear stress. At low shear rates relevant to the fluid muds, the shear stresses are hence underestimated (as a consequence the material flows too fast for acting shear stresses). A similar approach is proposed by Shakeel [41], where the wall slip branch is followed with a fit extending down to the origin. However, in application to field conditions, the first step in yielding (or commencement of wall slip) seems ultimately be skipped [45].

For CFD modelling, we need to have some viscosity (regularisation) at low shear rates. It is advised to have high viscosities here and at least follow the vane curve, but not the plate-plate, and certainly not the bob-cup concentric Couette results.

Implementations where particularly vane-type remoulded (**Figure 4**) branches are followed (fitted by Bingham & viscosity regularisation) are the TUDflow3D model in application to Water Injection Dredging of fluid mud [46, 47] for a schematised keel of vessels sailing through fluid mud. The authors were involved in associated rheometry. Bingham type of models [13], with added viscosity regularisation, are employed in the modelling of tailings deposition in the Delft3Ds model [48], and rheology is augmented by coarse solids. This model cannot be fitted to rheometric wall slip branches, and we never considered doing such.

5.2 Element usage

Given the complexity of mixtures, it is no surprise that manufacturers of rheometers offer a plurality of geometrical shapes for measuring elements. The search for good methods to circumvent problems arising from wall slip can be traced back for decades. Industries handling mixtures with high concentrations of solids often apply vane techniques. The vane-in-cup method and vane-in-bucket method have been developed at the end of the previous century and are since then applied in several studies, e.g. in oil sands [49]. We have found that the vane also reveals wall slip in a material of which one would not expect it at first sight. It is therefore that we advocate the usage of vane for non-Newtonian slurries with high concentrations of solids and recommend bob-cup in the absence of solids, but with a check for wall slip by utilising vane and act according to findings.

Concentric cylinder testing has the advantage that if settling occurs, it does not immediately jeopardise the measurement, contrary to horizontally orientated elements. The Couette inversion problem in concentric cylinder testing is mostly circumvented by applying thin gaps. This is, however, not always possible with solids-laden coarse mixtures and/or when flocs and/or aggregated structure are significantly large. Jamming and other confinement effects may occur, and the mixtures are also prone to wall slippage. In the case of grouts and mortars, dedicated testing devices have been built [50]. For solids-laden settling mixtures, vane testing/verification should be highly prioritised, without the need to revert to dedicated built devices.

Fluid muds are best first tested by concentric cylinder elements because of their good definition of shear rates and ability to accommodate small amounts of sand. Next is to verify for wall slip by vane testing. If samples contain too much sand, it is advised to test by vane and consider applying a transformation method depending on the size of the container. It should also be noted that rotoviscometers may output rotational velocity [rad/s] for vane instead of the shear rate [1/s] as is the case for other elements. Outputted viscosity is then based on rotational velocity.

The present tests reveal significant differences at low shear rates and coincidence at shear rates beyond wall slip. If segregation, i.e. the settling of sand, is essential to the flow problem, it is advised to test with sand (for a short duration, no extensive testing because sand settles under shearing), but also to test the material without sand in a concentric cylinder or similar. In the case of settling sand, the carrier fluid rheology determines the sand settling rate, and the mixture rheology determines the fluid flow. The same considerations regarding element usage apply if excessive wall slip may be expected, like with flocculated materials [49].

6. Conclusion

Wall slip of particulate systems is well known and is rather a rule than an exception. Here, we are encountering it also in a clay-only system, like natural fluid mud (with a sporadic settling solid, if any). The aggregate structure might similarly be a bit different at the wall and apparently also slips at low shear rates.

With complex mixtures, it is often not possible to apply the ideal measuring geometry: wider gaps are necessary and different (surface) geometries. In that case, direct outcomes of rotoviscometer need to be post-processed for rheological characterisation and/or vane testing is necessary complementary to testing with elements with better-defined shear rates.

Exploring in detail the low shear behaviour of yield shear thinning fluids by plotting the results as viscosity graphs accentuates measuring difficulties; care should be exercised not to interpret as (bulk) rheology.

It is unknown what is causing the wall slip of fluid muds, but whatever the cause, the first sign of yielding is not the static yield stress for application in rheological calculations.

Since wall slip of mixtures may constitute an efficient way of transport (pumping of fresh mortar is based on that), it would be worth systematically investigating if/how wall slip in rotoviscometers compares with wall slip in capillary viscometers, at least in the absence of coarse solids.

Acknowledgements

Thanks to Port of Rotterdam, Hamburg Port Authority and TKI for financing measurements such as described in Section 3, Pavan Goda MSc for measurements on Beerkanaal mud and Dr. Dennis Oberrecht of NLKWN Niedersachsen, for kindly providing the Batchelor reports of Franz and Oberrecht containing original rheometric data.

Author details

Arno Talmon[1*] and Ebi Meshkati[2]

1 Deltares, Delft University of Technology, Delft, The Netherlands

2 R&D Boskalis, (Former Deltares), Papendrecht, The Netherlands

*Address all correspondence to: arno.talmon@deltares.nl

References

[1] Cloitre M, Bonnecaze R. A review on wall slip in high solid dispersions. Rheologica Acta, Springer Verlag. 2017;**56**(3):283-305

[2] Mooney M. Explicit formulas for slip and fluidity. Journal of Rheology. 1931;**2**(2):210-222

[3] Goosen P, Paterson A. Trends in stationary deposition velocity with varying slurry concentration covering the turbulent and laminar flow regimes. In: proc. Hydrotransport 19; Golden, USA; 2014. Cranfield, UK: BHR Group Ltd; 2014

[4] Goosen P. An assessment of stationary versus moving bedload under laminar pipe-flow conditions. In: Proc. 15th International Freight Pipeline Society Symposium; Prague, Czech Republic; 2014. Prague: Institute of Hydromechanics AS CR; 2014

[5] Coussot P, Proust S. Slow, unconfined spreading of a mudflow. Journal of Geophysical Research. 1996;**101**(B11):25217-25229

[6] Swenson JB, Sheets B, Kolstad D, van Kesteren WGM. Semi-analytical modeling of thickened tailings flows. In: Proc. 4th Int. Oil Sand Tailings Conference. Lake Louise, Canada: IOSTC; 2014. pp. 415-423

[7] Li AL. Prediction of tailings beach slopes and tailings flow profiles. In: Proc. Paste; 2011; Perth. Crawley, Australia: ACG; 2011. pp. 307-322

[8] Lister JR. Viscous flow down an inclined plane from point and line sources. Journal of Fluid Mechanics. 1992;**242**:631-653

[9] Osmond DI, Griffiths RW. The static shape of yield strength fluids slowly emplaced on slopes. Journal of Geophysical Research. 2001;**106**(8):16241-16250

[10] GI McPhail. Beach prediction experience to date: Further development and review of the stream power-entropy approach. In: proc. Paste; 2018; Perth. Crawley, Australia: ACG; 2018

[11] Shakeel A, Kirichek A, Chassagne C. Yield stress measurements of mud sediments using different rheological methods and geometries: An evidence of two-step yielding. Marine Geology. 2020;**427**(September):106247

[12] Barnes HA. The ""yield stress myth?' paper – 21 years on. Applied Rheology. 2007;**17**(4):43110

[13] Talmon AM, Hanssen JLJ, Winterwerp JC, Sittoni L, van Rhee C. Implementation of tailings rheology in a predictive Open-Channel beaching model. In: proc. Paste. Chile: Santiago; 2016 ISBN 978.956.9393-47-1

[14] Jacobs W, van Kesteren WGM, Winterwerp JC. Strength of sediment mixtures as a function of sand content and clay mineralogy. In: Proc. 9th International Conference on Cohesive Sediment and Transport. Vol. 9. Saga, Japan: Proceedings in Marine Science, Elsevier; 2008. pp. 91-107

[15] Barnes HA, Carnali JO. The vane-in-cup as a novel rheometer geometry for shear thinning and thixotropic materials. Journal of Rheology. 1990;**34**(6):841-866

[16] Fisher DT, Clayton SA, Boger DV, Scales PJ. The bucket rheometer for shear stress-shear rate measurement of industrial suspensions. Journal of Rheology. 2007;**51**:821-831. DOI: 10.1122/1.2750657

[17] Slatter PT, Wasp EJ. The laminar/turbulent transition in large pipes. In: Proceedings 10th Int. Conf. On Transport & Sedimentation of Solids Particles; 2000; Wroclaw. Publishers of the Agricultural University of Wroclaw, Poland; 2000

[18] Talmon AM, Huisman M. Fall velocity of particles in shear flow of drilling fluids. Journal of Tunnelling and Underground Space Technology, including Horizontal Directional Drilling. 2005;**20**(2):193-201

[19] Talmon AM, van Kesteren WGM, Mastbergen DR, Pennekamp JGS, Sheets B. Calculation methodology for segregation of solids in non-Newtonian carrier fluids. In: proc. Paste 2014. Vancouver. Vancouver: InfoMine; 2014

[20] Cooke R. Laminar flow settling: The potential for unexpected problems. In: Proc. 15th International Conference on the Hydraulic Transport of Solids in Pipes (Hydrotransport 15); June 2002; Banff. June 2002. Cranfield, UK, BHR Group Ltd; 2002. pp. 121-133

[21] Chen L, Liu G, Cheng W, Pan G. Pipe flow of pumping wet shotcrete based on lubrication layer. Springerplus. 2016;**5**:495. DOI: 10.1186/s40064-016-2633-3

[22] Green MD, Boger DV. Yielding of suspensions in compression. Industrial and Engineering Chemistry Research. 1997;**36**(11):4984-4992

[23] Chryss AG, Monch A, Constanti-Carey K. Online rheology monitoring of a thickener underflow. In: Proc. 22nd International Conference on Paste, Thickened and Filtered Tailings; 2019; Cape Town. Crawley, Australia: ACG; 2019. pp. 495-504

[24] Boomsma W, van der Hoeven J, in 't Veld M, van Wijk JM, Talmon AM, Meshkati E. Autonomous online pipeline rheometer: Development and application to tailings slurry. In: Proc. Tailings; 2022. Santiago, Chile: Gecamin; 2022

[25] Bartosik AS, Shook CA. Prediction of vertical liquid-solid pipe flow using measured concentration distribution. Particulate Science and Technology. 1995;**13**:85-104

[26] van Wijk JM. Vertical Hydraulic Transport for Deep Sea Mining - a Study into Flow Assurance [PhD-thesis]. Delft University of Technology, The Netherlands; 2016

[27] Talmon AM. Analytical model for pipe wall friction of pseudo-homogenous sand-slurries. Particulate Science and Technology: An International Journal. 2013;**31**(3):264-270

[28] Boger DV, Scales PJ, Sofra F. Paste and thickened tailings and the impact on the development of new rheological techniques. In: Proc. Paste; 2008; Kasana. Crawley, Australia: ACG; 2008

[29] Boger DV. Rheology and the resource industries. Chemical Engineering Science. 2009;**64**:4525-4536

[30] Buscall R, McGowan JI, Morton-Jones AJ. The rheology of concentrated dispersions of weakly attracting colloidal particles with and without wall slip. Journal of Rheology. 1993;**37**(4):621-641

[31] Estellé P, Lanos C, Perrot A. Solving the Couette inverse problem using a Bingham model. In: AERC 3rd Annual European Rheology Conference; 2006. Hersonissos, Greece. HAL-00672923; 2006

[32] Papanastasiou TC. Flows of materials with yield. Journal of Rheology. 1987;**31**:385-404. DOI: 10.1122/1.549926

[33] Goda APK. Rheological and plate' 's Hydrodynamic Resistance in Fluid Mud Measurements for the Nautical Bottom Applications (MSc-thesis). Delft University of Technology, The Netherlands; 2021

[34] Dasch W, Wurpts R. Isoviscs as useful parameters for describing sedimentation. Terra et Aqua. 2001;**82**(March)3-7

[35] Wurpts R, Torn P. 15 years experience with fluid mud: Definition of the nautical bottom with rheological parameters. Terra et Aqua. 2005;**99**(June):22-32

[36] Oberrecht D. Rheologische Analyse von Flüssigschlicksuspension aus unterschiedlichen Lokationen entlang der Ems, Bachelorarbeit [thesis]. Hannover, Germany: LUH; 2009

[37] Seifert A. In Situ Detection and Characterisation of Fluid Mud and Soft Cohesive Sediments by Dynamic Piezocone Penetrometer Testing[PhD-thesis]. Germany: Univ. Bremen; 2011

[38] Ewoldt RH, Johnston MT, Caretta LM. Experimental challenges of shear rheology: How to avoid bad data. In: Spagnolie S, editor. Complex Fluids in Biological Systems. New York: Heidelberg. Dordrecht, London: Springer; 2015

[39] Yan Y, Zhang Z, Cheneler D,·Stokes JR, Adams MJ. The influence of flow confinement on the rheological properties of complex fluids. Rheologica Acta. 2009;**49**(3):255-266. DOI: 10.1007/s00397-009-0401-9

[40] Franz B. Rheologischer Vergleich von Flüssigschlicksuspension und synthetisher Tonsuspension, Bachelorarbeit [thesis]. Hannover, Germany: LUH; 2009

[41] Shakeel A. Rheological Analysis of Mud, Towards an Implementation of the Nautical Bottom Concept in the Port of Hamburg [PhD-thesis]. Delft University of Technology, The Netherlands; 2022

[42] Merckelbach L. Consolidation and Strength Evolution of Soft Mud Layers [PhD-thesis]. Delft University of Technology, The Netherlands; 2000

[43] Oberrecht D. Development of a Numerical Modeling Approach for Large-Scale Fluid Mud Flow in Estuarine Environment [PhD-thesis]. Hannover, Germany: LUH; 2021

[44] Worrall W, Tuliani S. Viscosity changes during the ageing of clay-water suspensions. Transactions and British Ceramic Society. 1964;**63**:167-185

[45] Ohle N, Thies T, Dlugosch J, Schmegel U. Das Projekt Nautische Tiefe im Hamburger Hafen und seine hydroakustischen Herausforderungen, Online-Vortrag im Rahmen des DHyG Hydrographentages "light" [internet]. 2021. Available from: https://www.dhyg.de/images/beitraege/2021/20210608_Projekt_NT_DHyG-Hydrographentag2021_fg_red.pdf

[46] de Wit L, ten Brummelhuis E, Talmon AM. 3D-CFD modelling of water injection dredging including mud rheology. In: proc. WODCON XXIII; 2022; Copenhagen, Denmark. Delft, The Netherlands: CEDA; 2022

[47] Lovato S, Kirichek A, Toxopeus A, Settels J, Talmon AM, Keetels GH. The resistance of a plate moving through mud: Towing tank experiments and numerical simulations. In: Proc. 23rd Numerical Towing Tank Symposium; Mülheim an der Ruhr, Germany. Red Hook, USA: Curran Associates Inc.; 2021

[48] Talmon AM, Sittoni L, Meshkati Shahmirzadi E, Hanssen JLJ. Shear settling in laminar open channel flow: Analytical solution, measurements and numerical simulation. In: proc. Paste; 2018; Perth. Crawley, Australia: ACG

[49] Mizani S. Experimental Study and Surface Deposition Modelling of Amended Oil Sands Tailings Products [PhD-Thesis]. Canada: Carleton University; 2016

[50] Koos E, Linares-Guerrero E, Hunt ML, Brennen CE. Rheological measurements of large particles in high shear rate flows. Physics of Fluids. 2012;**24**:013302

Chapter 6

Settling Slurry Transport: Effects of Solids Grading and Pipe Inclination

Václav Matoušek, Zdeněk Chára and Jiří Konfršt

Abstract

In many industrial applications, settling slurries composed of coarse solid particles (typically sand or gravel) and Newtonian-carrying fluid (typically water) are transported in pipelines. Turbulent flow of such slurries consumes significantly more energy than flow of the carrying fluid alone. A contribution of transported solids to the energy loss is sensitive to solids grading and to the related distribution of solids in a pipe. Also related to the solid's distribution are changes in energy losses caused by an inclination of a pipe transporting settling slurry. We report on recent advances in the description and modeling of pipe flows of settling slurries with a special focus on the effects that the solids grading and the flow inclination have on flow friction. The description includes results of laboratory experiments and model predictions.

Keywords: hydraulic conveying, multispecies slurry, flow friction, solids distribution, pipe experiment

1. Introduction

The size of a solid particle is one of the key parameters affecting the behavior of solid–liquid slurry flow in a pipe. The size determines the type of slurry and is responsible for prevailing mechanisms governing particle support and friction in slurry flow. A majority of predictive models for slurry flows consider just one characteristic size of transported particles and hence cannot take into account the profound effect a broad grading of solids can have on the slurry flow structure and energy loss due to friction.

For flows of settling slurries, it is well known that a considerable reduction of friction loss can be achieved if broadly graded solids are transported instead of uniformly graded solids of the same mass-median grain size [1–3]. Laboratory experiments on the effect of solids grading have been carried out primarily for bimodal slurries composed of two narrow-graded fractions of solids, each of different particle size [4–7].

Recent extensive experiments with various combinations of up to four different fractions of solids of the same density (each representing one type of settling slurry: fine, pseudo-homogeneous, heterogeneous, and stratified, respectively) [8] demonstrated a considerable effect that finer fractions added to coarse stratified flow have on the friction loss and enabled its quantification. An analysis of bimodal slurries tested in these experiments and composed of the coarse stratified fraction and one additional finer fraction (either the fine or pseudo-homogeneous or heterogeneous) showed that the effect of each of the added fractions on the friction loss is different and thus caused by a different mechanism [9]. Other laboratory experiments showed that the broad grading also affects the solids distribution in settling slurry flows [6, 7].

Our experimental investigation, combining observations of flow friction and solids distribution in settling slurry flows of various solids compositions, has aimed to identify mechanisms responsible for the effects that the particle size and the particle size distribution have on friction losses in horizontal and inclined flows. The first results have been published for a limited number of tested solids and flow conditions recently [10–15]. New results are discussed below.

2. Experimental work

The experiments were carried out in a laboratory loop at the Institute of Hydrodynamics in Prague.

2.1 Experimental setup and measuring techniques

The loop is composed of horizontal and vertical pipe sections, each with an internal diameter of 100 mm (**Figure 1**). The geometry of the loop, its measuring equipment, measuring techniques, and experimental procedures for slurry flow tests are described in detail in [15]. During tests, experimental data are collected from both the pipeline and the pump of the loop. Pipe measurements include the mean velocity of slurry V_m (defined as the ratio of the total volumetric discharge of slurry divided by the cross-sectional area of the pipe) by a magnetic flowmeter, the differential pressure over several measuring sections of a pipeline measured by a differential pressure transducer (DPT), and the chord-averaged vertical distributions of local volumetric concentration c by gamma-ray radiometric profilers mounted to some of the

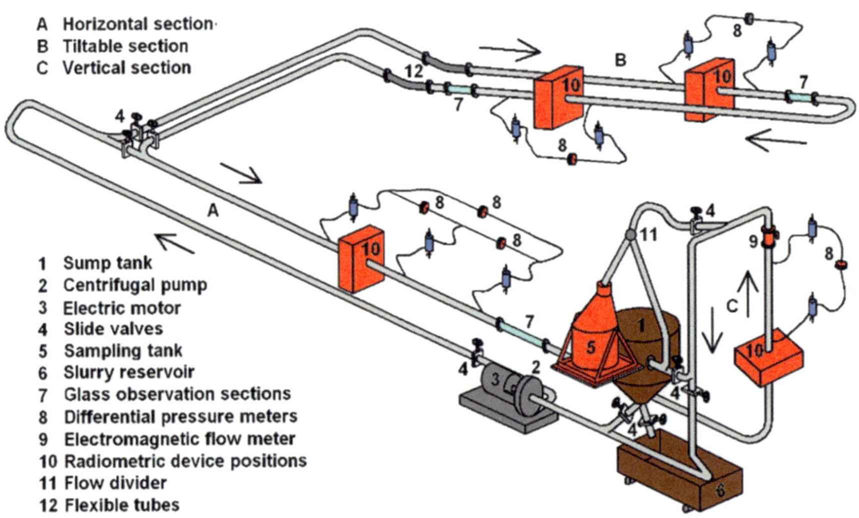

Figure 1.
Layout of experimental pipe loop at Institute of Hydrodynamics.

Fraction code	d_{50} [mm]	d_{85} [mm]	density [kg/m^3]
SS2030	2.19	2.49	2555
ST1040	1.56	2.41	2630
SP0612	0.87	1.20	2620
SP3031	0.55	0.78	2597
STJ25	0.22	0.35	2630

Table 1.
Properties of tested sand fractions.

pressure-drop measuring sections. The delivered concentration C_{vd} (defined as the ratio of the solids discharge and the total discharge) is obtained from the differential pressures measured either in the invert U-tube if it is set to the vertical position, or in the vertical pipe section below the flowmeter (**Figure 1**).

For horizontal-flow tests, local velocities of individual particles are measured at the bottom of the transparent pipe section (No. 7 in **Figure 1**) in the horizontal pipe section. The instantaneous velocities are obtained from images collected by a high-speed camera. The particle image velocimetry (PIV) method is used to analyze the motion of coarse particles in one-species-slurry flow and the motion of fine particles in bimodal slurry flow. The particle tracking velocimetry (PTV) method is used to determine the motion of coarse particles in the flow of bimodal slurry. More details on the velocity measuring techniques used are given in [15].

2.2 Solids fractions used in experiments

Five narrowly graded fractions of sand from fine-to-medium to very coarse (**Table 1**) were used to produce one-species (narrowly graded), bimodal, or multispecies (broadly graded) slurries for laboratory experiments.

3. Inclined flow of settling slurry

Our previous investigations focused on the effect of pipe inclination on partially stratified flow of narrow-graded medium (SP3031) sand [11–14]. The work reported here extends the investigation to inclined flows of narrow-graded coarse-sand (SP0612) slurry and broad-graded medium-sand slurry to test the effects of particle size and its distribution.

3.1 Experimental procedure

Inclined flow tests were carried out for slurries of constant mean delivered concentration C_{vd} flowing at constant mean flow velocity V_m through the ascending limb and the descending limb of the inclinable, invert U-tube of the laboratory loop at various inclination angles ω up to ±45 degrees from the horizontal. In test runs, V_m and C_{vd} are the same in both measuring sections irrespective of the inclination of the U-tube. The other measured parameters, manometric pressure gradient obtained from the installed DPTs and the mean spatial volumetric concentration C_{vi}, obtained by an integration of the solid's distribution over a cross-sectional area of the pipe, differ in the two measuring sections of the U-tube inclined to any angle different from zero. The manometric pressure gradient is composed of the static pressure gradient and the pressure gradient due to friction and both these gradients are affected by the flow inclination. The static gradient depends on the density of slurry in a measuring section and that density is determined from C_{vi}. If C_{vi} is not available, then C_{vd} is used as a less accurate alternative.

3.2 Effect of particle size on inclined flow

The previous experiments showed that the flow of aqueous slurry of narrow-graded medium SP3031-sand exhibited a very different degree of stratification in ascending and descending pipes inclined to the same slope between ±5 and ± 40 degrees. The partially stratified flow of the SP3031-sand produced higher friction than expected (and conventionally predicted) if inclined to slopes not steeper than approximately ±30 degrees [13, 14]. The frictional gradient reached the highest values at the mild negative slopes of say, −10 to −20 degrees. This anomalous trend was also seen in the course of the manometric gradient. It was demonstrated that the observed effect is associated with changes in solid's distribution across the pipe cross-section caused by a variation in the angle of inclination.

The slurry flow of a coarser sand (SP0612) tested in the same laboratory loop using the same procedure exhibits the same effects. Plots in **Figure 2** compare solids distributions (the local volumetric concentration, c, related to the vertical distance from the pipe bottom, y, relative to the internal diameter of a pipe, D) measured with the SP0612-sand slurry simultaneously in the ascending and descending limbs of the lab-loop U-tube set to 25 degrees. The flows of the same flow velocity V_m and delivered concentration C_{vd} differ significantly in the degree of stratification; the descending flow is fully stratified, while the ascending flow exhibits a gradual change in the local concentration across the pipe's entire cross-section. This effect can be predicted by a layered model [11], which captures the variation of the solid's distribution with the inclination angle as shown in **Figure 2**. The flow becomes fully stratified in the descending pipe because the bed slides faster (due to the submerged-weight component acting as an additional driving force in the flow direction) than in the ascending pipe. The top of the faster sliding bed is less eroded and hence the flow more stratified.

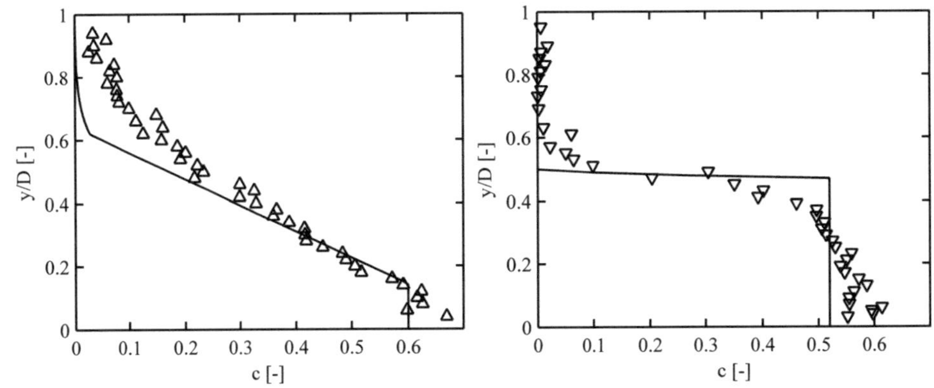

Figure 2.
Distribution of narrow-graded SP0612-sand in flow of $V_m \approx 1.84$ m/s and $C_{vd} \approx 0.17$ inclined at +25° (left) and −25° (right). Legend: Points = measurement, line = prediction by a layered model [12].

The variations in the thickness of the sliding bed cause considerable differences in the friction loss between the ascending limb and the descending limb of the U-tube when inclined up to ±45 degrees from the horizontal (**Figure 3**). Due to the significantly stronger stratification, the descending flow exhibits more resistance than the ascending flow at the same average velocity and delivered concentration if the flow is not very steep. This is particularly the case at mild slopes, where it may lead to a substantially larger frictional gradient in the descending flow than in the ascending flow.

Figure 3 compares different dimensionless pressure gradients ($i = \Delta p/\rho_w/g/L$, where Δp = measured pressure differential, ρ_w = density of standard water of 1000 kg/m^3, g = gravitational acceleration, L = length of measuring section) obtained from the U-tube measurements with the inclined flow of the SP0612-sand slurry. The manometric gradient exhibits both a general trend of an increase in the gradient with the increasing angle of inclination due to the increasing static part of the gradient and the local deviation from this trend for negatively sloped flow at the inclination angle ω of −25 degrees. The frictional gradient exhibits a peak at the same slope. Note that C_{vi} (obtained from measured solids distributions) in the ascending and descending pipes have been used to calculate the frictional gradient from the manometric gradient measurements in **Figure 3**.

The widely used Worster-Denny method [16] to predict the manometric and frictional gradients in inclined slurry flows is used to compare predictions with the experimental results (**Figure 3**). The method gives poor estimates of the inclination effect on the frictional pressure gradient as it does not account for the variable stratification that occurs as a result of variable bed shear in flow inclined to different angles. It gives also poor estimates of the manometric gradient if the measured C_{vi} is used to get the static term. If it uses C_{vd} instead of C_{vi}, the two contradictory trends affecting the manometric gradient compensate each other so that a successful prediction of the manometric gradient is reached for ascending partially stratified flow (but

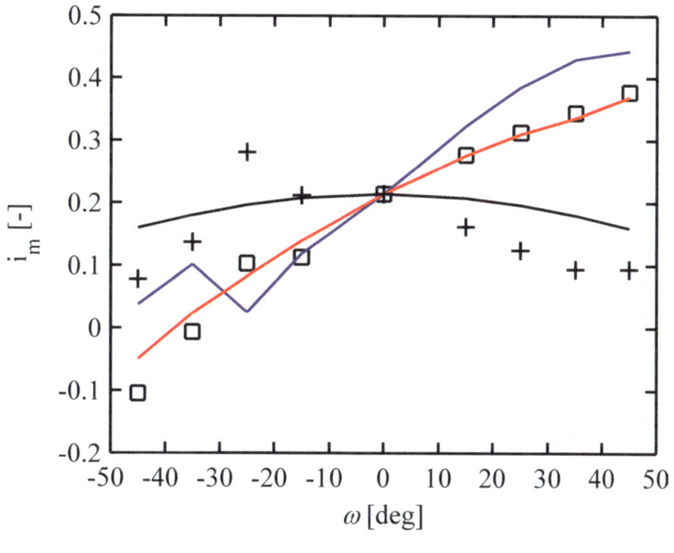

Figure 3.
Dimensionless pressure gradients at various angles of inclination for slurry flow of SP0612 sand at $V_m \approx 1.84$ m/s and $C_{vd} \approx 0.17$. Comparison is made with predictions by Woster-Denny method. Legend: Square = measured manometric gradient; black + = measured frictional gradient; red line = manometric gradient by Worster and Denny based on C_{vd}; blue line = manometric gradient by Worster and Denny based on C_{vi}; black line = frictional gradient by Worster and Denny.

not for descending flow). This case, however, is not general and the compensation effect can be considerably less successful in other stratified flows.

3.3 Effect of broad grading on inclined flow

In order to include the effect of broad grading of solids on inclined partially-stratified flow, an experiment was carried out with inclined flow of broad-graded sand slurry comparable with the previously tested inclined flow of narrow-graded SP3031-sand slurry. Both slurries had same mass median particle size d_{50}.

For the SP3031-slurry, the inclined flows were observed for the conditions given by the delivered concentration C_{vd} = 0.24 and flow velocity V_m = 2.5 m/s in the 100 mm pipe inclined to ±45 degrees [13, 14]. The same conditions were maintained in slurry tests with the broad-graded sand. It was made up by blending three sand fractions as shown in **Table 2**. The proportion of the individual fractions produced a smooth particle size distribution curve of the broadly graded sand which was significantly less steep than the curve for the SP3031 sand and provided the same mass-median size as the SP3031 fraction (d_{50} = 0.55 mm).

3.3.1 Dimensionless pressure gradients

The measured gradients are shown in **Figure 4**. The anomalous values of the manometric gradient occur in the range of angles between −5 degrees and − 25 degrees with a local peak at −15 degrees, which is consistent with the behavior of the narrow-graded slurry (**Figure 5**). The comparison shows that the sensitivity of the manometric gradient to the pipe slope is higher in the flow of the narrow-graded slurry than in the flow of the broad-graded slurry.

The frictional gradients are compared for both types of slurries in **Figure 6**. The results for the broad-graded slurry confirm the trend in the development of the gradient observed previously for the narrow-graded slurry. Furthermore, they give a clearer picture of the trends because of the larger number of data points (measurements at a larger number of inclination angles) and because of the smaller scatter of the data. The results show that the broad-graded slurry exhibits less friction losses than the narrow-graded slurry. The variation in the frictional gradient with the inclination angle is significantly smoother and exhibits smaller peaks in flow of the broad-graded slurry than in flow of the narrow-graded slurry, suggesting that the presence of broader solids grading diminishes effects of a pipe incline on settling-slurry flow.

The frictional gradient is higher than predicted by the Worster-Denny method at slopes milder than ±30 degrees (**Figure 4**). A comparison of the measured gradients (both manometric and frictional) at all flow inclinations confirms that the

Fraction code	Ratio in mixture [%]
SP0612	38
SP3031	31
STJ25	31
Mixture	100

Table 2.
Proportions of fractions of broadly graded sand mixture.

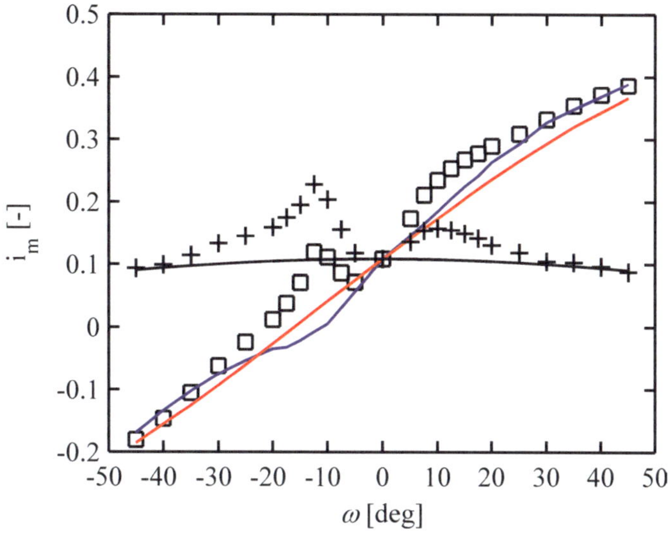

Figure 4.
Dimensionless pressure gradients at various angles of inclination for slurry flow of broad-graded sand at $V_m \approx 2.5$ m/s and $C_{vd} \approx 0.24$. Comparison is made with predictions by Woster-Denny method. Legend: as in **Figure 3**.

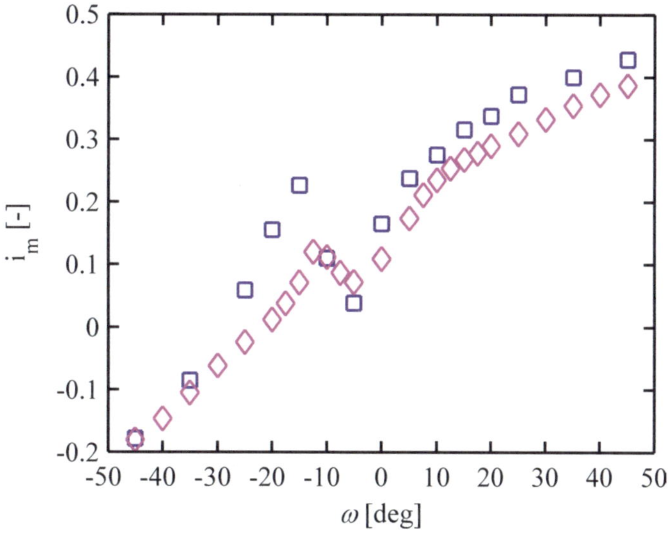

Figure 5.
Measured manometric gradient for broadly graded slurry and corresponding narrowly graded slurry. Legend: Blue square = narrow-graded slurry; magenta diamond = broad-graded slurry.

Worster-Denny method is reliable in predicting the gradients only if the slurry flow is not stratified. For our tested conditions, it is the case only at steep ascending and descending flows.

After examining the effect of the pipe inclination on the dimensionless pressure gradients, it is interesting to evaluate relation between the friction loss and the mean concentration of solids in a pipe and a relation between the friction loss and the solids distribution in the inclined flows.

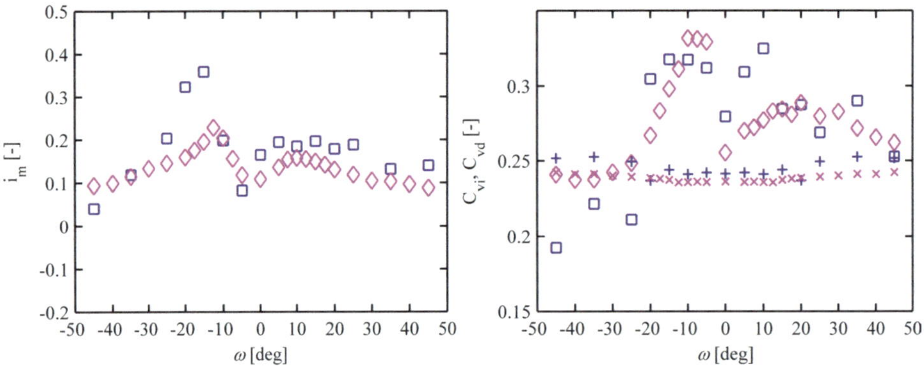

Figure 6.
Measured frictional gradient for broadly graded slurry and corresponding narrowly graded slurry (left). Measured mean concentrations for broadly graded slurry and corresponding narrowly graded slurry (right). Legend: Blue square = narrow-graded slurry (C_{vi}, i_m); magenta diamond = broad-graded slurry (C_{vi}, i_m); x and + = C_{vd}.

3.3.2 Mean concentrations and slip

Although C_{vd} was kept constant in the test runs for the broad-graded slurry at different inclination angles, corresponding values of C_{vi} varied with the inclination angle. **Figure 6** shows that the course of C_{vi} correlates tightly with the course of the frictional gradient and it is consistent with the courses for the narrow-graded slurry. The C_{vd} values tend to exceed the C_{vi} values in the descending flows steeper than −30 degrees, indicating a negative slip at which the mean velocity of particles is higher than the mean velocity of water in the flowing slurry.

3.3.3 Solids distribution

The shapes of concentration distributions differ in ascending flows and descending flows of the broad-graded slurry (**Figure 7**), which is consistent with the distributions in the previously observed flows of the narrow-graded sand.

The differences in the distribution of solids are quite small between the narrow-graded slurry and broad-graded slurry in ascending flows (**Figure 8**) where the

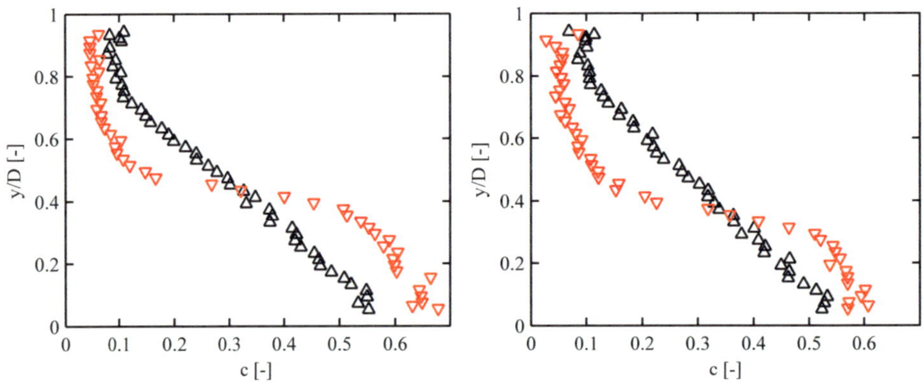

Figure 7.
Comparison of solids distribution of broadly graded sand (d_{50} = 0.55 mm) slurry flow at $V_m \approx$ 2.5 m/s and $C_{vd} \approx$ 0.24 in a 100 mm pipe inclined to ±15° (left) and ± 25° (right). Legend: Black = up; red = down.

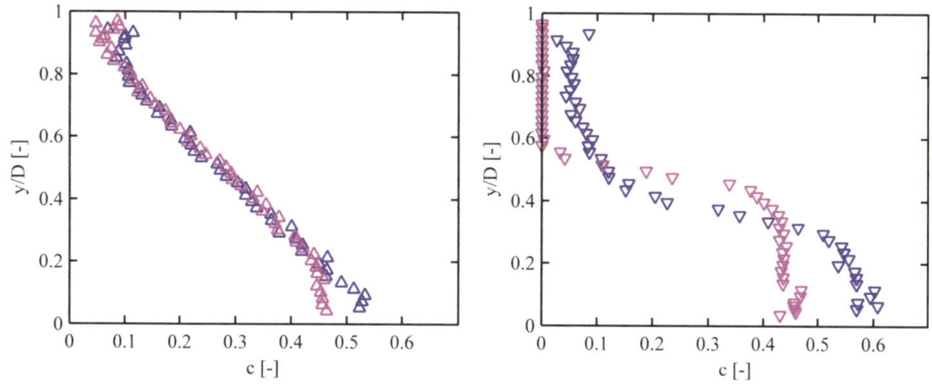

Figure 8.
Measured solids distributions in sand-water flow at $V_m \approx 2.5$ m/s and $C_{vd} \approx 0.24$ in a 100 mm pipe inclined to +25° (left) and −25° (right). Legend: Blue = narrow-graded slurry; magenta = broad-graded slurry.

degree of stratification is weak and the sliding bed thin. Contrary to ascending flows, descending flows exhibit distributions which are quite different in broad-graded slurry than in the corresponding narrow-graded slurry (**Figure 8**).

Comparisons of the developments in the solid's distribution and frictional gradient with the flow inclination angle confirm that more stratified flows produce higher frictional gradients than less stratified flows. Note that the flow of the broadly graded slurry tends to be more energy efficient (produces lower friction losses) than the flow of the narrow-graded slurry at the same flow condition, even though the degree of stratification seems to be very similar. This effect will be discussed further in connection with horizontal bimodal flows.

To summarize, the experimental comparison of inclined flows of narrow-graded and broad-graded sand-water slurries of the same d_{50} = 0.55 mm showed that the anomalous pressure gradient occurred at mild negative slopes in both slurries although it tended to be less pronounced in the broad-graded slurry. The reason for the anomalous gradient—a sharp stratification of descending flow—was the same too although the broad-graded slurry tended to produce a thinner and more concentrated sliding bed than the narrow-graded slurry at the same flow conditions. The friction loss tended to be smaller in the broad-graded flow than in the narrow-graded flow at various tested flow inclines between −45 to +45 degrees. The Worster-Denny method predicted friction loss successfully only if the flow was not stratified. For the stratified flows, the friction loss and other parameters should be predicted by a layered model.

4. Horizontal flow of settling slurry

Although the beneficial effect of a broad particle size distribution on friction loss has been experimentally observed in horizontal flows of settling slurries, for example [3, 6, 7], it has not been investigated systematically yet. Mechanisms through which an interaction of individual solids sub-fractions affects the overall flow resistance are not well understood. The simplest slurries with which to start an investigation on the interaction mechanisms are bimodal slurries. Our first results with horizontal flows of bimodal slurries were reported in [10, 15]. In this chapter, additional results for horizontal bimodal flows are discussed together with results for broad-graded slurries

Fraction code	Ratio in mixture [%]		
SS2030	70	22.5	18
ST1040	—	44.5	36
SP0612	—	33	27
STJ25	30	—	19
Mixture:	**2S**	**3S**	**4S**

Table 3.
Proportions of fractions of broadly graded sand mixtures.

composed of three or four fractions of sand. Results for slurry flows of individual narrow-graded fractions are also added for comparison.

4.1 Experimental procedure

Tests were carried out for different sand slurries at flow conditions allowing easy mutual comparisons. During testing, sand mixtures of different degrees of grading were produced by combining the individual narrow-graded sands at various proportions of each sand in a resulting mixture (**Table 3**).

In test runs, the differential pressures were measured over the measuring sections along the pipe loop and the mean delivered concentration C_{vd} was determined from the inverted U-tube or the other vertical-pipe section at various installed velocities V_m. The local quantities—the concentration of solids in different vertical positions in the pipe cross-section and the solid's velocity at the bottom of the pipe—were measured as well.

4.2 Bimodal slurry flow

The recent extensive broad-graded-slurry tests revealed that the flow of bimodal slurry composed of gravel and fine sand exhibited a considerably reduced friction loss compared to flow of gravel-slurry without the fine-sand addition [9]. It was hypothesized [10] that the major reason for the observed loss reduction was the reduction of mechanical friction between the sliding bed and the pipe wall and that this reduction was caused by a presence of a thin layer of fine-sand particles at the bottom of the pipe which at least partially separated the coarse sliding bed from the pipe wall. This hypothesis was indirectly supported by other results from the same experimental campaign, namely by those for bimodal slurry composed of medium-to-coarse sand and the same fine sand as in the former bimodal slurry. Flow of this bimodal slurry showed a negligible loss reduction by the fine sand. Since this flow did not contain a sliding bed, the result suggested that the friction reduction was effective only if the sliding bed was present. The actual presence of the fine separation layer could not be detected during the experiment due to the lack of flow visualization options.

A more detailed experiment was required to provide information about the internal structure of bimodal slurry flows. Such experiments had to include measurements of local concentrations and velocities of solids in the flow domain under investigation. The first runs from a series of such experiments were carried out for bimodal flows of ST1040-sand and STJ25 in our laboratory in 2020 [15]. Additional experiments followed with a different coarse-sand fraction (SS2030) and their results are discussed in this chapter.

The bimodal 2S-slurry was composed of the coarse SS2030-sand and the fine-to-medium sand STJ25 (**Table 3**). Tests were carried out for flow of the 2S-slurry at $C_{vd} \approx 0.27$ (0.19 of SS2030 and 0.08 of STJ25) and for flow of the corresponding one-species SS2030-slurry at $C_{vd} \approx 0.19$. Both flows were strongly stratified. The stratification was detected visually in the transparent section of the laboratory pipe and its degree was measured by a radiometric concentration meter in the measuring section of the laboratory pipe.

4.2.1 Visual observation

The visualization confirmed the presence of the thin layer composed of the STJ25 sand at the bottom of the pipe. Furthermore, images of a camera directed to the bottom of the transparent pipe captured an interaction of coarse particles and fine particles at the pipe wall and clearly recognized that the finer STJ25 particles reduced the contact of the coarse SS2030 particles with the wall (**Figure 9**).

4.2.2 Solids distribution and local velocity of solids at pipe bottom

Measured distributions of solids in the two comparable flows detected that the flow remained strongly stratified even when the finer sand fraction was added (**Figure 10**). Particles of the finer fraction increased the local concentration at all vertical positions in a pipe cross-section, including the positions in the sliding bed.

Developments in the longitudinal component of the instantaneous velocity of particles at the bottom of pipe were processed from high-speed-camera images over the period of a few seconds and then time-averaged. **Figure 11** compares time series of velocities of particles of the two fractions in the bimodal slurry at V_m = 3.0 m/s. It shows that the finer STJ25-particles (red line) of the thin layer covering the pipe wall move slower than the coarser SS2030-particles at the bottom of the sliding bed. This suggests that the faster coarse particles slide over the slower finer particles of the thin separation layer.

Figure 12 plots the development in the local velocity of coarse particles in the one-species SS2030-sand slurry corresponding with the bimodal slurry in **Figure 11**. **Figure 12** shows that the coarse particles at the bottom of the sliding bed are slower in this flow without the STJ25-additive than the same coarse particles in the bimodal slurry flow at the same flow velocity V_m = 3.0 m/s and the same concentration of the coarse sand. This suggests that the presence of the STJ25-particles at the bottom of the pipe promotes the sliding of the coarse bed.

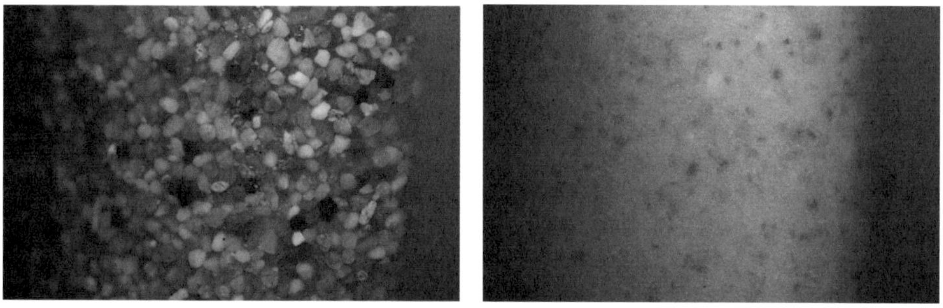

Figure 9.
Camera images (magnified) of slurry at the bottom of the transparent pipe section (flow at V_m = 3.0 m/s). Left: Coarse slurry (SS2030). Right: Corresponding bimodal 2S-slurry (SS2030 + STJ25).

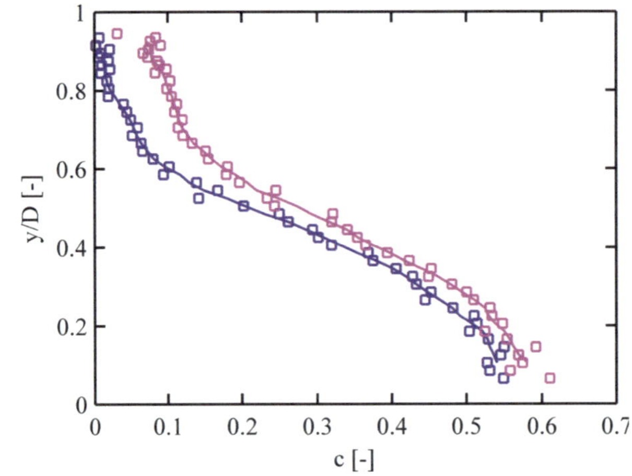

Figure 10.
Comparison of measured solids distributions in flow of coarse SS2030-slurry flow and of corresponding bimodal 2S-slurry at $V_m \approx 3.0$ m/s. Legend: Blue = SS2030-slurry, magenta = 2S-slurry.

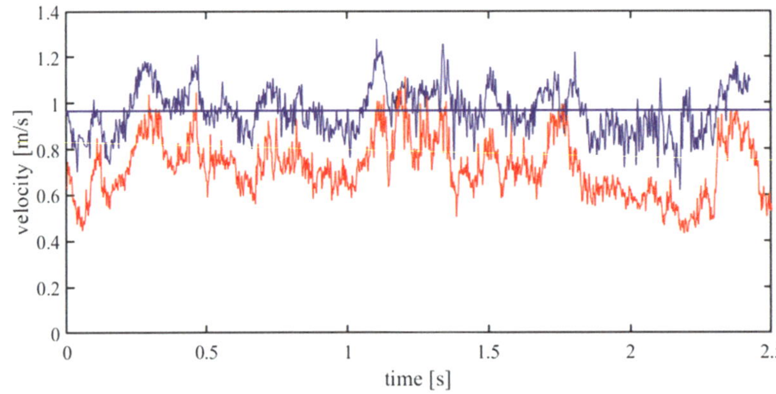

Figure 11.
Measured time series of local velocity of particles of two fractions at pipe bottom for 2S-slurry flow at $V_m = 3.0$ m/s. Legend: Blue = coarse particles in 2S-slurry (horizontal line gives mean value); red = fine particles in 2S-slurry.

Time-averaged longitudinal velocities, u, plotted as horizontal lines in **Figures 11** and **12** were collected at two more velocities additional to $V_m = 3.0$ m/s. The results are collected in **Figure 13** and give a more complete picture of the behavior of particles at the bottom of the pipe. **Figure 13** summarizes the velocities u_c of coarse particles (in the bimodal flow and corresponding one-species flow) and u_f of fine particles (in the bimodal flow). The plot shows that the coarse particles are faster than the fine particles at the bottom of the pipe ($u_c > u_f$) at all tested flow velocities V_m in the bimodal 2S-slurry flow. Moreover, the coarse particles in the 2S-slurry are faster than the same coarse particles in the corresponding one-species coarse slurry at the same flow velocity V_m.

4.2.3 Friction loss

The frictional gradients measured for flows of the bimodal 2S-slurry and of the corresponding coarse SS2030-slurry are compared in **Figure 14**. The bimodal slurry flow

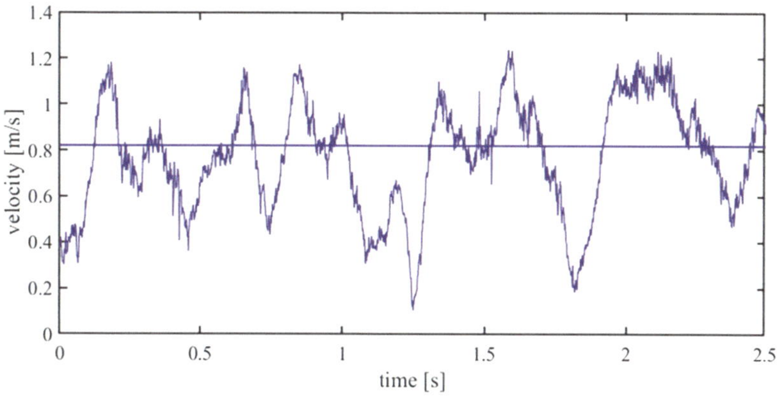

Figure 12.
Measured time series of local velocity of coarse particles at pipe bottom for SS2030-sand slurry flow at V_m = 3.0 m/s.

exhibits lower friction losses than the corresponding coarse-slurry flow and thus the addition of the STJ25-sand caused the loss reduction as in the ST1040-based bimodal slurry tested previously. Note that the STJ25-sand particles have little effect on the friction loss if they are transported in one-species STJ25-slurry at a low concentration similar to the concentration at which they were added to the ST2030-sand slurry (**Figure 14**).

4.2.4 Identification of friction-reduction mechanism

The collected experimental information about the bimodal slurry flow and about flow of the corresponding coarse slurry without the finer-sand additive provides sufficient support for reasonable identification of the prevailing mechanism responsible for the friction reduction in the observed bimodal flow. As shown in **Figure 10**, both flows are strongly stratified. Therefore, the solid's contribution to their friction loss must be due primarily to mechanical friction between the sliding bed and the pipe wall. Hence, the observed friction loss reduction (**Figure 14**) must result from the reduction of this mechanical friction. The detected presence of a thin layer of STJ25-particles (**Figure 9**) between the pipe wall and the bottom of the sliding bed composed preferably of coarse particles (**Figure 10**) suggests that this layer is responsible for the loss reduction.

The information on the local velocities of particles at the bottom of the pipe helps to clarify the role of the thin layer. The observations suggest that its role is as follows:

- the thin layer effectively reduces contacts of coarse particles of the sliding bed with the pipe wall,
- the coarse sliding bed slides over the moving thin layer ($u_c > u_f$), which itself slides over the pipe wall ($u_f > 0$),
- the thin layer makes sliding of the coarse bed easier (u_c in one-species slurry < u_c in the bimodal slurry) even though the pressure gradient, seen as the driving factor for bed sliding, is smaller in the bimodal slurry flow than in the coarse slurry flow (i_m in one-species slurry > i_m in bimodal slurry) at the same V_m.

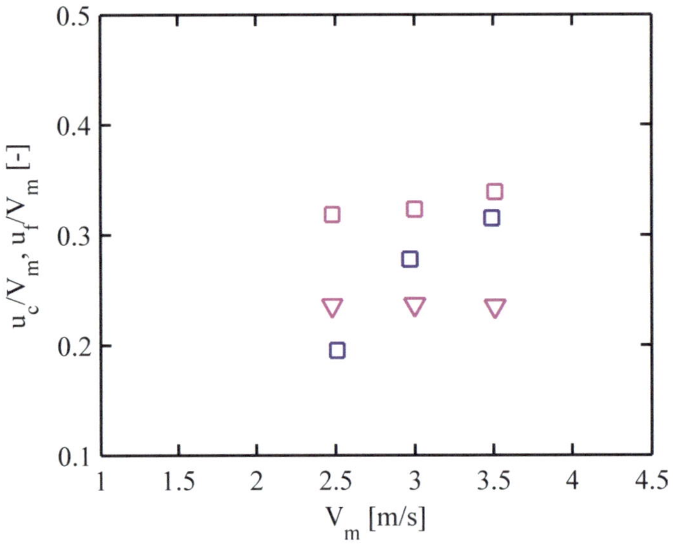

Figure 13.
Measured time-averaged local velocity (normalized by mean flow velocity) at pipe bottom for the flow of bimodal 2S-slurry and for flow corresponding SS2030-sand slurry. Legend: Magenta square = coarse particles in bimodal slurry (u_c/V_m), magenta triangle = fine particles in bimodal slurry (u_f/V_m), blue square - coarse particles in coarse slurry (u_c/V_m).

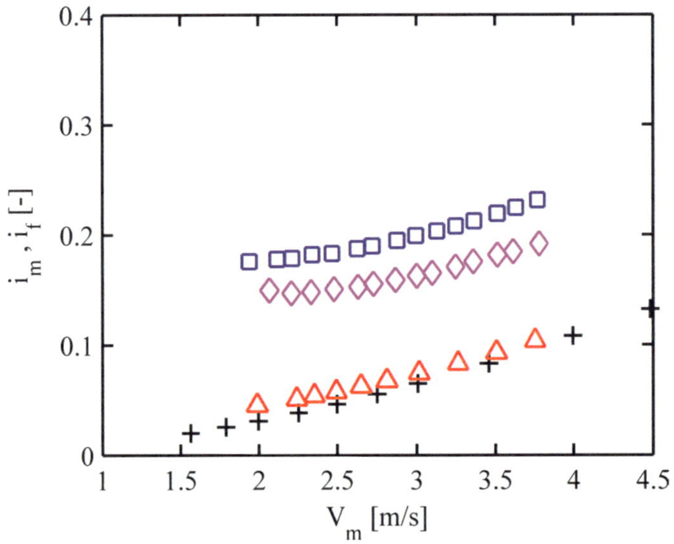

Figure 14.
Measured dimensionless pressure gradient for bimodal 2S-slurry (SS2030 + STJ25 at $C_{vd} \approx 0.19 + 0.08$) and corresponding one-species slurries of coarse sand (SS2030 at $C_{vd} \approx 0.19$) and medium to fine sand (STJ25 at $C_{vd} \approx 0.12$). Legend: Blue square = SS2030-sand slurry; red triangle = STJ25-sand slurry; magenta diamond = bimodal 2S-slurry; black + = water.

The coarse bed sliding easier and faster in the bimodal flow than the coarse bed of the same thickness (**Figure 10**) in the one-species flow, which also has a higher pressure drop, is a very strong indicator that there is a considerably smaller resisting force acting on the sliding bed from the pipe wall in the bimodal flow than in the coarse flow. This reduction of the wall resisting force must be due to the presence of the thin layer at the wall and, therefore the layer is responsible for the friction reduction. In summary, the thin fine layer reduces contacts of coarse particles of the sliding bed with the pipe wall and so reduces resistance and energy consumption associated with mechanical friction between the sliding bed and the pipe wall.

4.3 Broad-graded slurry flow

Besides the bimodal 2S-slurry, two more broad graded slurries were tested. The 3S-slurry contains a mixture of three sands, SS2030, ST1040, and SP0612 (**Table 3**), and its d_{50} = 1.48 mm is very similar to d_{50} = 1.56 mm of the narrow-graded ST1040-sand. Measured friction losses are compared between the 3S-slurry flow and the ST1040-slurry flow of similar values of C_{vd} in the left plot of **Figure 15**. The broader graded slurry obeys considerably less friction in the range of measured flow velocities.

The STJ25-sand is added to produce the 4S-slurry (**Table 3**) and to increase C_{vd} from 0.25 to 0.31. As shown in the right plot of **Figure 15**, the friction loss reduces further by the STJ25-addition, exhibiting the same effect that STJ25 exhibited in the previously discussed bimodal slurry flows.

4.4 Prediction of friction loss

There are several predictive models available for the frictional dimensionless pressure gradient in horizontal flow of settling slurry. As mentioned previously, settling slurry flows exhibit a wide spectrum of flow regimes from pseudo-homogeneous for fine slurries to fully stratified for very coarse slurries. Traditionally and pragmatically, a piecewise application of theories has been employed for each regime and different predictive models have been used for the different regimes. Examples of such models include the Vsm-model for the fully stratified flow, V50-model for the heterogeneous flow, and the equivalent liquid model (ELM) for the pseudo-homogeneous flow, for example, Ref. [17]. A 4-component model (4CM) was developed to predict friction loss over a range of settling-slurry compositions and flow regimes, for example, Ref. [8, 18]. In the 4-component methodology, friction losses are calculated by a weighted average approach of the standard Newtonian carrier-fluid flow model, combined with the ELM, V50-model, and Vsm-model. The broad-graded solids are partitioned into four volume fractions or "components" and each is assigned to one of the four sub-models. If the solids are narrowly graded and fall within one of the components, then the 4CM reduces to the sub-model for the specific flow regime.

4.4.1 Narrow-graded slurries

An example of the use of 4CM for a prediction of the friction loss in slurry flow of narrow-graded sand falling within one component of the 4-component pattern is shown in the left plot of **Figure 16**. The ST2030-sand matches the fully-stratified solids and its slurry flow can be predicted by both the 4CM and the Vsm-model. The plot shows an excellent agreement between the measured losses and the predictions for different concentrations of solids in the slurry.

The ST1040-sand is an interesting case of a narrowly graded sand, which does not fall within one component (in a 100 mm pipe), because its d_{50} is very close to the threshold size for the two components ($d_{\text{threshold}}$ = 0.015D = 1.5 mm; D is the internal

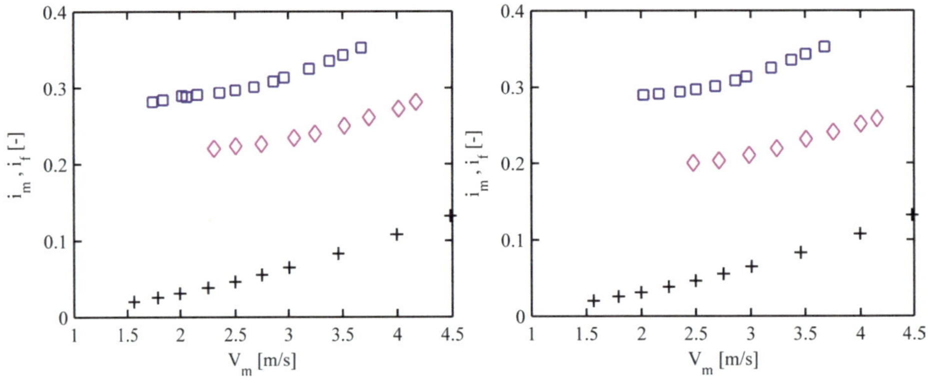

Figure 15.
Measured dimensionless pressure gradient for broad-graded slurry and comparable narrow-graded slurry (ST1040-sand slurry at $C_{vd} \approx 0.28$). Left: 3S-slurry of $d_{50} = 1.48$ mm at $C_{vd} \approx 0.25$. Right: 4S-slurry of $d_{50} = 1.28$ mm at $C_{vd} \approx 0.31$. Legend: Blue square = narrow-graded slurry; magenta diamond = broad-graded slurry; black + = water.

diameter of a pipe). Therefore, the friction loss prediction is not successful by using any of the two individual-component models (either the Vsm-model or the V50-model), and it is successful only if the 4CM is used (**Figure 16**, right plot).

4.4.2 Bimodal and broad-graded slurries

The individual-component models are not suitable for friction loss predictions in broad-graded slurry flows because they use the particle size only to identify the flow. Instead, the entire particle size distribution must be considered, as in the 4CM. As shown in **Figure 17**, an individual-component model can seriously overestimate the friction loss in the flow of bimodal slurry composed of coarse sand and medium-to-fine sand. The two plots of **Figure 17** compare the bimodal flows with flows of

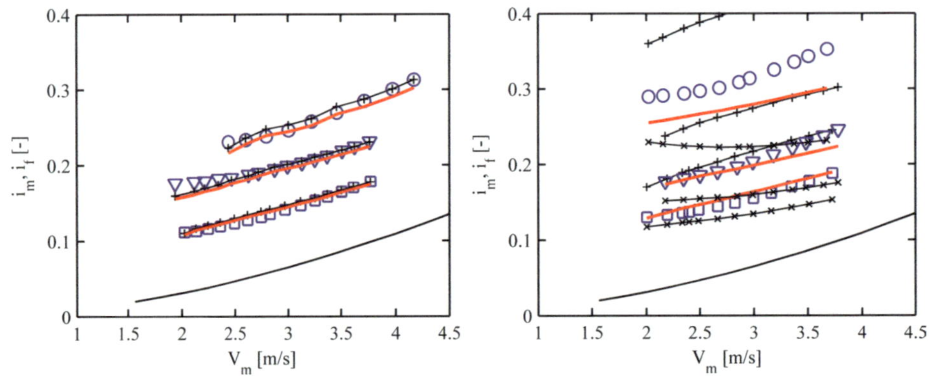

Figure 16.
Measured and predicted dimensionless pressure gradient for slurry flows of individual sand fractions. Left: SS2030-sand slurry at $C_{vd} \approx 0.12$, 0.19, and 0.28. Right: ST1040-sand slurry at $C_{vd} \approx 0.12$, 0.17, and 0.28. Legend: Blue points = measurements (square for C_{vd} of 0.12, triangle for 0.17 and 0.19, circle for 0.28); red line = prediction by 4CM; black line with + = prediction by Vsm-model, black line with x = prediction by V50-model, plain black line = prediction for water.

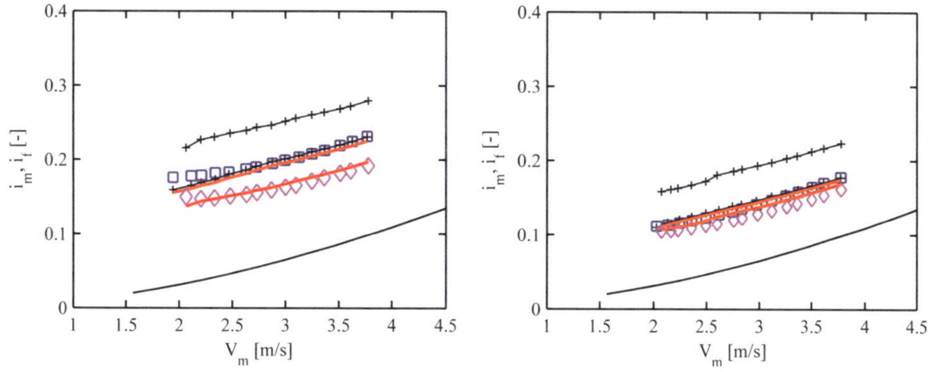

Figure 17.
Measured and predicted dimensionless pressure gradient for 2S-slurry (SS2030 + STJ25) and corresponding coarse slurry (SS2030). Left: as in **Figure 14***. Right: SS2030 + STJ25 at* $C_{vd} \approx 0.12 + 0.06$ *and corresponding SS2030 at* $C_{vd} \approx 0.12$*. Legend: Blue square = measurement for coarse slurry; magenta diamond = measurement for bimodal slurry; red line = prediction by 4CM; black line with + = prediction by Vsm-model; plain black line = prediction for water.*

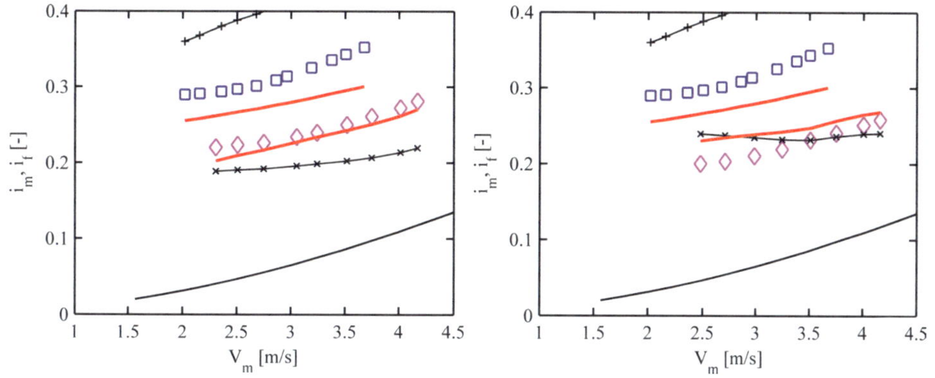

Figure 18.
Measured and predicted dimensionless pressure gradient for broad-graded slurry and comparable narrow-graded slurry as in **Figure 15***. Legend: blue square = measurement for narrow-graded slurry; magenta diamond = measurement for broad-graded slurry; red line = prediction by 4CM; black line with + = prediction for narrow-graded slurry by Vsm-model; black line with x = prediction for broad-graded slurry by V50-model; plain black line = prediction for water.*

their coarse-only counterparts at two different solids concentrations and show that, contrary to the Vsm-model, the 4CM predicts the effect of adding the STJ25-sand to the coarse SS2030-sand slurry very well.

The 3S-slurry, and 4S-slurry, have d_{50} < 1.5 mm (d_{50} = 1.48 mm for the 3S-slurry, d_{50} = 1.28 mm for the 4S-slurry) and thus their individual-component model is the V50-model. **Figure 18** shows that the V50-model prediction of the friction loss in the two broadly graded slurries is less successful than the prediction by the 4CM.

To conclude, a comparison of the new experimental results for various sand slurries in a horizontal 100-mm pipe with predictions of the 4-component model confirms that the 4CM is capable of very reasonable predictions of friction losses in bimodal and broad-graded settling slurry flows in horizontal pipes.

5. Summary conclusions

Extensive resources of experimental work have been called on to elucidate the effects of solids grading and pipe inclination on settling slurry transport. If flowing in horizontal and inclined pipes, broadly graded slurries exhibit lower friction losses than narrowly graded slurries of the same mean particle size, mean flow velocity, and slurry density. The difference in friction loss is particularly important in slurries that are stratified. In broad-graded slurries, fine particles are able to reduce mechanical friction associated with sliding of coarse particles over a pipe wall by developing a thin layer effectively separating the coarse particles from the pipe wall. Also associated with flow stratification and with a presence of a sliding bed is the observed anomalously high friction loss in mildly negatively sloped flows. This anomalous friction loss reduces but does not disappear if the slurry is broadly graded. The reason for the loss reduction is the same as in horizontal flows.

The observed variations of friction loss with the degree of solids grading can be predicted with reasonable success by the 4-component model. A prediction of the observed variation of friction loss with solids distribution, as in the tested inclined flows, requires a layered model.

Acknowledgements

The research has been supported by the Czech Science Foundation through grant project no. 20-13142S.

Author details

Václav Matoušek*, Zdeněk Chára and Jiří Konfršt
Institute of Hydrodynamics, Czech Academy of Sciences, Prague, Czech Republic

*Address all correspondence to: matousek@ih.cas.cz

References

[1] Wilson KC, Clift R, Addie GR, Maffett J. Effect of broad particle grading on slurry stratification ratio and scale-up. Powder Technology. 1990;**61**(2):165-172. DOI: 10.1016/0032-5910(90)80151-N

[2] Gillies RG, Shook CA. Modelling high concentration settling slurry flows. Canadian Journal of Chemical Engineering. 2000;**33**:709-716. DOI: 10.1002/cjce.5450780413

[3] Wilson KC, Clift R, Sellgren A. Operating points for pipelines carrying concentrated heterogeneous slurries. Powder Technology. 2002;**123**:19-24. DOI: 10.1016/S0032-5910(01)00423-5

[4] Shook CA, Gillies R, Haas DB, Husband WHW, Small M. Flow of coarse and fine sand slurries in pipelines. Journal of Pipelines. 1982;**3**:13-21

[5] Maciejewski W, Oxenford J, Shook CA. Transport of coarse rock with sand and clay slurries. In: Proceedings of the 12th Hydrotransport; 28-30 September 1993. Brugge, Belgium: BHR Group; 1993. pp. 705-724

[6] Matoušek V. Pressure drops and flow patterns in sand-mixture pipes. Experimental Thermal and Fluid Science. 2002;**26**:693-702. DOI: 10.1016/S0894-1777(02)00176-0

[7] Kaushal DR, Sato K, Toyota T, Funatsu K, Tomita Y. Effect of particle size distribution on pressure drop and concentration profile in pipeline flow of highly concentrated slurry. International Journal of Multiphase Flow. 2005;**31**:809-823. DOI: 10.1016/j.ijmultiphaseflow.2005.03.003

[8] Visintainer R, Furlan J, McCall G, Sellgren A, Matoušek V. Comprehensive loop testing of a broadly graded (4-component) slurry. In: Proceedings of the 20th Hydrotransport; 3-5 May 2017; Melbourne, Australia: BHR Group; 2017. p. 866-870

[9] Matoušek V, Visintainer R, Furlan J, Sellgren A. Frictional head loss of various bimodal settling slurry flows in pipe. In: Proceedings of the ASME-JSME-KSME 2019 Joint Fluids Engineering Conference (AJKFLUIDS2019); 28 July – 1 August 2019. San Francisco, USA: ASME; 2019. paper No. AJKFLUIDS2019-5395. DOI: 10.1115/AJKFluids2019-5395

[10] Matoušek V, Kesely M, Visintainer R, Furlan J, Sellgren A. Pipe friction of bimodal settling slurry flow. In: Proceedings of the 9th International Conference on Conveying and Handling of Particulate Solids (CHoPS 2018); 2018; London, UK: University of Greenwich; paper No. 44

[11] Matoušek V, Krupička J, Kesely M. A layered model for inclined pipe flow of settling slurry. Powder Technology. 2018;**333**:317-326. DOI: 10.1016/j.powtec.2018.04.021

[12] Matoušek V, Kesely M, Chára Z. Effect of pipe inclination on internal structure of settling slurry flow at and close to deposition limit. Powder Technology. 2019;**343**:533-541. DOI: 10.1016/j.powtec.2018.11.035

[13] Matoušek V, Krupička J, Konfršt J, Vlasák P. Effect of pipe inclination on solids distribution in partially stratified slurry flow. In: Proceedings of the ASME-JSME-KSME 2019 Joint Fluids Engineering Conference (AJKFLUIDS2019); 28 July – 1 August 2019. San Francisco, USA: ASME; 2019. paper No. AJKFLUIDS2019-5397. DOI: 10.1115/AJKFluids2019-5397

[14] Matoušek V, Krupička J, Konfršt J, Vlasák P. Anomalous pressure drop in settling slurry flow through pipe of mild negative slope. In: Proceedings of the 19th International Conference on Transport and Sedimentation of Solid Particles; 24-27 September 2019. Cape Town, RSA: Wroclaw University of Environmental and Life Sciences; 2019. pp. 161-168

[15] Matoušek V, Chára Z, Konfršt J, Novotný J. Experimental investigation on effect of stratification of bimodal settling slurry on slurry flow friction in pipe. Experimental Thermal and Fluid Science. 2022;**132**:110561. DOI: 10.1016/j.expthermflusci.2021.110561

[16] Worster RC, Denny DF. Hydraulic transport of solid materials in pipelines. Proceedings of the Institution of Mechanical Engineers. 1955;**169**:563-586

[17] Wilson KC, Addie G, Sellgren A, Clift R. Slurry Transport Using Centrifugal Pumps. 3rd ed. New York: Springer; 2006. p. 432. DOI: 10.1007/b101079

[18] Visintainer R, McCall G II, Sellgren A, Matoušek V. Large scale, 4-component, settling slurry tests for validation of pipeline friction loss and pump head derate models. WEDA Journal of Dredging. 2022;**20**(1):16-37. In press

Section 3

Instrumentation and Measurement of Slurry Systems

Chapter 7

Electrical Resistance Tomography Applied to Slurry Flows

Lachlan Graham

Abstract

Electrical resistance tomography (ERT) is used to investigate a variety of slurry flow applications including pipe flow, mixing tanks, and thickener feed wells. Transparent liquids such as Carbopol polymer solutions and water are often used to allow for visualization of slurry flows, but ERT can provide data about solids behavior when the liquid phase is transparent or when it is opaque. The state of suspension of solids using ERT is often useful even when the technique is not a primary requirement of a test. The chapter introduces ERT from the point of view of a user in a research environment, but with flow scenarios relevant to industrial applications in mineral processing. Relevant literature concerning slurry flow applications of ERT is reviewed. The basic theory of ERT will be presented together with a discussion of the image reconstruction problem which is a topic of research activity in the slurry transport community. An overview of ERT applications in slurry pipe flow and mixing tanks will be presented. Examples of the application of ERT to pipe flow and tanks will be discussed in detail, including practical experiences with integrating ERT into slurry pipe and tank rigs.

Keywords: electrical resistance tomography, slurry flow, pipe flow, visualization, slurry pipe applications

1. Introduction

Electrical resistance tomography (ERT) is a well-established technique for obtaining the cross-sectional distributions of solids in slurry pipe flows and tanks, among other uses. Basic details of the ERT technique are given in [1] and many other publications. ERT for process applications was discussed in [2]. Previously, ERT had been extensively used in geophysical applications as well as being explored for use in biomedical imaging. The basics of design and implementation of ERT technology suitable for process applications are presented in the paper. The authors specifically mention mixing scale-up as an application for ERT and introduced the 1.5-m diameter tank at UMIST (University of Manchester Institute of Science and Technology), which was equipped with a full set of ERT electrodes covering most of the tank wall. A recent book describing many forms of tomography for industrial applications, including ERT, is [3].

The present contribution describes the basic principle of ERT as applied to slurries focusing on pipe flow and mixing tanks as conducted by the Fluids Engineering Team at CSIRO.

2. Basic principle of ERT

The principle of operation of electrical resistance tomography (ERT) is to inject a known electrical current into a pair of the (usually) 16 electrodes in a plane equi-spaced around a vessel or pipe wall and measure the voltages present on the remaining electrodes. The process is cycled through the remaining possible pairs of injection current locations (15 pairs) to give an extensive data set for the measurement plane. The complete set of measured voltages is then used to reconstruct an image of the conductivity in the vessel's cross section from which the solids concentration or gas fraction can be obtained in principle, if the liquid- and solid-phase conductivities are known (gas and most solids in slurries would have zero conductivity). A basic schematic of the measurement and reconstruction process is shown in **Figure 1**.

ERT requires an inverse problem algorithm to calculate the conductivity distribution from the voltage measurements. If the conductivity distribution is known from such a calculation, the volume concentration of the nonconductive solids or gas can be calculated from the measured conductivity via the reduced Maxwell equation:

$$\phi = \frac{2(\sigma_1 - \sigma_{mc})}{\sigma_{mc} + 2\sigma_1} \tag{1}$$

where.

σ_1 = continuous phase or background conductivity (typically water or another homogenous supernatant such as a carrier fluid or fine particle slurry).

σ_{mc} = measured reconstructed conductivity.

ϕ = volume fraction of the nonconductive phase.

Note that the aforementioned equation is applicable for zero conductivity solids only with a more complex version applicable if the solids exhibit some level of conductivity. The equation is also applicable for a gas phase which can also be considered having zero conductivity. The volume fraction may be readily converted to other measures of concentration if the solids and liquids densities are known.

Areas of an image with a lower conductivity indicate the presence of solids to be higher as the particles present in many slurries are nonconductive. The data acquisition process is repeated across multiple planes in the vessel or pipe; however,

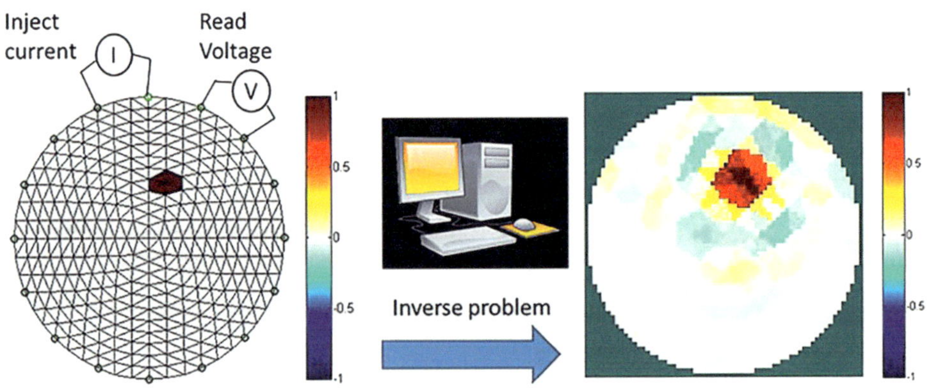

Figure 1.
Basic operation principle of ERT. Differential reconstruction assumed.

usually only one plane can be measured at any one time with most commercial hardware and software.

3. Slurry ERT literature review

Improving the accuracy and utility of ERT for slurry applications has been the subject of many articles over the years, and a selection of these is reviewed here. A recent comprehensive overall review of slurry applications of ERT is given in [4].

Ref. [5] has presented a general iterative algorithm to improve the quantitative accuracy of ERT. This used a 2D model for the forward problem and was shown to be superior to the linear backprojection (LBP) algorithm used for rapid image reconstruction.

A further paper from the same group demonstrated ERT in use to understand the differing flow regimes in pipe flows [6]. They used slurry concentrations up to 20% by volume in a pipe loop with diameter 3 inches. The ERT was shown to readily visualize the flow regimes from homogenous flow to stratified flow. The transitions between these flow regimes could also be readily detected.

Ref. [7] examined the solids distribution in suspension flows with ERT. They used both neutrally buoyant, low- and high-density particles. Their algorithm used a 2D inverse problem and a 3D forward problem called a "pseudo three-dimensional algorithm." They attempted to model the observed particle distributions with limited success.

Ref. [8] examined bidispersed suspensions of negatively buoyant particles in a low Reynolds number pressure-driven pipe flow. A nonlinear ERT reconstruction algorithm was used. They used PMMA particles and silver particles. Due to the conductivity of the silver particles, the two types of particles were able to be imaged separately. These data were used for comparison with a suspension model, and another interesting result was the observation of the hindering of particle settling of one phase by the other phase.

Ref. [9] used a high-speed ERT system to measure concentration and velocity profiles in pipe flow. An 80-mm diameter pipe rig was used for all the tests. Two electrode planes of 100 mm apart were used for a cross-correlation technique to measure velocities. Kaolin carrier fluids and silica sand coarse particles were used to make the slurries.

Ref. [10] described one of the earliest ERT results for pipe flow. They used 60-mm and 100-mm diameter pipe loops with slurries made from water and sand or glass particles. Solids concentrations ranged from 6.8 to 13.7% by weight. Among other results, they were able to demonstrate ERT detection of a dispersed suspension compared with a saltating suspension. They proposed that a deposition velocity could be determined from the ERT image.

A recent example of ERT in conjunction with CFD applied to slurry tank flows is [11] where the mixing performance of a coaxial system comprises a wall scraper and a pitch blade central impeller. It was found that the coaxial mixer system provided better particle suspension than a single-impeller system.

A combination of ERT and magnetic flow meter has recently become commercially available as discussed in [12, 13]. The device was trialed in a dredging application. A significant advantage of the new device is that it eliminates the safety concerns of nuclear sources on board dredging vessels. The ERT is integrated into a single spool together with the magnetic flow meter.

Ref. [13] also describes other industrial applications of ERT in slurry flows, including mineral processing, tunneling, and deep-sea mining. Again, the motivation for much of this work is replacement of nuclear density gauges.

4. CSIRO slurry research facilities

CSIRO Mineral Resources has a 100-mm diameter pipe rig in several versions which has been equipped with ERT since 2002. The rig also is equipped with conventional instrumentation including a magnetic flow meter and pressure transducers as shown in the schematic diagram in **Figure 2**. This rig can also be inclined if required as shown in **Figure 3**. Transparent sections allowed for visualization. The sampling point shown allows for carrier fluid/slurry to be taken off the top of the flow in

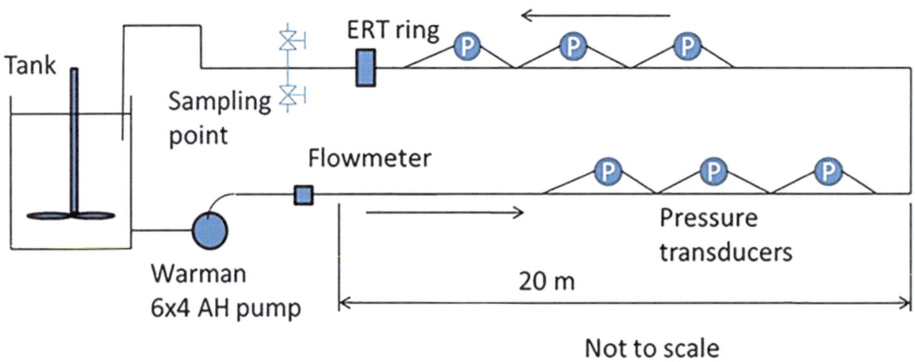

Figure 2.
Schematic diagram of CSIRO mineral resources pipe rig.

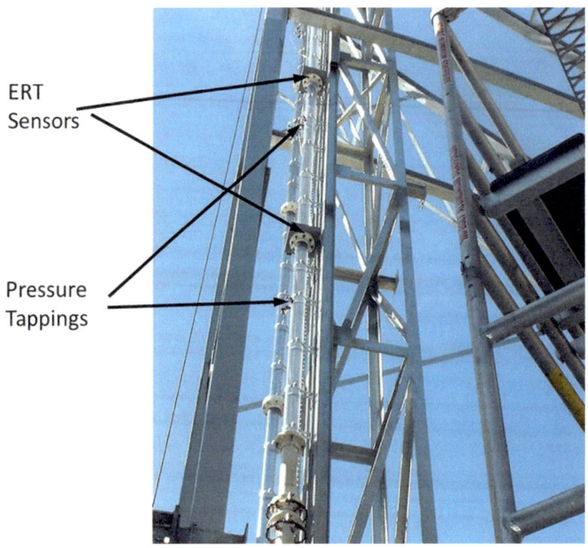

Figure 3.
View of ERT sensors on pipe rig when pipe is in the vertical orientation.

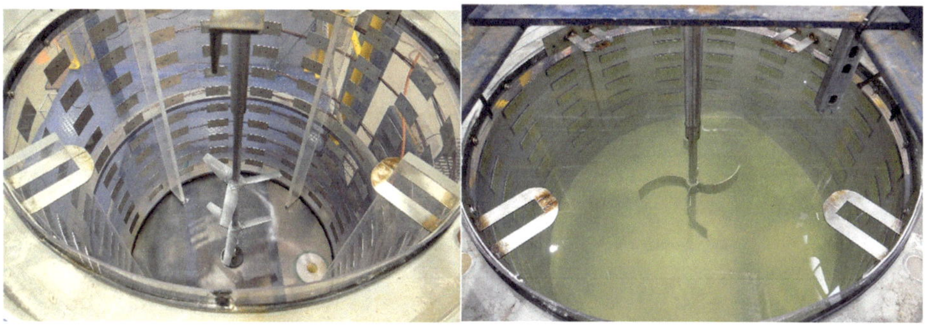

Figure 4.
Photographs of a 1-m diameter tank equipped with ERT electrodes. Two different impeller configurations shown: Baffled and unbaffled.

laminar flow to allow for rheology measurements as well as conductivity measurements without having to fully screen the complete slurry samples. Further rig details are given in [14].

The slurry mixing tanks at CSIRO typically include impeller torque and speed measurement capability and are made from transparent acrylic to allow for flow visualization, particularly in order to examine particle suspension behavior. Selected tanks have recently been equipped with ERT electrode sets to allow for imaging of concentration distributions and particularly to explore solids concentration variations within the tank which cannot be discerned from video recordings or other means. **Figure 4** shows photographs of two tank configurations used at CSIRO for slurry research.

CSIRO Mineral Resources primarily uses ITS ERT equipment including 2x ITS P2000 and 1x p2+ instruments together with the data acquisition and reconstruction software provided with these instruments. The P2000 was the primary instrument for the pipe rig and was placed in a remote weatherproof box on the rig to minimize the analog signal cable lengths. Similarly, the ERT electrode rings and cables were weather-proofed.

5. Image reconstruction for slurry applications

5.1 Background

Image reconstruction is one of the major challenges in ERT applications as it is an ill-posed problem, as noted in [15], and is still an active research area. An in-depth analysis of research work in the area of image reconstruction will not be discussed here; however, relevant points for slurry applications will be illustrated.

An overall principle of ERT is that image reconstruction is an inverse problem; it is required to calculate the conductivity distribution in a defined space based on boundary measurements. The calculation of the measurements based on a known conductivity distribution within the space and electrode injection current is relatively straightforward and is referred to as the "forward problem."

Early reconstruction methods were based around a backprojection algorithm as described in [16]. Algorithms based on this concept are still in use at the time of writing as the usual reconstruction technique supplied with commercial ERT systems.

Typically, this is a linear backprojection (LBP) algorithm. It has the advantage of speed, allowing for near real-time imaging and relative simplicity. The backprojection has the disadvantage of being qualitative and also suffers from blurring in instances where high-conductivity gradients are present as noted by [17]. However, in many circumstances, it is sufficient for investigating slurry flows and is widely used. Usually, the ERT process begins with collecting a homogenous reference data set in the vessel of interest. A data set is then obtained with the solids or gas added to the vessel and the reconstruction performed using a differential approach relative to the reference.

Alternative algorithms are available to overcome some of the shortcomings of the LBP in situations where there would be a benefit such as sharp concentration gradients and rapid images are not required. These algorithms have grown in popularity, especially as computational power has increased, thus allowing more complex computational processing in a reasonable time.

Ref. [18] presented a sensitivity conjugate gradient (SCG) method for ERT which was also an early commercial offering. This technique was shown to decrease the blurring or smearing inherent in the LBP for sharp discontinuities and thereby provide improved contrast recognition than the backprojection algorithm tested on synthesized data. Examples using real data were also presented including imaging a human hand. The real data results showed that the SCG was able to provide much more detail than other contemporary alternatives.

Ref. [19] describes a MATLAB toolkit, EIDORS, which provides a framework for developing and testing tomography reconstruction algorithms. Simulations of ERT measurements can be made in the toolkit and various reconstruction approaches tested. Experimental data can also be processed in EIDORS using a wider variety of algorithms. Further details of EIDORS are given in [20].

The commercial ERT suppliers are also continuing to develop their offerings for postprocessing of ERT data. An example of this is described in [21]. A variety of algorithms were presented which were stated to be suitable for various scenarios in ERT. A recent state of the art is described in [12].

Most ERT data acquisition and reconstruction are performed assuming two-dimensional behavior of the electric fields. This is a simplification as noted by [22] as the actual electric fields are three-dimensional. The effects can be mitigated in some circumstances by using a 2.5D approach as described in [23]. While the 2.5D approach was successfully used for slurry pipe imaging by [24], it is more difficult to apply the concept to a mixing tank as the invariance of the slurry condition along the axis of the vessel is not necessarily present, unlike for the case for pipe flow. Judicious choice of the injection current for the ERT test and the spacing between electrode rings may reduce the 3D effects. A full 3D data acquisition and reconstruction is also possible in principle to avoid these issues but is not available in the presently available commercial hardware, since the planes are usually measured separately in sequence. However, if the flow timescales are long relative to the data acquisition time, the data from the separate planes can be combined to provide three-dimensional information. This approach can be useful for tanks or gas/liquid systems and for the cross-correlation velocity measurements. High-speed versions (500 frames per second or more) of the commercial ERT systems are available for these applications.

5.2 Comparison with other imaging techniques

Other imaging techniques have been applied for slurry flows. An example is gamma-ray tomography which is an extension of the industrially used gamma-ray density instrument. This technique relies on the attenuation of the gamma-ray varying as varying density slurry flows through the measurement section as described in [25]. Tomography applications require multiple sources and detectors or a single source and detector that can be rotated or translated across the measurement section. More details of the technique are given in [26]. Disadvantages of the method were the time taken to acquire the data (tens of minutes using a single source/detector) and an increase in errors near the pipe wall. The acquisition time can be a concern given that laboratory slurry tests are usually carried out in recirculating rigs, thus leading to potential change of the properties of the slurry due to particle attrition and temperature rise. A multiple source/detector system was described in [27] based on a system described in [28] and the errors of the system evaluated for water/clay/sand slurries in a 100-mm pipe up to 20% v/v of sand. Further work by the SRC group is given in [29], where they use the gamma-ray technique to assist with correcting ERT for conductivity changes in the carrier fluid. The device used was capable of rapid imaging (up to 100 Hz) unlike single source/detector systems.

The present author and his colleagues have used MRI imaging to investigate slurry flows, prior to using ERT. Ref. [30] describes the basic principles of NMR/MRI together with its application to flows. A useful property of NMR is that there is a velocity sensitivity inherent in the physics, which is manifested in the phase image. While it was possible to obtain velocity and concentration data from MRI for synthetic polymer solution-based slurries, the rapid decay of the NMR signal due to the short T2 relaxation time prevented application to industrial slurries in larger pipes where rapid gradient switching is difficult, although smaller systems such as the rheological application discussed in [31] are possible. A further update of MRI possibilities for rheology and fluid dynamic applications is given in [32]. Another consideration is that the MRI equipment is often larger and more expensive than ERT, although permanent magnet systems are available which are more economical than cryogenic systems, whereas ERT is more usable industrially as described in [13]. It is possible to obtain velocity information from ERT data via a cross-correlation technique using two electrode planes. This technique was used by [9] with a high-speed ERT data acquisition system to obtain velocity data in slurry pipe flow.

Figure 5 from [33] shows a comparison between a photograph, MRI and ERT from the CSIRO pipe rig where a bed of solids was present in the pipe flow. The ERT data includes LBP as well as a more advanced SCG processing [18] of the same data. This algorithm was one of the early postprocessing options available commercially, and the results are in better qualitative agreement with the MRI and photograph than the LBP. Slurry velocity images obtained by MRI over a range of velocities are shown in **Figure 6**. These flows were all in the laminar regime. Unfortunately, the MRI system was not usable with industrial slurries or the later development of the pipe rig which had a steel structure.

5.3 ERT image reconstruction for pipe flow

The commercial ERT systems (ITS P2000 and p2+) used at CSIRO for slurry flow research were supplied with the LBP reconstruction as the default option. In practice, when operating the pipe rig and mixing tanks, the real-time LBP images are very useful in monitoring the state of suspension in the flow and adequate for determining the effect of pipe velocity or impeller speed on particle suspension.

An early comparison between LBP and a more advanced algorithm (SCG) for a settled bed of solids was given previously in **Figure 5**.

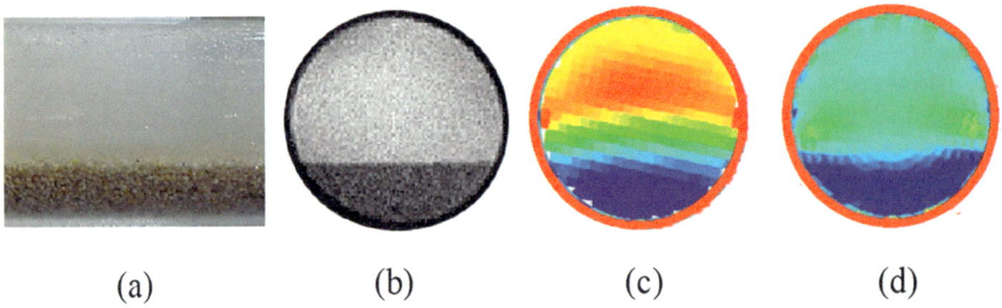

Figure 5.
Comparison between (a) photograph, (b) MRI and ERT algorithms, (c) LBP, and (d) SCG ([18]). As originally published and presented at the BHR 15th International conference on Hydrotransport, Banff, Canada, 3rd-5th, June 2002, [33].

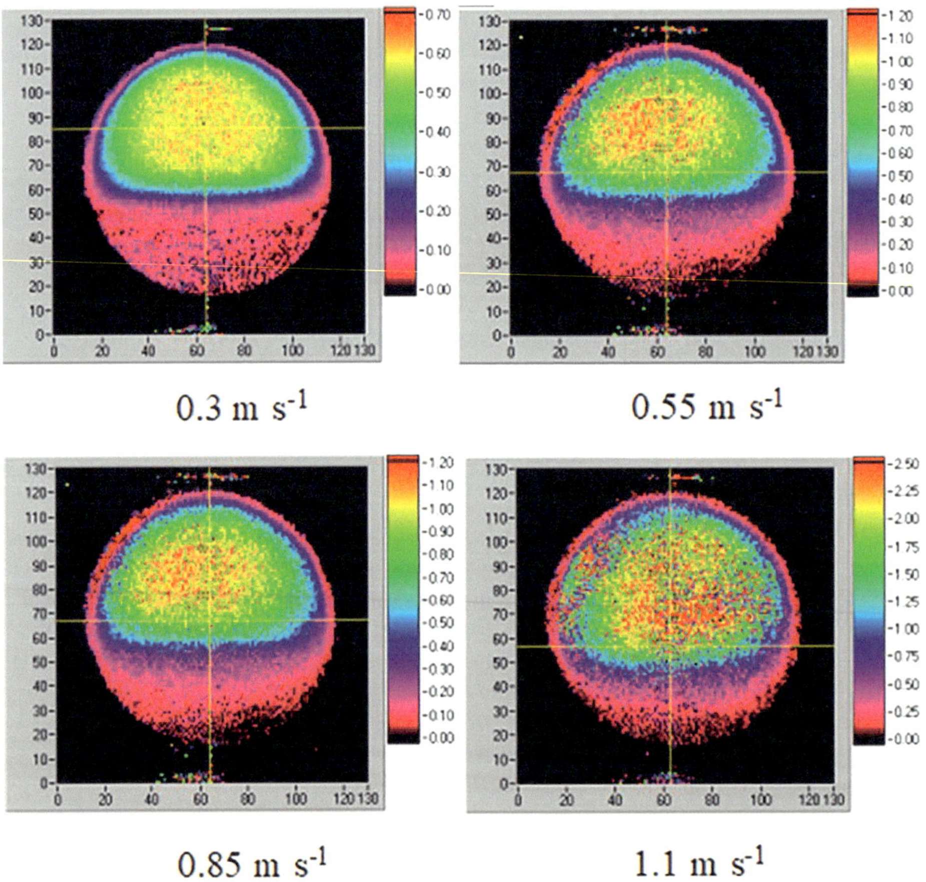

Figure 6.
MRI velocity images (5% v/v solids in Ultrez 10 (Carbopol polymer solution)) at superficial velocities from 0.3 to 1.1 m s^{-1}. The distortion in the velocity images is due to the bed of solids.

The author and his colleagues also use a 2.5D approach as described in more detail in [24] which describes the application of an absolute image reconstruction approach which does not require a reference image other than for data acquisition. The essential

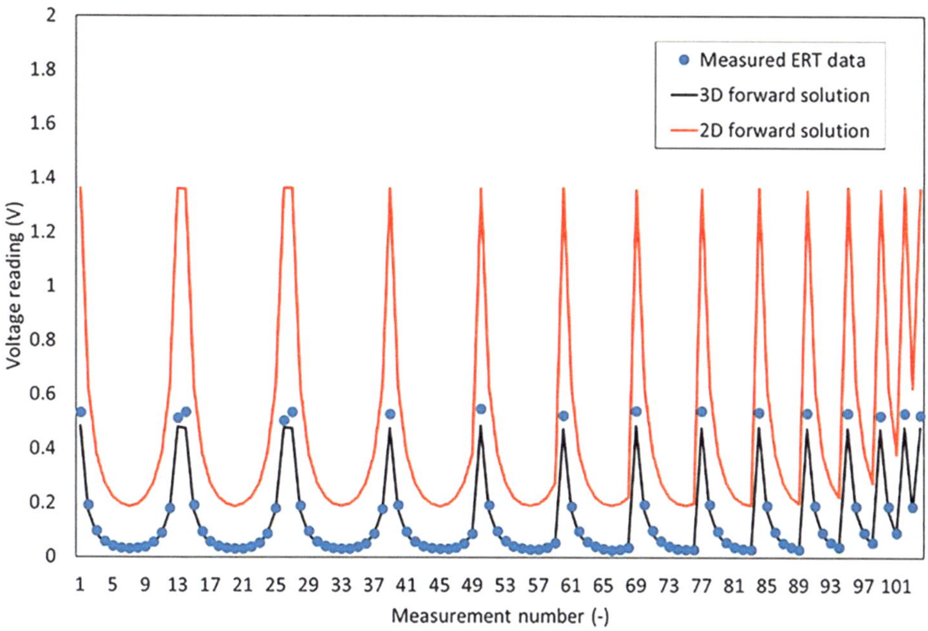

Figure 7.
ERT voltages from experiment and simulation of a homogenous fluid in a pipe asssuming 2D and 3D behavior. As originally published and presented at the BHR 20th International conference on Hydrotransport, Melbourne, Australia, 3rd–5th may 2017, [24].

feature of this approach is to conduct the forward problem in 3D (assuming that the pipe flow is invariant along the pipe axis) and the inverse problem as a 2D slice through the center of the electrodes. The significance of the 3D forward problem is shown in **Figure 7** where measured ERT from a pipe with a homogenous fluid is shown compared with 2D and 3D forward solutions. It is clear the 3D forward problem is the most appropriate.

The results from conventional LBP differential processing and 2.5D absolute processing are shown in **Figures 8** and **9**, respectively, for a high-conductivity tailings sample in a 100-mm pipe. In this case, the reference data were taken from a homogenized sample of the slurry. It should be noted that both approaches adequately detect the stratification of the flow, but the absolute processing allows for the case where obtaining a suitable carrier fluid reference image is difficult. The author's colleagues are continuing research into image reconstruction approaches for pipe flow at the time of writing.

6. Slurry pipe applications and challenges

This section discusses application examples of ERT in slurry pipe flow over a variety of slurries ranging from synthetic laboratory slurries to industrial tailings samples.

Figure 10 shows LBP images from a CSIRO test in a 50-mm NB pipe rig examining the transition from horizontal to vertical flow for a polymer solution/crushed glass-based suspension based on data presented in [34]. The sample results here showed that the stratification could be maintained, change side, or be destroyed in the pipe depending on flow conditions which, in the case of constant carrier fluid rheology,

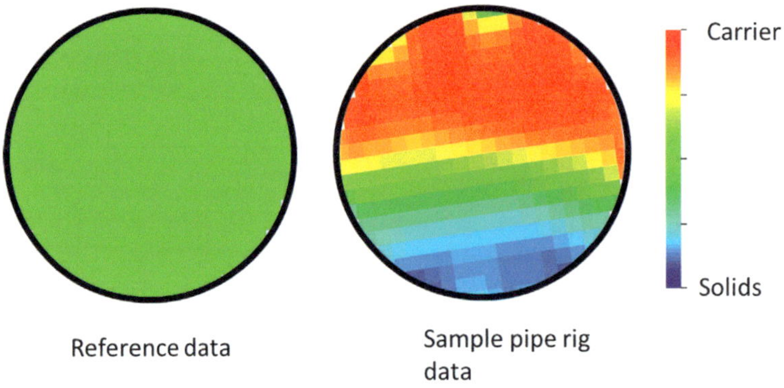

Figure 8.
Comparison between reference data and sample pipe rig data for high-conductivity tailings. Conventional differential 2D LBP processing. Both images are at the same (arbitrary) scale. As originally published and presented at the BHR 20th International conference on Hydrotransport, Melbourne, Australia, 3rd–5th may 2017, [24].

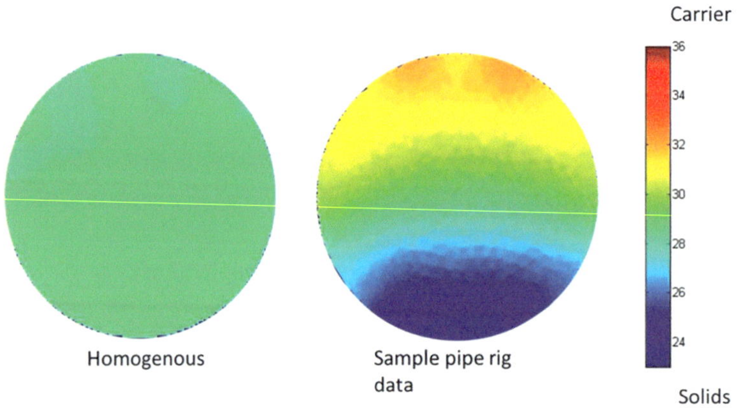

Figure 9.
Comparison between homogenous and stratified ERT images using absolute 2.5D processing on the same data as **Figure 8**. *Conductivity images shown. As originally published and presented at the BHR 20th International conference on Hydrotransport, Melbourne, Australia, 3rd–5th may 2017, [24].*

could be superficial velocity. Further results from [34] showed that the distribution of solids in the vertical pipe was a function of the rheology of the carrier fluid and the pipe velocity for a fixed 4x diameter bend as the transition element from horizontal to vertical, with some conditions leading to the stratification being maintained in the vertical pipe. It should be noted that the yield stress of the carrier fluid could statically support the dispersed coarse particles in the vertical pipe, but not a bed of solid particles thus leading to particle settling on shutdown. Hence, the design of a system to vertically convey coarse solids would need to take account of the observed behavior and ideally guarantee particle dispersion.

Figure 11 shows LPB images taken from a pipe test with a synthetic clay/sand/gravel slurry during a pipe test for evaluating rheology additives [14]. The effect of the pipe velocity on the degree of suspension is clear from the ERT images.

An industrial slurry was supplied to CSIRO for pipe tests as a complete slurry; thus, it was not possible to obtain a separate reference from a homogenous carrier fluid. Thus, a reference had to be obtained from a homogenous mix of the slurry as

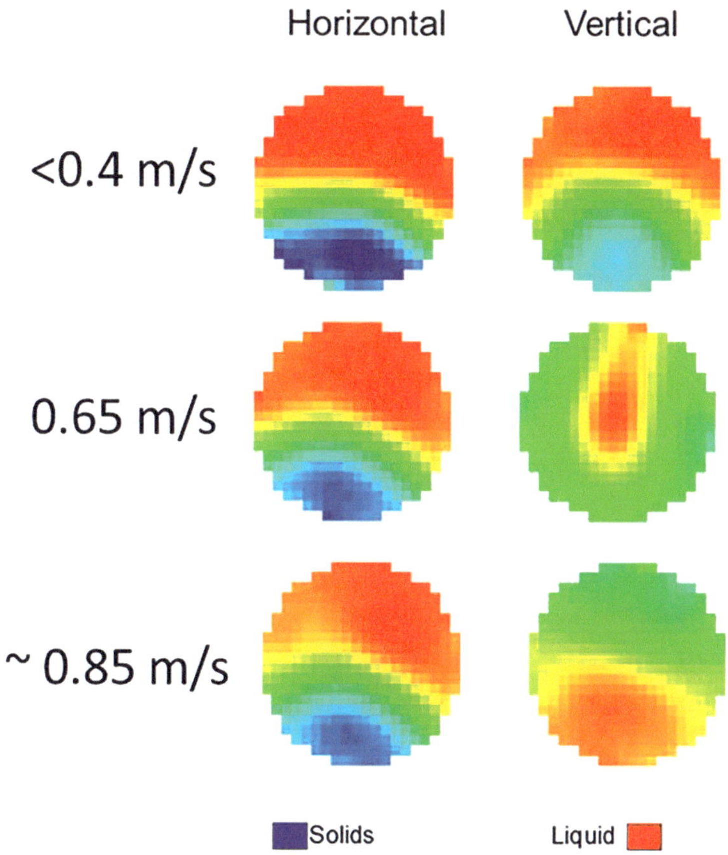

Figure 10.
ERT images for flow around a vertical pipe bend. Adapted from data presented in [34].

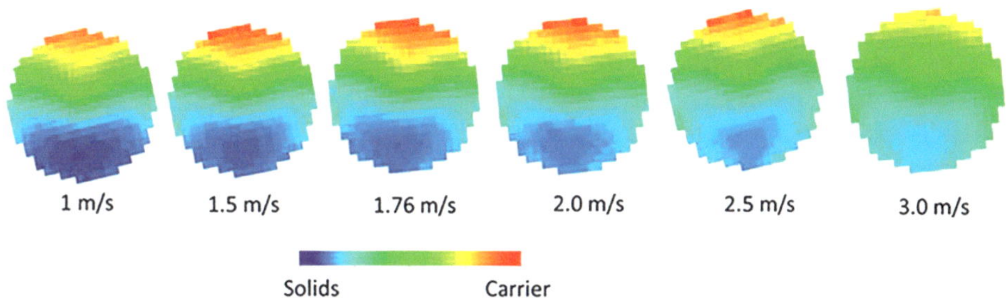

Figure 11.
Synthetic clay/sand/gravel slurry at 80% w/w solids.

supplied in order for the data acquisition to occur. It was known that there were coarse particles in the slurry, but the slurry overall had the appearance of a high-yield-stress-based suspension. A view of the slurry slump test together with ERT results obtained from the 2.5D absolute imaging approach as described in Section 5.3 are shown in **Figure 12**, showing stratified behavior, even with a high yield stress carrier fluid.

A data set for very high-conductivity tailings is shown in **Figure 13** which shows ERT images plotted on the flow curve for two concentrations of the tailings from [24].

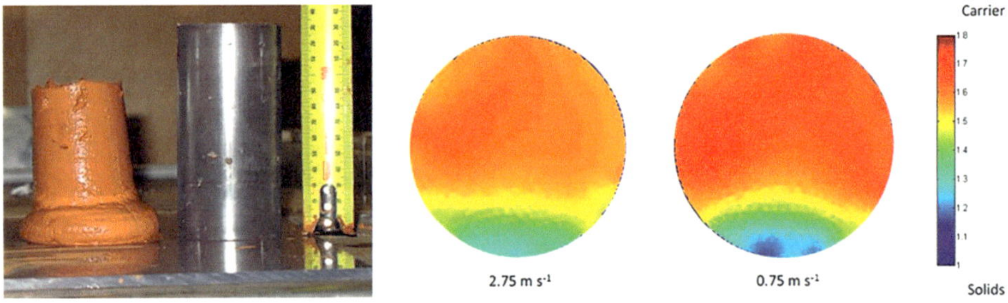

Figure 12.
High yield stress slurry conductivity images showing stratification. As originally published and presented at the BHR 20th International conference on Hydrotransport, Melbourne, Australia, 3rd–5th may 2017, [24].

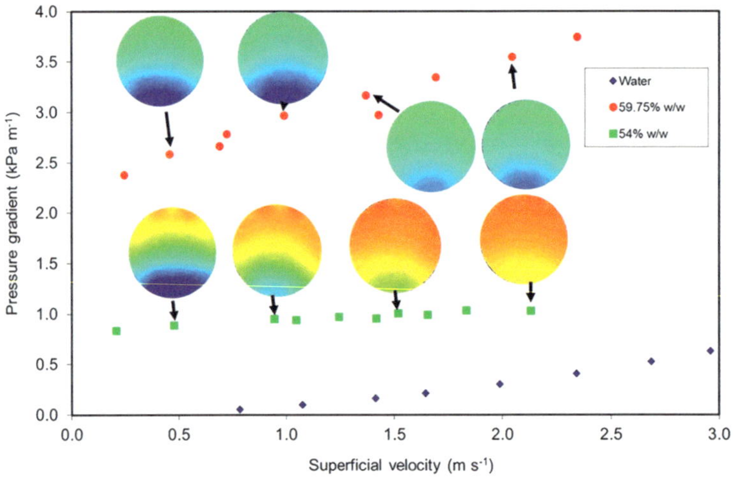

Figure 13.
Flow curve and ERT for high-conductivity tailings at two concentrations in a 100-NB pipe. Color represents conductivity. As originally published and presented at the BHR 20th International conference on Hydrotransport, Melbourne, Australia, 3rd–5th may 2017, [24].

The ERT data shown were processed using the absolute 2.5D ERT approach. The ERT system had to be operated at its highest possible current setting (75 mA) to obtain usable data in the 100-mm diameter pipe rig.

The slurries tested in **Figures 12** and **13** were supplied as complete slurries; thus, there was no possibility to separately obtain a reference image from a homogenous carrier fluid. The procedure was then to use a dummy section of pipe with an ERT sensor to obtain a reference from a homogenized sample of the slurry as shown in **Figure 14**. It is conceded that this approach involves a compromise; however, it was possible to obtain data sufficient to demonstrate that the slurry flows were stratified under shear in the pipe which was the primary objective of the tests. The significance of the stratified flow is that predictive models are required to take this behavior into account for correct predictions of industrially sized pipe flows as discussed in [35] and subsequent publications up to [36].

While many of the results described earlier are in the laminar flow regime, the CSIRO group has also investigated the turbulent pipe flow regime using ERT as described recently in [37]. For this work, ERT was used to obtain solids concentration

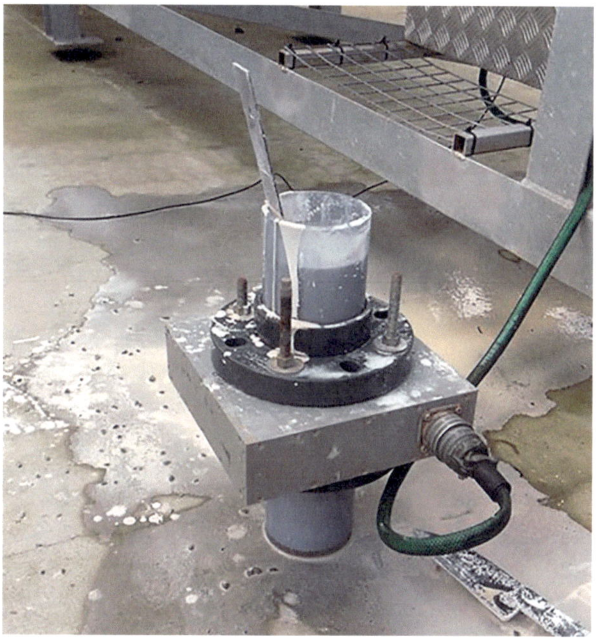

Figure 14.
Dummy pipe section for obtaining ERT references of homogenous slurries.

data for comparison with a DNS-DEM model for weakly turbulent coarse-particle non-Newtonian suspensions.

Other practical challenges relevant to the use of ERT in pipe flow were as follows:

- The ERT required short cables (3 m or less), especially when high-conductivity slurries were used. This restricted the number of ERT rings that could be used on the pipe rig to one installed adjacent to the ERT electronics rather than distributed along the pipe rig. For lower-conductivity carrier fluids, (<0.5 ms/cm) 10-m cables provided satisfactory results, thus allowing the electrode sets to be distributed along the pipe rig.

- Since the rig was outside, care was taken to enclose the electrodes in a waterproof box and the cables in a waterproof covering with a military specification connector. The electronics was located in a weatherproof box approximately halfway along the pipe rig in order to minimize the maximum cable length needed to cover the entire rig.

- The carrier fluid conductivity needed to be monitored and any changes taken into account if accurate concentration values are required.

- The choice of injection current required some consideration as the bulk resistivity increased as the solids were introduced into the slurry. The resistivity increase could lead to clipping of the ERT signals when polymer solution carrier fluids were used (e.g. ~0.3 ms/cm conductivity). It was found that reducing the injection current overcame this issue with a typical satisfactory value of 6 mA used for the 100-mm pipe rig. Higher injection currents (30–75 mA) were used with industrial slurries of higher conductivity to obtain usable data. In practice, it was found to be useful to obtain reference data at several different injection currents before introducing coarse solids. This procedure allowed choice of a suitable current for the majority of the test campaign, once initial slurry measurements had been made.

- Any air in the fluid/slurry must be eliminated as much as practicable. Air bubbles cause difficulties with obtaining satisfactory reference data as they pass by electrodes and can also lead to incorrect concentration data at the top of the pipe. References were normally taken with the pipe flow running in order to avoid the case where an air bubble was trapped against an electrode. The author and his colleagues also preferred to operate pipe tests with the return pipe to the holding tank submerged in the carrier liquid or slurry to minimize air entrainment due to the plunging jet effect. They also filled the pipe system with water and eliminated air from the rig before adding polymer powder or clay whenever possible, since air bubbles were difficult to remove from slurries with high yield stress carrier fluids.

- Adjustment of carrier fluid conductivities was usually not possible as addition of salt, etc., ran the risk of significantly changing the carrier fluid rheology which was fundamental to the flow behavior.

- The solids conductivity was not always known, especially for minerals or tailings slurries from sites. In these cases, a relative stratification may be the only obtainable data from ERT which is used in conjunction with rheology, flow curves, etc., to interpret the flow behavior.

7. Slurry tank applications

CSIRO has a long history of mixing tank research as shown in [38] and has recently started to apply ERT to this area of slurry flow dynamics. ERT allows for a deeper exploration of concentration inhomogeneities as a function of the agitation type. These inhomogeneities have been observed in unbaffled tanks under certain agitation conditions and have recently started to be investigated by ERT by [39] using a 1-m diameter tank at CSIRO and water/sand slurry.

A time series of ERT images from a single plane of the 1-m diameter tank are shown in **Figure 15**, and stills from a video are shown in **Figure 16**. A low concentration region is evident, traveling around the tank near the slurry surface. These concentration transients can then be correlated with other aspects of tank performance such as impeller torque and particle suspension. This research activity is continuing at CSIRO at the time of writing.

Further recent ERT work has commenced at CSIRO in a smaller (390 mm diameter) tank which is unbaffled. A photograph of the tank with the impeller turned off and particles settled is shown in **Figure 17**. This tank is used for fundamental research into impeller suspension performance before scaling up to the larger 1-m diameter tanks.

The object of the initial work with the tank was to investigate the performance of the various options for ERT processing using the ITS Reconstruction Tool Suite [21]

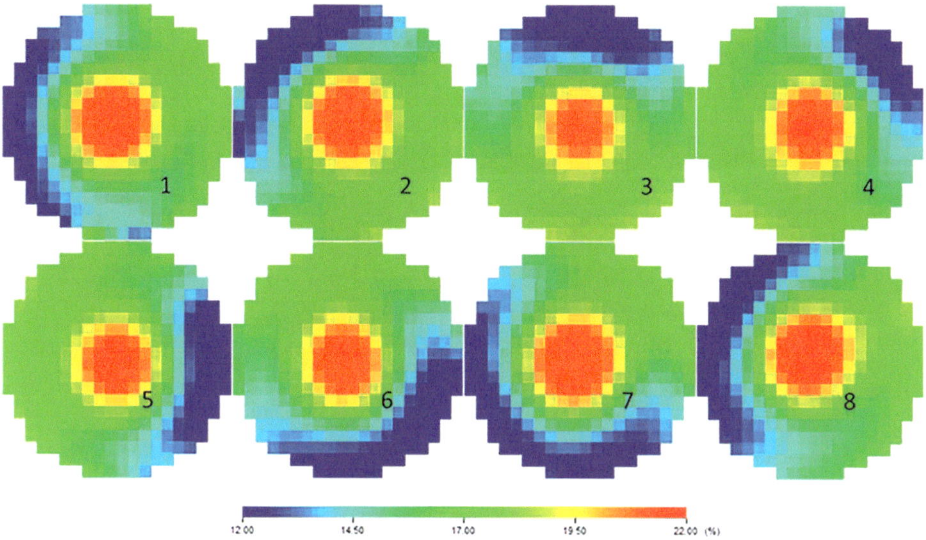

Figure 15.
Time-dependent concentration in unbaffled tank. Electrode plane near the top of the tank.

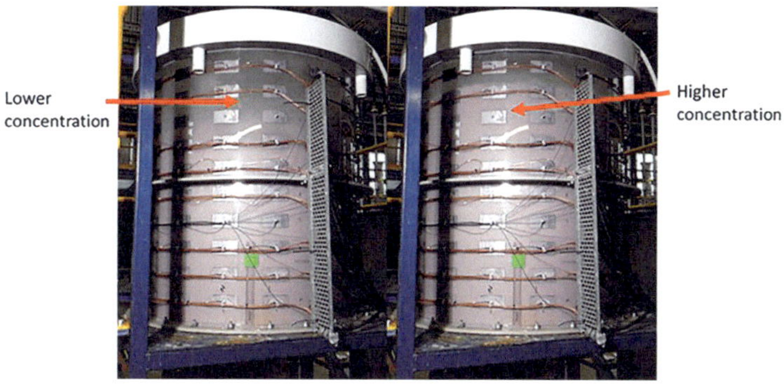

Figure 16.
Stills from video taken at the same time as ***Figure 15****.*

for tank applications, especially when settled solids were present. **Figure 18** shows a comparison between the LBP and the Laplace option where it is seen that the Laplace option performs significantly better in capturing the settled solids without the artifacts in the center of the images from the LBP. Work is ongoing at the time of writing to further optimize the imaging of the suspension in the tank as well as obtain data on the effect of different impellers, etc.

8. Conclusions

ERT has been a part of CSIRO's research into slurry pipe flows for nearly 20 years and is now being extended to mixing tanks.

The insight that ERT offers into the state of suspension of the flow is difficult to obtain by other means, especially given the opaque nature of industrial slurries.

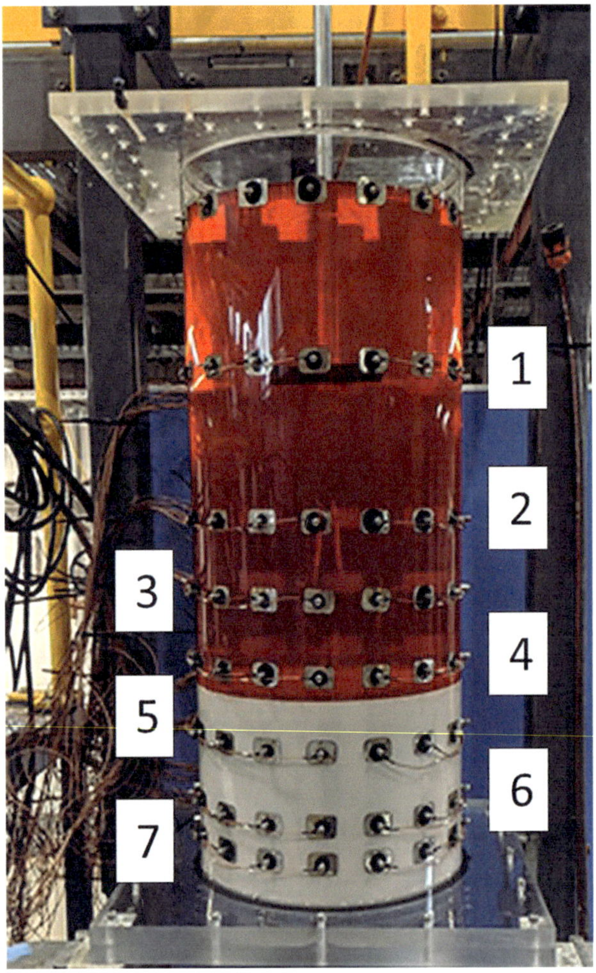

Figure 17.
Photograph of tank with settled solids. Plane 7 is the lower-most electrode ring, with plane 1 at approximately the impeller height.

A variety of image processing options are available for ERT, both commercial and open source, and both approaches are useful in a slurry flow research environment.

At CSIRO the preferred approaches are currently:

- linear backprojection for online live imaging using the ITS data acquisition software;
- absolute 2.5D for pipe flow postprocessing using EIDORS [20], especially where the conductivities of the constituents are unknown;
- the ITS Reconstruction Tool Suite for further off-line data analysis.

There are continuing developments in reconstruction algorithms both in the literature and commercially available which are aimed at improving the quantitative accuracy of ERT for slurry applications.

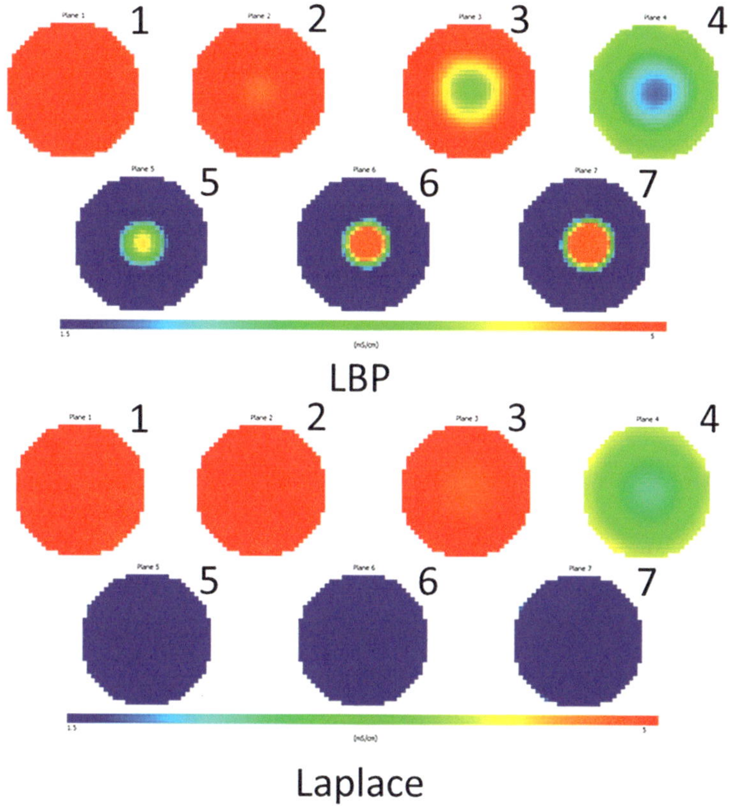

Figure 18.
Images from seven planes of the 390-mm tank with settled solids lower image set processed with the ITS reconstruction tool suite, Laplace algorithm. 50-mA injection current, 9600 Hz. Threshold set to 1.5–5.0 ms/cm. Liquid conductivity of 4.99 ms/cm. Photograph and ERT images courtesy of Michael Hurley, CSIRO mineral resources.

The significance of ERT (and previously MRI) for CSIRO was that the data demonstrated the regimes of flow in cases where visual observation or other diagnostic instruments were not usable. These results were then used to feed back into development of slurry pipe flow prediction models which were based on correct flow mechanisms rather than purely empirical methods. The demonstration of stratification of high yield stress carrier fluid-based slurries in laminar pipe flow was of particular significance in gaining acceptance of stratified flow models for that flow regime.

Acknowledgements

The author is grateful for the collaborations and support of Dr. Jie Wu, Dr. Lionel Pullum, Bon Nguyen, Kosta Simic, Dr. Andrew Chryss, Dr. Enzu Zheng, Jeremy Kieruj, Michael Hurley, Greg Short, Prof. Murray Rudman, and Dean Harris. The support of previous AMIRA research projects as well as industrial clients for the slurry research activities is also acknowledged.

Author details

Lachlan Graham
CSIRO Mineral Resources, Clayton, Victoria, Australia

*Address all correspondence to: lachlan.graham@csiro.au

References

[1] Williams RA, Beck ME. Process Tomography - Principles, Techniques and Applications. Oxford, United Kingdom: Butterworth-Heinemann; 1995

[2] Dickin F, Wang M. Electrical resistance tomography for process applications. Measurement Science and Technology. 1996;7(3):247-260

[3] Wang M. In: Wang M, editor. Industrial Tomography. 2nd ed. Cambridge, MA, United States: Woodhead Publishing; 2022. 2022/01/01

[4] Faraj Y. 20 - measurement and characterization of slurry flow using electrical resistance tomography. In: Wang M, editor. Industrial Tomography. 2nd ed. Cambridge, MA, United States: Woodhead Publishing; 2022. pp. 647-673

[5] Giguere R, Fradette L, Mignon D, Tanguy PA. ERT algorithms for quantitative concentration measurement of multiphase flows. Chemical Engineering Journal. 2008;**141**(1-3):305-317

[6] Giguere R, Fradette L, Mignon D, Tanguy PA. Characterization of slurry flow regime transitions by ERT. Chemical Engineering Research and Design. 2008;**86**(9A):989-996

[7] Norman JT, Bonnecaze RT. Measurement of solids distribution in suspension flows using electrical resistance tomography. Canadian Journal of Chemical Engineering. 2005;**83**(1):24-36

[8] Norman JT, Oguntade BO, Bonnecaze RT. Particle-phase distributions of pressure-driven flows of bidisperse suspensions. Journal of Fluid Mechanics. 2008;**594**:1-28

[9] Sutherland APN, Long TM, Randall EW, Wilkinson AJ. Determining concentration and velocity profiles of non-Newtonian settling slurries using electrical resistance tomography. Journal of the Southern African Institute of Mining and Metallurgy. 2008;**108**(10):583-590

[10] Fangary YS, Williams RA, Neil WA, Bond J, Faulks I. Application of electrical resistance tomography to detect deposition in hydraulic conveying systems. Powder Technology. 1998;**95**(1):61-66

[11] Mishra P, Ein-Mozaffari F. Using flow visualization and numerical methods to investigate the suspension of highly concentrated slurries with the coaxial mixers. Powder Technology. 2021;**390**:159-173

[12] Wei K, Qiu CH, Primrose K. Super-sensing technology: Industrial applications and future challenges of electrical tomography. Philosophical Transactions of the Royal Society a-Mathematical Physical and Engineering Sciences. 2016;**374**(2070). DOI: 10.1098/rsta.2015.0328

[13] Primrose K. 16 - from process understanding to process control—Applications in industry. In: Wang M, editor. Industrial Tomography. 2nd ed. Cambridge, MA, United States: Woodhead Publishing; 2022. pp. 519-544

[14] Graham LJW, Short G, Chryss A, Constanti-Carey K, Wu J. Effect of additives on suspension pipe flow. In: Jewell RJ, Fourie AB, editors. Paste 2018: Proceedings of the 21st International Seminar on Paste and Thickened Tailings; 11-13 April; Perth. Perth:

Australian Centre for Geomechanics; 2018. pp. 169-180

[15] Cui ZQ, Wang Q, Xue Q, Fan WR, Zhang LL, Cao Z, et al. A review on image reconstruction algorithms for electrical capacitance/resistance tomography. Sensor Review. 2016;**36**(4):429-445

[16] Barber DC, Brown BH. Applied potential tomography. Journal of Physics E: Scientific Instruments. 1984;**17**(9):723-733

[17] Dyakowski T, Jeanmeure LFC, Jaworski AJ. Applications of electrical tomography for gas–solids and liquid–solids flows — A review. Powder Technology. 2000;**112**:174-192

[18] Wang M. Inverse solutions for electrical impedance tomography based on conjugate gradients methods. Measurement Science & Technology. 2002;**13**(1):101-117

[19] Polydorides N, Lionheart WRB. A Matlab toolkit for three-dimensional electrical impedance tomography: A contribution to the electrical impedance and diffuse optical reconstruction software project. Measurement Science & Technology. 2002;**13**(12):1871-1883

[20] Adler A, Lionheart WRB. Uses and abuses of EIDORS: An extensible software base for EIT. Physiological Measurement. 2006;**27**(5):S25-S42

[21] Wei K, Qiu CH, Soleimani M, Primrose K. ITS reconstruction tool-suite: An inverse algorithm package for industrial process tomography. Flow Measurement and Instrumentation. 2015;**46**:292-302

[22] Wang M. Three-dimensional effects in electrical impedance tomography. In: Proceedings of 1st World Congress on Industrial Process Tomography. Manchester, UK: International Society for Industrial Process Tomography; 1999. pp. 410-415

[23] Bahrani N, Adler A. 2.5D finite element method for electrical impedance tomography considering the complete electrode model. In: 25th IEEE Canadian Conference on Electrical & Computer Engineering. 2012

[24] Graham L, Pullum L, Chryss A. Absolute 2.5D electrical resistance tomography in pipe systems. In: Hydrotransport 2017 - 20th International Conference on Hydrotransport; 3-5 May 2017. Melbourne, Australia: BHR Group; 2017. pp. 387-398

[25] Shook CA, Roco MC. Slurry Flow Principles and Practice. Stoneham, MA, USA: Butterworth-Heinemann; 1991

[26] Krupička J, Matoušek V. Gamma-ray-based measurement of concentration distribution in pipe flow of settling slurry: Vertical profiles and tomographic maps. Journal of Hydrology and Hydromechanics. 2014;**62**(2):126-132

[27] Spelay RB, Hashemi SA, Sanders RS, Hjertaker BT. Improved scatter correction model for high attenuation gamma-ray tomography measurements. Measurement Science and Technology. 2021;**32**(8). DOI: 10.1088/1361-6501/abfddf

[28] Johansen GA, Froystein T, Hjertaker BT, Olsen O. A dual sensor flow imaging tomographic system. Measurement Science and Technology. 1996;**7**(3):297-307

[29] Hashemi SA, Spelay RB, Sanders RS, Hjertaker BT. A novel method to improve electrical resistance tomography measurements on slurries containing

clays. Flow Measurement and Instrumentation. 2021;**80**:101973

[30] Callaghan PT. Principles of Nuclear Magnetic Resonance Microscopy. Oxford: Oxford University Press; 1991

[31] Jarny S, Roussel N, Rodts S, Bertrand F, Le Roy R, Coussot P. Rheological behavior of cement pastes from MRI velocimetry. Cement and Concrete Research. 2005;**35**(10):1873-1881

[32] Coussot P. Progress in rheology and hydrodynamics allowed by NMR or MRI techniques. Experiments in Fluids. 2020;**61**(9):1-20

[33] Graham L, Hamilton R, Rudman M, Strode P, Pullum L. Coarse solids concentration profiles in laminar pipe flows. In: 15th International Conference on Slurry Handling and Pipeline Transport HYDROTRANSPORT 15. Banff, Canada: British Hydromechanics Research Group; 2002. pp. 149-158

[34] Graham LJW, Wu J, Pullum L. Transition from horizontal to vertical conveying of complex slurry suspensions IN laminar flow. Canadian Journal of Chemical Engineering. 2011;**89**(4):817-824

[35] Pullum L, Graham LJW, Slatter P. A non-Newtonian two-layer model and its application to high density hydrotransport. In: Hydrotransport 16. BHR Group: Santiago, Chile; 2004

[36] Matoušek V, Chryss A, Pullum L. Modelling vertical concentration distributions of solids suspended in turbulent visco-plastic fluid. Journal of Hydrology and Hydromechanics. 2021;**69**(3):255-262

[37] Zheng EZ, Rudman M, Kuang SB, Chryss A. Turbulent coarse-particle non-Newtonian suspension flow in a pipe. International Journal of Multiphase Flow. 2021;**142**. DOI: 10.1016/j.ijmultiphaseflow.2021.103698

[38] Wu J, Nguyen B, Graham L, Hurley M, Harris D, Short G, et al. Increased agitation reliability for slurry suspension in mineral processing. Minerals Engineering. 2021;**170**:1-11

[39] Kieruj J, Graham L, Short G, Harris D. Electrical Resistance Tomography Tank Commissioning. CSIRO. 2020. pp. 1-53. Report No.: EP 207635

Section 4

Advances in Pipe Wear

Chapter 8

Erosion-Corrosion in Pipe Flows of Particle-Laden Liquids

Robert J.K. Wood and Alexander D.C. Cook

Abstract

The transmission of particle-bearing liquids in pipes has motivated continuing research into erosion mechanisms and the distribution of erosion rates over wetted surfaces. This chapter covers these initiatives with particular reference to erosion-corrosion modelling within bends and straight sections of cylindrical pipes manufactured in a variety of materials and transporting a variety of liquids. Erosion-corrosion modelling techniques such as submerged slurry jets and rotating cylinder electrodes have been used to study factors influencing material degradation. Improvements in computational fluid dynamics (CFD), such as the development of a moving deforming mesh (MDM) have improved the accuracy of CFD models in predicting pipe wall erosion rates. Combined discrete phase tracking approaches such as the CFD-DPM-DEM (discrete phase-discrete element model) have helped improve computational efficiency. Wall impact erosion models are calibrated using laboratory scale tests. Validation of CFD models using full-scale test data is rare, meaning their accuracy is still largely unreported. Material testing has helped to identify the resilience of prospective pipeline materials to erosion-corrosion, while modifications to internal geometry and pipe section have shown potential to improve erosion-corrosion resistance.

Keywords: erosion-corrosion, computational fluid dynamics, pipelines, slurry, modelling, state-of-the-art

1. Introduction

Erosion-corrosion (E-C) is recognised as one of the most significant threats to the integrity of pipelines carrying fluids mixed with solid particles. It affects numerous industries including mining, oil and gas, power generation and sediment transport. Marine, aero and food production industries are also affected [1]. Pipework, turbines, pump components and valves can all become heavily damaged by E-C. Improper management can lead to loss of productivity, unplanned downtime, or complete component failure, with obvious environmental and safety concerns. Erosion-corrosion is said to be the primary cause of fluid leakage in pipelines and is estimated to cost the Canadian oil sands industry $1bn a year in damages [2, 3]. Owing to its importance within industry, the field of erosion-corrosion has enjoyed plentiful research over several decades.

Material type	Angle of impingement		
	<20°	45°	90°
Elastic	No effect	Negligible	Surface deformed
Ductile	"Cutting" wear dominates	Mixed regime	Deformation wear dominates
Brittle	Negligible	Intermediate	Maximum

Table 1.
Material response to solid particle impact (adapted from [7]).

Since the first focused work on theoretical mechanisms at least 28 different erosion equations have been proposed, including a total of 33 different parameters [4]. Erosion rate is defined as the rate of mass loss from a surface due to particle impingements. The response of pipeline materials to solid particle impacts depends on the nature of the target material and the treatments to which that material has been subjected. Environmental parameters such as flow velocity [5], pressure [6], temperature, impact angle, solid particle concentration, size and shape are also known to influence erosion [7]. The influence of impact angle depends on the mechanical characteristics of the pipe material. Brittle materials such as ceramics experience maximum erosion at impact angles of 90°. In ductile materials, cutting wear dominates at low impact angles (<20°) while deformation wear is most prominent at high impact angles [7]. This is summarised in **Table 1**.

Finnie [8] suggested that the volume loss due to erosion was proportional to the square of velocity. This comes because kinetic energy is likely the dominant factor governing erosion. Despite this, values of the exponent have been reported between 0.34 and 4.83 [9]. This variation has likely come in part due to difficulties accurately determining the impact velocities of particles in laboratory experiments. Other parameters that affect this number are particle size and its shape. The roundness of particles is often described using the circularity factor (CF). In perfectly spherical particles this factor is equal to 1, reducing as particles become more angular. It has been found that the circularity factor and erosion rate hold an inverse power law relationship [10]. A similar relationship has been found for particle size, with the exponent value quoted ranging between 0.2–4.0 depending on test conditions [9]. The behaviour of particles entrained within a flow is described by the Stokes number. Particles with Stokes numbers close to 1 tend to follow streamlines of the continuous phase. In flows with higher stokes numbers, particle motion is largely inertia-dominated and wall collisions are more likely, leading to increased erosion rates [11]. Particles of higher hardness are known to cause higher erosive wear, although the ratio of particle to pipe hardness is perhaps the more important factor governing erosion rate [12].

Corrosion is an electrochemical process, caused by the interaction of the conveying fluid with the pipe material. As was the case with erosion, corrosion strongly depends on the nature of the pipe material. It has been found that the combined effects of erosion and corrosion can lead to significantly higher material loss rates than the summation of both processes separately [13, 14]. In the past decade, most erosion-corrosion research has been driven by the oil and gas industry. However, additional sectors have also been subject to investigation. In recent years, erosion-corrosion has been studied in concentrating solar power systems [15], engine cooling systems [16], fertiliser/mineral processing [14, 17] and geothermal power generation

[18] to name a few. The focus of research in these fields has been varied. Influencing factors such as pipe material, geometry and flow conditions have been studied. Methods of studying E-C due to particle-laden fluids can be broken down into pipeline tests, laboratory simulations and numerical simulations. The first two methods were reviewed in by Vahid Javaheri et al. [9]. Numerical simulation using computational fluid dynamics (CFD) was reviewed in 2014 by Mazdak Parsi et al. [19], and later by Messa et al. [20] in 2021. Recent developments in erosion-corrosion research were reviewed in 2017 [1]. This chapter will review developments in the modelling and management of erosion-corrosion subsequent to these works. The scope of this work will be limited to E-C of pipelines containing liquid-solid flows. Three-phase, gas-liquid or gas-solid flows will not be considered.

2. Numerical and laboratory scale modelling

2.1 Laboratory techniques

After the review in [1], various researchers have published work in which the erosion-corrosion behaviour of pipeline materials has been tested. Owing to their existing popularity, pipeline steels have been the focus of the majority. Due to their low cost, compact size, easy setup and short test durations, bench-scale laboratory tests are the most popular method for investigating E-C. Of these, the jet impingement test and slurry pot testers are the most popular techniques used today [9]. Other techniques used include the submerged jet impingement test [17, 21], pin-on-disk test [22], electrode cells [23] and rotating cylinder electrode [24] to name a few. Aside from the latter two techniques, these experimental methods have been recently reviewed in [9, 25].

Submerged jet impingement tests are a popular means of testing different materials. Results from jet tests are commonly used to calibrate erosion models in CFD packages, as will be discussed later in this chapter. While the high velocities required make the method unsuitable for simulating erosion in real pipelines, they are a valuable tool for evaluating material performance [9]. For example, Karafyllias et al. [17] used a submerged direct impact jet to investigate the performance of two stainless steels (UNS S31600 and UNS S42000) and two white cast irons (27WCI and 37WCI). Tests were carried out in a neutral and acidic (pH 3) environment. They found that the austenitic grain structure of the UNS S31600 and WCI37 samples better-resisted corrosion at pH 3. At neutral pH, the increased hardness of both WCI alloys led to increased erosion resistance over the softer stainless steels. Their tests were carried out at 90° impact angles and 21 m/s jet velocities. This limits the applicability of the results to real-world scenarios where a wide range of slurry velocities and impact angles are common. Using a similar methodology, Brownlie et al. [18] investigated the performance of various engineering materials for use in geothermal power generation. The performance of three grades of stainless steel, a carbon and low-alloy steel, Inconel 625 and Ti-6Al-4 V were evaluated. They found that low-carbon and low-alloy steels are especially vulnerable to erosion-corrosion at shallow impingement angles. Inconel 625 and super austenitic stainless steel UNS S31254 exhibited the greatest E-C resistance. Cathodic protection was employed and found to have a profound effect on erosion rate, reducing volume loss due to E-C of low alloyed ATSM A470 Grade C steel by nearly 6 times. Mostafa et al. [26] investigated the wear rate of HDPE as a function of impact velocity and angle using slurry impingement tests.

Impact angles between 30 and 90° were studied at velocities of 4, 5 and 6 m/s. The erodent particles were silica sand. Mass change measurements were used to quantify material loss from target samples. Erosion was found to peak at impact angles around 45–50° and increased proportionally with slurry velocity.

The popularity of the slurry pot apparatus is owed to the ease at which the influence of slurry velocity, concentration and impact angle can be studied on sample materials. By substituting test specimens, the performance of different materials can be easily evaluated. However, hydrodynamic differences limit this method's ability to predict erosion rates within real-world pipe flows [9].

Chung et al. [27] used a slurry pot tester to study E-C in a variety of different pipeline steels. API 5 L X65, X70 and X80 steels were compared with ASTM A1053 dual phase stainless steel and AR400 hard plate. Tests were carried out at two speeds and dissolved oxygen levels. The steels were characterised using electron microscopy, X-ray, micro-mechanical probing, and electrochemical testing techniques. At the lowest oxygen level (0.6 ppm) corrosion was mainly suppressed. At high oxygen levels and slurry velocities, dual-phase stainless steel suffered enhanced damage to its passive film and E-C resistance decreased. They concluded that E-C resistance is a function of a combination of mechanical properties including hardness, strain hardening capability, ductility, toughness, and deformation before failure. The high E-C resistance exhibited by AR400 was attributed to its finer microstructure (when compared to the X series steels) obtained after the tempering and quenching process. The author recommended the use of fine micro-structured steels for slurry transport.

A slurry pot tester was also used by Singh et al. [28]. They investigated the influence of particle type and circularity factor on erosion wear of stainless steel (SS 316L). Samples of fly ash, bottom ash and sand were compared. Particle characteristics were measured using digital image processing on SEM images. It was discovered that the value of erosion wear decreased with the circularity factor. The relationship between erosion rate and circularity factor appeared to follow the inverse power law. The exponent value was predicted as 2.668 for multisized slurry.

Rotating disk/cylinder electrode systems are a popular choice for those wishing to establish the effect of flow velocity and solid concentration on corrosion in pipeline steels. Aguirre et al. [24] used a rotating cylinder electrode (RCE) to investigate the mechanism of corrosion-accelerated erosion in carbon steel API 5 L X65 in alumina slurry doped with mineral quartz. Tests were carried out at different fluid velocities and dissolved oxygen (DO) concentrations. SEM and electron backscatter diffraction (EBSD) inspection was used to analyse surface wear patterns. DO availability increased the wear rate of steel. It was proposed that plastic deformation due to particle impingements increased the formation of anodic/cathodic sites to an order of magnitude larger than the original impact site. This led to further increases in corrosion rate.

A multifactorial study by the same author [29] used similar apparatus to investigate the influence of velocity, particle concentration, temperature, pH, dissolved oxygen, and copper ion content on E-C in pipes of the same material. Sample degradation was measured using a combination of gravimetric techniques and surface morphology measurement using SEM imaging and energy dispersive X-Ray spectroscopy (EDX). Also using an RCE, Molina et al. [30] assessed the directionality of wear scars at different velocities when API 5 L X65 steel is exposed to quartz slurry. This was done by applying Fast Fourier Transform (FFT) to SEM images. They found that patterns in erosion wear scars could be successfully identified. Implementation of this technique could be used to enhance understanding of erosion wear.

Using combined wire beam and coupon electrodes, Xu et al. [23] investigated the influence of pre-corrosion on E-C in X65 pipeline steel. Pre-corrosion is common in pipelines where residual moisture is present following pressure testing. While they found that the E-C rate was similar in pre-corroded and non-pre-corroded samples, their findings cannot be extended beyond X65 steel.

2.2 Numerical methods

Computational fluid dynamics (CFD) is a popular method of wall impact erosion modelling in particle-laden fluids. Erosion modelling procedures generally follow three steps: First, the continuous phase is resolved. The motion of elements within the discrete phase is then calculated. Finally, by using element motion in the near wall region estimates of material removal due to collisions can be generated at each wall node. By following this procedure, detailed erosion maps can be generated for geometry analysis [2]. While CFD simulations can yield highly detailed results, their accuracy has come under scrutiny in many papers [31]. The main sources of uncertainty lie within accurately modelling particle wall impact behaviour and estimating the material loss due to particle wall impingement. Particle tracking has also proven difficult and computationally expensive. Two main methods of multiphase modelling exist in CFD packages today. An overview of each is provided below.

2.2.1 Eulerian-Eulerian approach

The Eulerian-Eulerian methodology, often referred to as the two-fluid model, treats both phases equally. This approach is computationally efficient and allows models containing numerous phases to be resolved. The downside of the Eulerian approach is that individual particle motion cannot be calculated. This limits the use of the Eulerian-Eulerian approach in erosion modelling. Despite this, the approach remains useful in applications where high solid concentrations are present or when the coupling between the fluid-particle or particle-particle is important [3].

2.2.2 Eulerian-Lagrangian approach

The Eulerian-Lagrangian formulation allows the trajectories of particles within the discrete phase to be tracked. As before, the carrier fluid (continuous phase) is modelled following the Eulerian framework. To model the erosion process in turbulent flows, steady state Reynolds-averaged Navier-Stokes (RANS) equations have been combined with a variety of turbulence models to simulate fluid flows [32]. This approach has been used somewhat successfully over the past couple of decades [2, 33]. While the RANS approach can be used to establish the time-averaged erosion characteristics of a particle-laden fluid, it is unable to establish the unsteady nature of turbulent flows being modelled. To simulate unsteady properties of pipe flows such as the evolution of vortices and recirculation, large eddy simulation (LES) algorithms have been developed. A detailed description of LES can be found in [32]. The performance of both algorithms has been evaluated. Wang et al. [34] studied erosion in pipe elbows using an LES Euler-Lagrange model. Results obtained using the RANS and LES were compared. Results were verified using experimental results taken from [35]. Good agreement between velocity profiles predicted by the LES method and experimental values was noted. In comparison, the RANS method was found to overpredict the fluid velocity in the near-wall region. The increased accuracy of the LES model was attributed to its ability to model the unsteady secondary flow at the inner radius.

The Lagrangian framework resolves the motion of particles based on a translational force balance for each entity. The Discrete Phase Model (DPM) tracks the movement of particles through the continuous phase. In the DPM each modelled entity represents a 'parcel' of particles having similar dynamic properties [36]. Another approach to particle tracking is the Discrete Element Method (DEM). Unlike the DPM, individual particles are tracked and their equations of motion solved. The benefit of this method is that information related to inter-particle collisions can be calculated using the 'soft sphere' approach, making the DEM suitable for flows with high solid concentrations. The applicability of the DPM is limited to solid concentrations where the influence of inter-particle collisions can be neglected. Wang et al. [2] found the influence of inter-particle collisions to be negligible at solid concentrations up to 5.37% wt., while Kloss et al. [37] limited their use of DPM modelling to below 5% by volume. Lagrangian inter-particle collision models have been used in [38, 39] to extend the range of applicability to higher concentrations of solid particles. However, their use remains limited due to the increased computational burden and the number of difficult-to-estimate parameters these models rely on [40].

Coupling between the DEM and DPM has been proposed to improve the accuracy of the CFD-DPM approach without the full computational expense of the CFD-DEM method. Kloss et al. [37] used the CFD-DPM-DEM approach to model the dispersed phase in air-particle flows. They showed that the simulation speed of various systems using DEM could be significantly increased by switching to the DPM methodology in regions of low particle concentration without a significant effect on the results of the simulation. By extending this technique to solid-liquid flows the ability of CFD packages to model regions of high concentration could be improved.

2.3 Advancements in CFD

2.3.1 Flow modelling

It is widely accepted that erosion is a time-dependent process. The formation of wear scars takes time to develop and is most severe in areas with highly disturbed flows (such as in elbows, contractions, and tees). It is known that deformations to wall geometry can modify the flow field and cause changes to the local erosion rate. Despite this, most CFD packages assume that cavities formed are insignificant to the flow field. This assumption can lead to significant errors in erosion field calculations, especially in areas with sharp geometrical changes. López [41], Dong [42] and Agrawal et al. [43] all proposed modifications to CFD solvers to dynamically change wall geometry based on the local erosion rate.

A López et al. [41] utilised open source CFD software OpenFOAM. Surface erosion was calculated using built-in functions to establish an erosion vector for each point on the surface. This material loss was used to calculate the change in the shape of the solid surface. The geometry of the solid surface was modified by moving points of the mesh depending on the material loss magnitude. This process was repeated at regular intervals, with the flow field being re-calculated at each instance.

Using commercial CFD software Ansys Fluent, Dong et al. [42] proposed a methodology using a dynamically deforming mesh to model the deformed surface profile due to material erosion. Material removal was converted into a wall deformation using a user-defined function (UDF) within Fluent. As in [41], the mesh was updated at regular time intervals. The flow field was updated according to the new deformed wall shape. Their methodology was implemented in the erosion modelling of an economizer bank used in coal-fired power plants. A good agreement between the erosion profile predicted using the CFD model and the on-site test sample was noted. By utilising the CFD model, the evolution of erosion profile and particle trajectories could be seen. While their results appeared promising, no comparison to CFD models without the moving mesh approach was made, meaning the accuracy increase with their methodology cannot be quantified.

Similarly, Agrawal et al. [43] developed a moving-deforming-mesh (MDM) model within CFD software Ansys Fluent. The mesh deformation was calculated using UDFs within the software. Based on the local erosion rate, the geometry of the solid wall and its computational mesh were updated at regular time intervals. The flow field was recalculated following each update. It was found that the dynamically changing flow fields were able to capture the development of flow features which were not present in the undeformed model. Their approach proved capable of predicting secondary erosion features not present in non-MDM CFD models. Agrawal concluded that the effect of the MDM was most pronounced at sharp geometrical features (such as changes in section or elbows) where erosion caused significant changes to the flow field. A case study of a mitre-bend was used to illustrate the differences between models with and without the MDM algorithm.

Additional challenges in CFD modelling come when trying to calculate particle motion near solid boundaries. For erosion estimates to be accurate, the motion of the particle must be equivalent to that found in real-world scenarios. Different researchers have tried to investigate near wall effects and rebound characteristics of the discrete phase. Issues in particle motion and rebound modelling were demonstrated by Karimi et al. [31]. From their review of literature, it was found that CFD packages over-estimated the true rate of erosion. They found that modelling errors led to small particles becoming trapped in eddies in the near wall region, leading to multiple wall impacts. This non-physical behaviour was thought to contribute to some of the over-estimates commonly seen in CFD modelling. It was found that more realistic erosion estimates could be obtained by limiting the number of impacts a given particle to one. It was concluded that current rebound models are not simulating small particle behaviour after wall impacts correctly. More work is therefore required in this area.

2.3.2 Wall erosion modelling

Accurately turning wall impingements into an estimate of material loss is perhaps the biggest challenge in CFD erosion modelling. The process is highly complex, and research is still ongoing to understand the exact mechanisms behind erosion. Since the 1990s computational methods have been used to simulate erosive wear [44]. Erosion modelling using the Finite Element Method (FEM) has been successfully implemented to produce fairly accurate results [44–47]. The advantage of FEM is that erosion is calculated directly from material properties and the underlying physics. The drawback of this method is that it is limited to domain sizes at the same scale of the particles and for only a handful of collisions. This limits its use in CFD packages where both the scale and number of collisions are orders of magnitude higher.

The approach taken by CFD modellers is to disregard the physics at the micro-scale, instead focusing on the macroscale model encompassing the domain of interest. Trajectories and velocities of particles are calculated. Material removal due to wall impingements is estimated using empirical relationships derived from jet impact test results. While popular due to the ease at which such relations can be incorporated into CFD packages, the validity of the results is limited. Empirical relations fail to account for the variation of particle size in naturally occurring materials and the non-linearity of the erosion process. Jet impact tests are carried out at higher velocities than most fluid flows, meaning that relationships drawn are often outside of the experiment's calibration range. Also, as was noted in the introduction, relations derived from experiments vary massively depending on methodology and test conditions. Even with careful application, it is not certain that test results are representative of the environment to be modelled.

Leguizamón et al. [47] proposed a multi-scale approach to surface erosion modelling. They created a database of physically determined micro-scale erosion results, calculated using the FEM approach. Particle collisions were modelled under a variety of conditions. These results were used to calculate material loss due to collisions within a macroscale model. The main benefit of this method is that erosion rates are based on detailed impact simulations as opposed to experimentally determined erosion correlations. To ensure the accuracy of this method a reliable and comprehensive set of erosion tests were carried out at the microscale. Validation results proved encouraging with significant improvements in accuracy over correlation-based approaches. Unfortunately, the proposed approach comes at a massive computational expense meaning that the method is unfeasible for full-scale modelling.

An alternative approach to improve the accuracy of wall material removal models was proposed by Mansouri [48] and later modified by Messa et al. [40]. Their solution consisted of an upgraded CFD/experimental methodology to calibrate coefficients used in the empirical erosion models based on slurry jet impingement tests. The slurry jet tests were performed on aluminium and curved glass reinforced epoxy samples. One-way coupling was used in the simulation owing to the relatively low volume fraction of solid. This was done to reduce the computation time as the trajectories of fluid parcels could be decoupled from the solution of the carrier fluid flow. The CFD simulation was carried out using ANSYS FLUENT and particle trajectories were calculated using the Lagrangian method. Modifications to the CFD code were implemented to account for the influence of particle shape on particle-wall impingement characteristics. Additionally, to reduce uncertainty due to the point-particle approximation, impact characteristics were evaluated at half of the particle diameter from the wall. This methodology was originally proposed by Messa and Wang [49], who found that a region of high drag near the wall resulted in an underestimation of impact velocity. An improvement in the reliability of CFD-based erosion predictions was noted. It was concluded that the method represented a practical compromise in the prediction of erosion using empirical models without the need for modelling at the micro-scale.

Wee et al. [11] sought to improve erosion damage prediction of CFD approaches by implementing the Rosin Rammler particle size distribution model. Simulations were carried out using Ansys Fluent 17.2. Two-phase flow and particle wall interactions were solved using the Euler-Lagrange model. Simulations were carried out using both water-sand and air-sand flows, to compare the influence of carrier-fluid on erosion rate. Results from the CFD simulation were compared with experimental results. Implementation of the Rosin Rammler particle size model reduced the error in CFD results from between 6.81–24.31% and below 5% for all test cases. Erosion wear was found to be up to 97.44% lower when using water as the carrier fluid. This is because sand particles follow the streamlines in the water much better than air, as characterised by their respective Stokes numbers.

2.4 Studies using CFD

To reduce costs associated with erosion damage in sections of pipeline, many have turned their attention to optimising pipe geometry. Changes in cross-section, curvature and internal profile have all been suggested as methods of reducing E-C [50]. Internal ribs, a vortex chamber and twisting sections have been found to reduce erosion in elbows by modifying flow conditions within the pipe. However, in all these studies only gas-solid mixtures were considered. Li et al. [50] used a CFD-DEM simulation to model the influence of wall shape on wear rates in the vicinity of a pipe bend. The working environment consisted of a two-phase flow with particle concentrations of 1–10% and 1–3 mm in diameter. By adding a solid protrusion to the internal surface of the bends outer radius at the region at which particles first contact the wall it was found that the wear rate could be reduced significantly. The 'bump' reduced the kinetic energy of particles entrained in the flow and the number of times particles collide with the wall. The effectiveness of the bump in reducing wall wear was subject to other factors, including particle size, flow velocity and mass flow rate of particles.

Okhovat et al. [51] used a combined mathematical and CFD approach to model erosion-corrosion in straight and contracted pipe sections. COMSOL Multiphysics v3.5a was used to model fluid flow, while corrosion rate was determined as a function of oxygen concentration in the near wall regions. The pipe geometry used was a converging-diverging section, with an inlet diameter of 38.6 mm, contraction diameter of 21.2 mm and outlet diameter of 42.5 mm. When compared with experimental results, erosion estimates using the CFD model offered reasonably good agreements in the inlet and contracted region, but significantly underpredicted E-C in the expanded (downstream) section. This was put down to the momentum model used. Although the effects of both erosion and corrosion were predicted, their synergism was assumed negligible, which would likely have led to an underprediction of the true material loss rate.

It is not uncommon for the results of CFD simulations to be combined with experimental work. Many have used this approach to verify results from experimental tests. For example, More et al. [52] investigated the influence of impact angle on erosion wear in mild steel pipelines handling coal ash slurry. Findings from CFD simulations were verified against slurry pot test results. Impact angles ranged between 7 and 90°. All tests were carried out at slurry velocities of 4 m/s. While similar trends between impact angle and erosion rate were noted, CFD simulations were found to underpredict erosion rate by an average of 21%. The author suggested that difficulties exactly replicating the nature of coal ash particles in the CFD simulation may have attributed to this error. An underprediction of impingement velocity, or miscalculation of flow regime could have also attributed to this error. Speculatively, it could in part be due to inaccuracies in fluid models used by the CFD solver.

CFD has been used to model the influence of particle size on erosion rate. As part of his PhD thesis, Braut [36] studied the influence of nano-sized particles on erosion. CFD studies were carried out using commercial software STAR-CCM+ and verified using experimental data. Particle size varied between 1 and 500 μm. Erosion rate was found to increase with particle diameter, despite a larger number of particles at smaller diameters. This was put down to higher kinetic energies of larger particles. Erosion pattern was also found to change with particle size. It was suggested that this was because smaller particles were more affected by the fluid flow, as they had lower inertia.

Li et al. [53] used combined results from CFD and experimental testing to establish the effect of large particles on pipe erosion. The particles used were 3 mm in diameter at mass concentrations from 1 to 15%. An aluminium sheet was fixed to the inside of the test bend to establish the erosion profile. The resulting profile was found to be corrugated, a result of the 'bouncing' of the particles along the bends outer radius. The size of this 'erosion ripple' was found to be dominated by the concentration of solid particles. The observed periodic wave pattern was found to be consistent with that predicted by the numerical model.

Using a submerged impingement jet, Owen et al. [21] investigated the influence of impingement conditions on erosion-corrosion of X65 carbon steel. Particle trajectories within the jet were predicted using COMSOL Multiphysics CFD software. Impact angles and velocities of particles in the jet were predicted. Within the impingement zone, sites with differing degradation mechanisms were identified. The synergy between erosion and corrosion was investigated. Under these test conditions (60°C, pH 4.7 2% NaCl solution, 1 g/L sand particles at 20 m/s) corrosion-enhanced erosion was found to be much more significant than erosion-enhanced corrosion.

3. Full scale experimental and *in-situ* monitoring techniques

3.1 Recirculation tests

Closed loop pipeline recirculation rigs are a popular choice for those looking to accurately replicate industrial conditions. Tests are conducted within specimen sections which can be inspected periodically. Various techniques have been used to investigate E-C damage within the specimen section. For example, Wood et al. [54] used a combination of gravimetric, ultrasonic thickness and diameter measurements taken using a ball-ended micrometre to quantify material loss within stainless steel test sections. The latter two measurements allowed for damage mapping across the wetted area, which showed good agreement with results from a CFD model, demonstrating that their method could be used to predict erosion damage patterns within pipe sections.

Owen et al. [55] developed a 3D printed pipe elbow to aid with prototyping and flow mapping within pipe sections. Multiple samples of X65 carbon steel were inserted into the elbow. Mass loss measurements at each sample location were used to map erosion damage across the sample section. While their results showed reasonable agreement with those expected from existing literature, it is questionable if their methodology provides any benefit over that used by Wood et al. [54] for the following reasons: the samples were only installed on the inner and outer radius of the elbow, so are incapable of detecting erosion to the elbows sides; it is not certain that the 3D housing, its material, and the geometry of the samples in the housing accurately replicate the flow in real elbows. No measurement of material loss from the housing was provided, so changes in flow condition due to housing erosion could not be ruled out. Rebound characteristics from the 3D printed housing may also be different to a full steel elbow and could affect erosion rates downstream of the first particle-wall impingement. With this being said, due to the ease of 3D printing, this method may be of use in rapid prototyping applications. It also allows for rapid substitution of test material samples for comparison tests.

Elemuren et al. [14] used a continuous recirculation rig with four 1018 steel 90° elbows to investigate the influence of slurry velocity on E-C. A slurry of potash brine with silica sand was used. Gravimetric measurement was used to quantify mass loss from each elbow. The synergy between erosion and corrosion was investigated by comparing results from separate erosion (deoxygenated potash brine w/10% wt. solid) and corrosion (saturated potash brine w/0% wt. solid) tests. It was found that the synergy decreased with slurry velocity, reducing by 45% between 2.5 m/s to 4 m/s. At high velocities, surface impingement became the dominant mechanism of material loss. Erosion-corrosion was found to be a function of solid concentration and flow velocity.

Regions in which flow trajectories are severely altered are found to be the most prone to erosion damage. Such areas include tees, elbows, and contractions, where changes in flow direction mean entrained particles are more likely to cross streamlines and contact the solid walls. Bilal et al. [56] investigated the influence of pipe geometry on wear due to water-sand and water-air-sand flows in pipe bends. They aimed to investigate alternative geometries to standard 90° elbows, where the curvature radius is equal to 1.5 times the pipe diameter, D. Geometries of 2.5D and 5D along with a 45° elbow with a radius of 1.5D were investigated. Numerical studies were carried out using commercial CFD code ANSYS FLUENT. Results from the CFD study were compared against experimental results. The inner surfaces of acrylic pipe bends/elbows were painted with black paint primer. Solid particles entrained in the flow remove the paint from the internal surfaces and allow erosion patterns to be observed. The tests were run until no further change occurred in the paint pattern. This gave a qualitative indication of which pipe geometry is least susceptible to erosion. It was found that smoother transitions in pipe geometry reduced erosion rates as particles are less susceptible to hitting pipe walls. Additionally, smaller changes in direction (45°) led to lower erosion. Generally, CFD results were found to corroborate the experimental paint removal study. An exception to this was that CFD failed to predict some of the secondary erosion patterns downstream of elbows. Wall function (modelling of flow in the near wall boundary region) was also found to affect the observed erosion patterns, producing a secondary hotspot on the inside of the elbow that wasn't present in the paint removal study. This was put down to be an artefact of the turbulence model used.

In industry, a wide range of pipe geometries are used in a variety of orientations. It is known that erosion properties can be quite different depending on the orientation of a section. Reportedly, most studies examining erosion in elbows have placed the sections in the horizontal-vertical configuration. Wang et al. [2] studied the effect of orientation on erosion in pipe elbows in the horizontal-horizontal configuration. Two elbows connected in series were analysed. Additionally, the effect of particle concentration and inlet conditions were also examined. CFD simulations were verified against experimental results. The effect of gravity became less noticeable, and the erosion profile became more symmetric across the pipe section as inlet velocity increased. The downstream elbow was found to be severely influenced by the flow profile exiting the previous elbow. The distance between the two had a significant influence on this effect.

To accurately model pipeline decay in real-world operation, factors outside those discussed above should be considered. External factors such as human, geotechnical, and natural hazards are all known to pose a risk to pipeline integrity [57]. External corrosion related to environmental conditions is known to be one of the most significant factors governing pipe life. Methods of monitoring and inspecting pipelines were reviewed in [58]. The same article proposed a risk-based integrity management model.

Yang et al. [6] carried out a performance investigation for slurry erosion in high-pressure hydraulic fracturing pipelines. Unlike other papers which studied slurry erosion, the effects of tensile stress induced due to internal/external pressure was considered. Additionally, the effects of impact angle, particle velocity and concentration, and target material were also considered. Results from an experimental study were used to develop a random forest regression (RFR) algorithm to develop an erosion prediction model for fracturing pipelines. A jetting circulating erosion test rig was used to apply adjustable tensile stress on the specimen during erosion. Test samples consisted of 4 different hypereutectoid steels. The effect of impact angle was evaluated on a sample of unstressed 42CrMo steel. Erosion wear was found to reach its maximum at an impact angle of 30°. At low angles, micro-cutting was found to be the prominent erosion mechanism, while plastic deformation caused erosion at higher impact angles. Erosion rate was found to be proportional to tensile stress. At 30° the increase was approximately 70% between 0 and 500 MPa, while it nearly doubled for the same stress range at impact angles of 90°. This is due to a lower yield force under high stresses being more easily overcome by the kinetic energy of impacting particles.

3.2 *In-situ* damage monitoring

Online condition monitoring (OCM) allows for the health of critical components to be continuously monitored. OCM systems generally rely on an array of sensors linked to a processing device to display output parameters to the user. Readings can be used to schedule repairs and detect early signs of failure, reducing costs of manual inspection and safety/economic implications of unplanned downtime. The benefits of OCM are numerous and its implementation has become common practice in several industries. Liu et al. [59] proposed a system to allow for the online monitoring of metal loss in pipelines. Ring pair electrical resistance sensor (RPERS) arrays were used to monitor erosion loss around the diameter of the pipe, while linear polarisation resistance (LPR) was used to measure the corrosion rate in a pipe ring. Electronic measurements were compared to weight loss measurements. The X65 steel test pipe was embedded in a recirculation rig, and CFD studies were used to calculate flow distribution and sand concentration in the section. LPR, RPERS and gravimetric measurements showed good agreement for this configuration. It should be noted that the results cannot be generalised as they only relate to the specific configuration and conditions used.

4. Conclusion

Erosion-corrosion research in the past decade has been dominated by application-specific studies. Most of these papers have focused on comparing different materials or pipe geometries under specific flow conditions. Laboratory testing techniques such as slurry pot testers or electrode cells can be used to provide an understanding of factors influencing E-C within several materials. Due to the differences between laboratory and in-service conditions, the applicability of results obtained to real-world scenarios should be checked.

It is well known that pipe geometry has a significant effect on erosion rate. Despite this, relatively little research has been done to investigate alternative pipe geometries. Work by Li et al. [50] exploring the influence of internal bumps in a pipe elbow showed that erosion rate could be reduced with well-designed internal surface modifications. This could be implemented in particularly vulnerable pipe sections and should be explored further. As demonstrated by Wang et al. [2] pipe orientation and flow conditions entering pipe elbows can heavily influence the resulting erosion pattern. Despite this, few papers focus on the role of pipe geometry upstream of subject sections on erosion. By altering the upstream configuration, it is conceivable that one could alter the erosion pattern to increase component lifetime with relatively little difficulty. Perhaps this could be the subject of future work.

Recent improvements in the area indicate a promising future for CFD erosion modelling. Improved impact models, dynamically deforming geometry and more accurate particle tracking have all helped improve the accuracy of CFD erosion predictions. Despite these advancements, more work is required before CFD can be heavily relied upon. Errors in near-wall erosion models have been identified and require rectification. Loosely representative empirical erosion models are still heavily relied upon for wall erosion modelling and limit the applicability of the technique for a wide range of materials. While CFD-DEM allows the modelling of more dense slurry flows, the computational expense limits its use to small-scale modelling. To reduce computational expense, coupled DEM-DPM appears promising, but its application to liquid-solid flows is yet to be thoroughly explored.

List of abbreviations

E-C	erosion corrosion
DO	dissolved oxygen
CFD	computational fluid dynamics
EBSD	electron backscatter diffraction
SEM	scanning electron microscopy
EDX	energy dispersive X-ray spectroscopy
RCE	rotating cylinder electrode
RANS	Reynolds averaged Navier-Stokes
LES	large eddy simulation
DPM	discrete phase model
DEM	discrete element model
MDM	moving-deforming-mesh
UDF	user defined function
FEM	finite element model
CF	circularity factor
FFT	fast Fourier transform
OCM	online condition monitoring

Author details

Robert J.K. Wood* and Alexander D.C. Cook
National Centre for Advanced Tribology, Department of Mechanical Engineering, University of Southampton, Southampton, United Kingdom

*Address all correspondence to: r.wood@soton.ac.uk

References

[1] Burson-Thomas C, Wood R. Developments in erosion–corrosion over the past 10 years. Journal of Bio- and Tribo-Corrosion. 2017;**3**(2):14

[2] Wang Q, Huang Q, Wang N, Wen Y, Wen Y, Ba X, et al. An experimental and numerical study of slurry erosion behavior in a horizontal elbow and elbows in series. Engineering Failure Analysis. 2021;**30**:105779

[3] Adedeji OE. Development of Prediction Tools for Improved Wear Assessment of Pipelines and Complex Geometries. Edmonton, Alberta: University of Alberta; 2021

[4] Wood R. Erosion/corrosion. In: Erosion Corrosion Fundamental. Amsterdam: Elsevier Ltd.; 2007. pp. 395-427

[5] Stack M, Abdelrahman S, Jana B. Some perspectives on modelling the effect of temperature on the erosion–corrosion of Fe in aqueous conditions. Tribology International. 2010;**43**(12):2279-2297

[6] Yang S, Zhang L, Fan J, Sun B. Experimental study on erosion behavior of fracturing pipeline involving tensile stress and erosion prediction using random forest regression. Journal of Natural Gas Science and Engineering. 2021;**87**:103760

[7] Bhushan B, Gupta B. Friction, wear and lubrication. In: Handbook of Tribology. New York: McGraw-Hill Inc; 1991. pp. 2.1-2.41

[8] Finnie I. Erosion of surfaces by solid particles. Wear. 1960;**3**(2):87-103

[9] Javaheri V, Porter D, Kuokkala V-T. Slurry erosion of steel—Review of tests, mechanisms and materials. Wear. 2018;**408-409**(1):248-273

[10] Walker C, Hambe M. Influence of particle shape on slurry wear of white iron. Wear. 2015;**332-333**:1021-1027

[11] Wee SK, Yap YJ. CFD study of sand erosion in pipeline. Journal of Petroleum Science and Engineering. 2019;**176**:269-278

[12] Stachowiak GW, Batchelor AW. Abrasive, erosive and cavitation Wear. In: Engineering Tribology. 3rd ed. Burlington, MA: Elsevier Inc.; 2005. pp. 501-547

[13] Shang T, Zhong X-K, Zhang C-F, Hu J-Y, Medgyes B. Erosion-corrosion and its mitigation on the internal surface of the expansion segment of N80 steel tube. International Journal of Minerals, Metallurgy and Materials. 2021;**28**(1):98-111

[14] Elemuren R, Evitts R, Oguocha I, Kennell G, Gerspacher R, Odeshi A. Slurry erosion-corrosion of 90° AISI 1018 steel elbow in saturated potash brine containing abrasive silica particles. Wear. 2018;**410-411**(1):149-155

[15] Gietzen E, Karimi S, Goel N, Shirazi SA, Keller M, Otanicar T. Experimental investigation of low velocity and high temperature solid particle impact erosion wear. Wear. 2022;**506-507**:204441

[16] Niu L, Cheng Y. Synergistic effects of fluid flow and sand particles on erosion–corrosion of aluminum in ethylene glycol–water solutions. Wear. 2008;**265**(3-4):367-374

[17] Karafyllias G, Galloway A, Humphries E. The effect of low pH in

erosion-corrosion resistance of high chromium cast irons and stainless steels. Wear. 2019;**420-421**:79-86

[18] Brownlie F, Hodgkiess T, Pearson A, Galloway A. A study on the erosion-corrosion behaviour of engineering materials used in the geothermal industry. Wear. 2021;**477**:203821

[19] Parsi M, Najmi K, Najafifard F, Hassani S, McLaury BS, Shirazi SA. A comprehensive review of solid particle erosion modeling for oil and gas wells and pipelines applications. Journal of Natural Gas Science and Engineering. 2014;**21**(1):850-873

[20] Messa G, Yang Q, Adedeji O, Chara Z, Duarte C, Matousek V, et al. Computational fluid dynamics modelling of liquid–solid slurry flows in pipelines: State-of-the-art and future perspectives. PRO. 2021;**9**(9):1566

[21] Owen J, Ramsey C, Barker R, Neville A. Erosion-corrosion interactions of X65 carbon steel in aqueous CO_2 environments. Wear. 2018;**414-415**:376-389

[22] Stachowiak G. Particle angularity and its relationship to abrasive and erosive wear. Wear. 2000;**241**(2):214-219

[23] Xu Y, Liu L, Zhou Q, Wang X, Huang Y. Understanding the influences of pre-corrosion on the erosion-corrosion performance of pipeline steel. Wear. 2020;**442-443**(1):203151

[24] Aguirre J, Walczak M, Rohwerder M. The mechanism of erosion-corrosion of API X65 steel under turbulent slurry flow: Effect of nominal flow velocity and oxygen content. Wear. 2019;**432-439**:203053

[25] Shinde SM, Kawadekar DM, Patil PA, Bhojwani VK. Analysis of micro and nano particle erosion by analytical, numerical and experimental methods: A review. Journal of Mechanical Science and Technology. 2019;**33**(5):2319-2329

[26] Mostafa A, El-badia TMA, El-Rab RMG. Effect of impact angle and impact velocity on the slurry erosion behavior of high density polyethylene (HDPE). Engineering Research Journal. 2021;**171**(0):269-281

[27] Chung R, Jiang J, Pang C, Yu B, Eadie R, Li D. Erosion-corrosion behaviour of steels used in slurry pipelines. Wear. 2021;**477**:203771

[28] Singh J, Kumar S, Mohapatra S. Study on role of particle shape in erosion wear of austenitic steel using image processing analysis technique. Journal of Engineering Tribology. 2018;**233**(5):712-725

[29] Aguirre J, Walczak M. Multifactorial study of erosion–corrosion wear of a X65 steel by slurry of simulated copper tailing. Tribology International. 2018;**126**:177-185

[30] Molina N, Aguirre J, Walczak M. Application of FFT analysis for the study of directionality of wear scars in exposure to slurry flow of varying velocity. Wear. 2019;**426-427**:589-595

[31] Karimi S, Shirazi SA, McLaury BS. Predicting fine particle erosion utilizing computational fluid dynamics. Wear. 2017;**376-377**:1130-1137

[32] Piomelli U. Large-eddy simulation: Achievements and challenges. Progress in Aerospace Sciences. 1999;**35**(4):335-362

[33] Mansouri A, Arabnejad H, Shirazi SA, McLaury BS. A combined CFD/experimental methodology for erosion prediction. Wear. 2015;**332-333**:1090-1097

[34] Wang Q , Ba X, Huang Q, Wang N, Wen Y, Zhang Z, et al. Modeling erosion process in elbows of petroleum pipelines using large eddy simulation. Journal of Petroleum Science and Engineering. 2022;**211**:110216

[35] Enayet M, Gibson M, Taylor A, Yianneskis M. Laser-doppler measurements of laminar and turbulent flow in a pipe bend. International Journal of Heat and Fluid Flow. 1982;**3**(4):213-219

[36] Braut M. Experimental and Numerical Investigation of the Erosive Effects of Micro- and Nanometer-Sized Particles in Water Flow. Bergen: Dept. of Phys. and Tech University of Bergen; 2020

[37] Kloss C, Goniva C, Aichinger G, Pirker S. Comprehensive DEM-DPM-CFD simulations—Model synthesis, experimental validation and scalability. In: Seventh International Conference on CFD in the Minerals and Process Industries. Melbourne, Australia: CSIRO; 2009

[38] Duarte CAR, Souza FJD, Salvo RDV, Santos VFD. The role of inter-particle collisions on elbow erosion. International Journal of Multiphase Flow. 2017;**89**:1-22

[39] Lain S, Sommerfield M. Numerical prediction of particle erosion of pipe bends. Advanced Powder Technology. 2019;**30**(2):366-383

[40] Messa G, Wang Y, Negri M, Malavasi S. An improved CFD/experimental combined methodology for the calibration of empirical erosion models. Wear. 2021;**476**:203734

[41] López A, Stickland MT, Dempster WM. CFD study of fluid flow changes with erosion. Computer Physics Communications. 2018;**227**:27-41

[42] Dong Y, Qiao Z, Si F, Zhang B, Yu C, Jiang X. A novel method for the prediction of erosion evolution process based on dynamic mesh and its applications. Catalysts. 2018;**8**(10):432-448

[43] Agrawal M, Khanna S, Kopliku A, Lockett T. Prediction of sand erosion in CFD with dynamically deforming pipe geometry and implementing proper treatment of turbulence dispersion in particle tracking. Wear. 2019; **426-427**(Part A):596-604

[44] Wang Y-F, Yang Z-G. Finite element model of erosive wear on ductile and brittle materials. Wear. 2008;**265**(5-6): 871-878. Available from: https://www.sciencedirect.com/science/article/pii/S0043164808000215

[45] Zheng C, Liu Y, Chen C, Qin J, Zhang S. Finite element analysis on the dynamic erosion process using multiple-particle impact model. Powder Technology. 2017;**315**:163-170

[46] ElTobgy M, Ng E, Elbestawi M. Finite element modeling of erosive wear. International Journal of Machine Tools and Manufacture. 2005;**45**(11):1337-1346

[47] Leguizamón S, Jahanbakhsh E, Maertens A, Alimirzazadeh S, Avellan F. A multiscale model for sediment impact erosion simulation using the finite volume particle method. Wear. 2017;**392-393**:202-212

[48] Mansouri A. A Combined CFD-Experimental Method for Developing an Erosion Equation for both Gas-Sand and Liquid-Sand Flows. Ann Arbour, Michigan: ProQuest LLC; 2016

[49] Messa G, Wang Y. Importance of accounting for finite particle size in CFD-based erosion prediction. In: Proceedings of the ASME 2018 Pressure Vessels and Piping Conference, Fluid-Structure Interaction. Vol. 4. Prague, Czech Republic; 2018

[50] Li Y, Cao J, Xie C. Research on the Wear characteristics of a bend pipe with a bump based on the coupled CFD-DEM. Journal of Marine Science and Engineering. 2021;**9**(6):672-691

[51] Okhovat A, Heris SZ, Asgarkhani MAH, Fard KM. Modeling and simulation of erosion–corrosion in disturbed two-phase flow through fluid transport pipelines. Arabian Journal for Science and Engineering. 2014;**39**:1497-1505

[52] More SR, Bhatt DV, Menghani JV, Jagtap RK. CFD simulation and experimental results validation of slurry erosion wear using slurry pot testing. Trends in Sciences. 2022;**19**(11):4524

[53] Li Y, Zhang H, Lin Z, He Z, Xiang J, Su X. Relationship between wear formation and large-particle motion in a pipe bend. Royal Society Open Science. 2019;**6**(1):181254

[54] Wood R, Jones T, Ganeshalingam J, Miles N. Comparison of predicted and experimental erosion estimates in slurry ducts. Wear. 2004;**256**:937-947

[55] Owen J, Ducker E, Huggan M, Ramsey C, Neville A, Barker R. Design of an elbow for integrated gravimetric, electrochemical and acoustic emission measurements in erosion-corrosion pipe flow environments. Wear. 2019;**428-429**:76-84

[56] Bilal FS, Sendrez TA, Shirazi SA. Experimental and CFD investigations of 45 and 90 degrees bends and various elbow curvature radii effects on solid particle erosion. Wear. 2021;**476**:203646

[57] Tesfamariam S, Woldesellasse H, Xu M, Asselin E. General corrosion vulnerability assessment using a Bayesian belief network model incorporating experimental corrosion data for X60 pipe steel. Journal of Pipeline Science and Engineering. 2021;**1**(3):329-338

[58] Khan F, Yarveisy R, Abbassi R. Risk-based pipeline integrity management: A road map for the resilient pipelines. Journal of Pipeline Science and Engineering. 2021;**1**(1):74-87

[59] Liu L, Xu Y, Xu C, Wang X, Huang Y. Detecting and monitoring erosion-corrosion using ring pair electrical resistance sensor in conjunction with electrochemical measurements. Wear. 2019;**248-429**(1):328-339

Section 5

Wastewater Systems

Chapter 9

Optimization of Polymer Dosing for Improved Belt Press Performance in Wastewater Treatment Plants

Veruscha Fester and Rössle Werner

Abstract

A factorial trial approach was used to determine the relationship between process parameters and filtrate suspended solids, solids capture, cake solids, and yield stress. The work was conducted in a large-scale wastewater treatment plant where there is sludge thickening on a linear screen before filter press. The work demonstrated that there is a relationship between filtrate suspended solids, the rheology of sludge, and the optimum dewatering of the filter belt press. A relationship between the yield stress of the sludge on the BFP and the filtrate suspended solids was found. The sludge flow rate was the most influential parameter on the filtrate suspended solids and solids capture as well as yield stress. The linear screen speed was a significant main parameter for cake solids. The results showed clearly that the interaction between sludge flow rate and either polymer dosing rate or polymer concentration was consistently more significant than polymer concentration and polymer dosing rate individually. An important outcome from this work is that it shows that changes in polymer concentration rather than polymer dosing rate are more important for optimization and control.

Keywords: belt filter press, filtrate suspended solids, rheology, sludge, wastewater treatment plants

1. Introduction

Belt filter presses (BFPs) are mechanical dewatering equipment commonly used in municipal wastewater treatment plants (WWTP)[1]. The main reasons for sludge dewatering are to reduce the volume as it relates to the cost of sludge handling, especially transportation cost, increase in sludge heating capacity[2], and reduction of leachate [1].

---

[1] Plate Filter Press installations present a greater capital cost, but have comparatively low running costs. The high running costs of belt presses are mainly attributable to the cost of polymer dosing, and it is the optimization of this cost that is the predominant motive for this chapter.

[2] Dewatered sludge is sometimes incinerated to provide heat energy.

The mechanical components of a BFP include dewatering belts, rollers and bearings, belt tracking and tensioning system, controls and drives, and a belt washing system. The operation of the BFP includes a polymer conditioning zone, gravity drainage zone, low-pressure zone, and high-pressure zone [2]. A schematic diagram of a BFP is provided in **Figure 1** [1].

The water is released in three stages: (a) free water is allowed to drain through belt pores in the gravity zone and then it is passed through (b) the low-pressure zone where it is gently compressed, and (c) the interstitial water is released in the high-pressure zone where it is further compressed through a series of rollers of different sizes [3]. The dewatered sludge also known as the cake is removed by scrapers. The belts are washed by high-pressure jets to remove sludge and polymer deposits from the belt.

The process parameters that affect the BFP performance, that is, the final cake solids concentration and filtrate suspended solids, are the influent sludge characteristics and flow rate, solid feed rate, polymer concentration, dosage and mixing energy, belt speed, and belt tension [4]. There are no fundamental models relating the process conditions to the final cake solid concentration, filtrate suspended solids, or cake solids.

Johnson and coworkers conducted tests to evaluate the effect of process conditions on BFP performance [4]. They evaluated the effect of sludge flow, solid feed, polymer dosage, belt speed, belt tension, and polymer mixing energy. Their tests were conducted over a 6-month period.

The solid feed rate was found to be one of the most critical variables for the optimization of BFP performance. They also emphasized the importance of using polymer prepared at plant scale as mixing energy influences the performance of the polymer. They used both cationic and nonionic polymers. Under-dosing resulted in poor flocculation causing a thin, dry cake. Johnson and coworkers determined the optimum value for each parameter individually and then ran the BFP at the optimized value for each condition. They found that there was no correlation between the

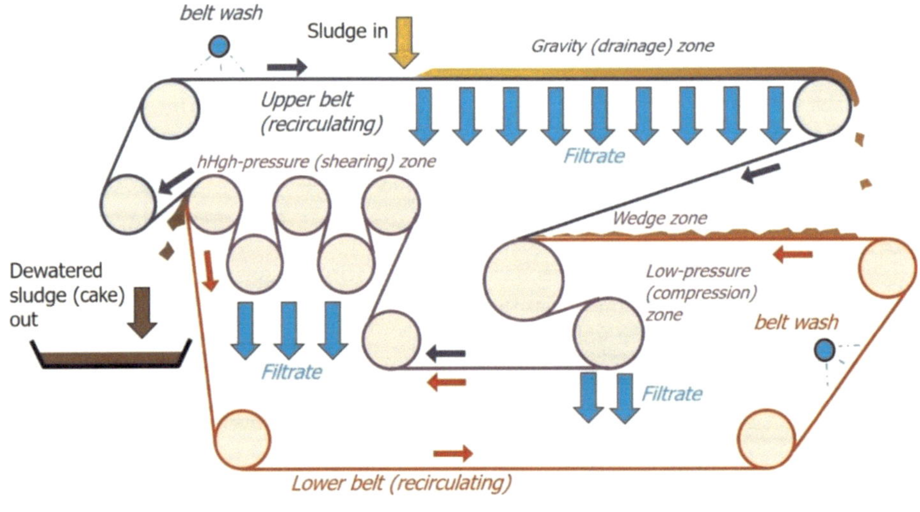

Figure 1.
Schematic diagram of the operation of a BFP [1].

process parameters and the sludge production or cake solids and that it was not predictable and that similar optimization studies should be done when parameters need to change.

Kholisa and coworkers used a factorial trial design and response surface methodology to evaluate the interaction between process parameters for BFP optimization [5]. The work was also conducted at the WWTP at full scale. The plant co-thickens secondary sludge using a cationic poly-electrolyte Flopam 4800, holds it in an aerated holding tank, and dewaters using belt filter press. A four-factor three-level Box–Behnken response surface experimental design (BBD) was used to determine the effect of process conditions on BFP performance. The operating parameters were polymer concentration, polymer dosing, sludge flow rate, and belt speed. The performance measures were sludge cake solid percentage, filtrate suspended solids, and solid capture. The sludge cake solid concentration was found to be constant over the wide range of experimental conditions tested. They found that the sludge flow rate was the most important parameter affecting the filtrate suspended solids and solid capture while the belt speed was insignificant. The results showed clearly that the interaction between sludge flow rate and either polymer dosing rate or polymer concentration was consistently more significant than polymer concentration and polymer dosing rate individually. This was important information that cannot be established by varying single parameters at a time, as in the work of Johnson et al. [4].

Kholisa and coworkers [5] proposed quadratic models to describe the relationship between operating parameters and the filtrate suspended solids (FSSs) and solid capture (SC) based on response surface model as shown in Eqs. (1) and (2)

$$\sqrt{\text{FSS}} = -5.805 - 29.906 * A + 17.013 * B + 0.5495 * C - 1.286 * AC \\ -1.325 * BC + 87.184 * A^2 + 0.034 * C^2 \tag{1}$$

$$SC = 81.03 + 855.42^* A - 85.85^* B - 8.35^* C - 592.68^* AB + 21.96^* AC \\ + 18.14^* BC - 1274.35^* A^2 - 0.47^* C^2 \tag{2}$$

Where

A = polymer concentration g/L; B = polymer dosing m^3/hr; C = sludge feed m^3/hr; D = belt speed Hz; and E = linear screen speed Hz

In addition, Kholisa et al. [5] found a relationship between the yield stress of the sludge and the filtrate suspended solids. An optimum yield stress of 90Pa of sludge was found that was suitable to produce filtrate suspended solid concentrations that were within acceptable limits.

It is important to verify the trend with other filter belt presses and another WWTP especially a plant where there is sludge thickening on linear screen before filter press, which was the objective of this work.

2. Experimental work

2.1 Experimental facility

The experimental work was conducted on a large scale at the WWTP. The municipal wastewater treatment works are designed for an average dry weather flow (ADWF) capacity of 24 Ml/d, with the current flow of about 14 M/l/d, mostly of domestic origin. All inflow is pumped from the catchment to the inlet works, consisting of screening, degritting, and flow division. The plant is equipped with two biological reactors, which are arranged in the University of Cape Town (UCT) process configuration for enhanced biological phosphorus removal (EBPR). The mixed liquor is thereafter distributed to four secondary settling tanks (SSTs). The SST overflow gravitates to maturation ponds followed by Ultraviolet (UV) disinfection, and the underflow gravitates to the return activated sludge (RAS) pump station where it is pumped back to the anoxic zone in the reactors. Two variable-speed-driven pumps (duty/standby) pump the waste-activated sludge (WAS) directly out of each reactor's final zone to the sludge dewatering building, where the WAS is thickened in two linear screens (Siemens Gravity table GTN 2500), followed by dewatering in two belt filter presses (Siemens BPF 2000 CMF Optima S11 Cascade). The filtrate and wash water from the thickening/dewatering trains gravitate back to the RAS division box where it is mixed with the RAS before entering the anoxic zones of the bioreactors. The pressed sludge (cake) is discharged via a centerless screw conveyor to a reinforced concrete hopper, from which sludge is discharged to trucks for removal from site for beneficial agricultural reuse application. A schematic diagram of the WWTP is given in **Figure 2**.

The loading on the belt presses can be controlled according to solids or flow loading. Control using solid loading is the preferred operation and is managed based on the output from the total suspended solids (TSSs) meter in the reactor aeration

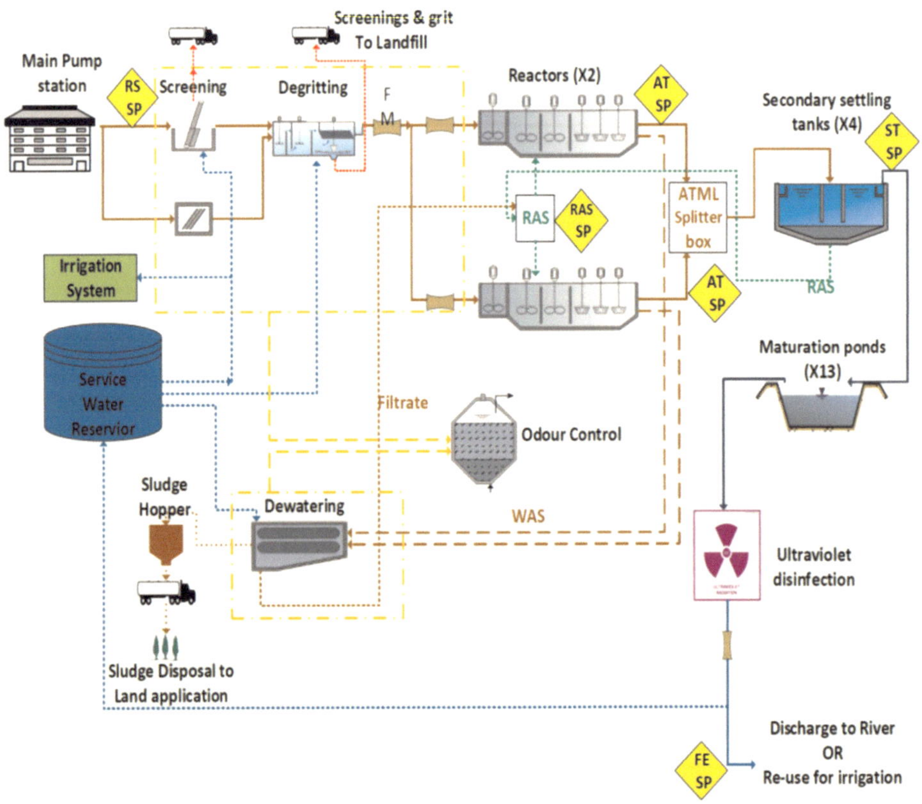

Figure 2.
Schematic diagram of the WWTP.

basin. The design parameters of the Linear Screens require a minimum WAS feed of 4500 mg/l mixed liquor suspended solids (MLSSs) from the reactors. Treated effluent is reused with an automated in-line filtration stage and is available as process water in the dewatering building, both for belt washing and polymer makeup purposes. The sludge-conditioning polymer (Flopam FO4650) is provided in 25kg bags in powder form, and powder is pneumatically transferred and wetted for blending and storage in two makeup tanks. This polymer solution flows into a sump from where it is withdrawn by the polymer dosing pumps and dosed in-line into the WAS before it is fed to the linear screens. The dosing rate is set at the supervisory control and data acquisition (SCADA), based on analysis data and visual observations. The dewatering performance is guided by a minimum cake solid content of 14% and a solid recovery of 95%, respectively, which is affected by the ageing infrastructure that is due for a major refurbishment.

2.2 Experimental design

In this work, a Box-Behnken response surface experimental design (BBD with five factors at three levels was used to examine the effect of process operating parameters on the BFP performance measures. The process conditions were polymer concentration (%) [**A**], polymer dosing rate (m^3/hr) [**B**], sludge feed rate (m^3/hr) [**C**], filter belt speed (Hz) [**D**], and linear screen speed (Hz) [**E**]. The BFP performance measures were sludge cake, filtrate suspended solids, and solid capture, and these were selected as responses with the addition of the yield stress. The range of the operating parameters investigated was chosen based on the preliminary trials. The ranges and levels of the selected operating parameters are presented in **Table 1**. The final design matrix consisted of 31 experiments including five center points. Due to difficulty in changing the polymer concentration according to the normal randomization of results, a grouped approach was selected to run a polymer concentration per day (The polymer concentration was defined as "hard to change" in the Design-Expert V11 software). Random repeats and intermediate conditions were selected by the Design-Expert software to ensure randomization.

2.3 Experimental procedure

The complete Box-Behnken design parameters are provided in **Table 2**. The trials were run over a period of 6 days to allow for the required polymer concentration to be

Factors	Factorial label	Levels used		
		Low	Medium	high
Polymer concentration (%)	A	0.2 (−1)	0.25 (0)	0.30 (+1)
Polymer dosing (m^3/hr)	B	0.4 (−1)	0.5 (0)	0.6 (+1)
Sludge feed (m^3/hr)	C	40 (−1)	50 (0)	60 (+1)
Belt speed (Hz)	D	40 (−1)	45 (0)	50 (+1)
Linear screen speed (Hz)	E	60 (−1)	65 (0)	70 (+1)

Table 1.
Factors in Box-Behnken experimental design.

Group	Run	Factor 1	Factor 2	Factor 3	Factor 4	Factor 5
		A: Polymer concentration	B: Polymer dosing	C: Sludge feed	D: Belt speed	E: Linear screen speed
		%	m^3/hr	m^3/hr	Hz	Hz
1	1	0.25	0.50	50.00	45.00	65.00
	2	0.25	0.50	50.00	45.00	65.00
	3	0.25	0.50	50.00	45.00	65.00
2	4	0.20	0.40	60.00	50.00	70.00
	5	0.20	0.60	60.00	40.00	66.10
	6	0.20	0.56	60.00	50.00	60.00
	7	0.20	0.60	40.00	43.20	65.00
	8	0.20	0.40	55.00	40.00	60.00
	9	0.20	0.41	40.00	50.00	61.75
	10	0.20	0.50	48.60	44.55	70.00
3	11	0.30	0.60	40.00	50.00	60.00
	12	0.30	0.40	46.00	50.00	70.00
	13	0.30	0.60	60.00	49.75	70.00
	14	0.30	0.40	51.00	40.00	60.00
	15	0.30	0.52	50.80	50.00	65.00
	16	0.30	0.52	40.00	44.85	70.00
4	17	0.24	0.54	40.00	40.00	60.00
	18	0.24	0.60	50.20	46.40	60.00
	19	0.24	0.60	40.00	50.00	70.00
	20	0.24	0.40	40.00	40.00	70.00
	21	0.24	0.40	60.00	45.10	64.43
	22	0.24	0.51	60.00	40.00	70.00
5	23	0.30	0.40	40.00	45.40	60.00
	24	0.30	0.40	60.00	41.20	70.00
	25	0.30	0.47	44.00	40.00	64.95
	26	0.30	0.60	47.35	40.00	70.00
	27	0.30	0.40	60.00	50.00	60.00
	28	0.30	0.59	60.00	41.00	60.00
6	29	0.25	0.50	50.00	45.00	65.00
	30	0.25	0.50	50.00	45.00	65.00
	31	0.25	0.50	50.00	45.00	65.00

Table 2.
Complete Box-Behnken design parameters.

prepared for each day in the plant at large scale. Each experiment was run for 30 min to reach steady state before samples were collected. The responses were measured three times, and the average value was recorded.

The response variables measured were the sludge cake solids, the filtrate suspended solids, solid capture, and the yield stress. The solids were measured using the standard oven drying technique for the cake, filtrate suspended solids, and the feed. The percentage solid capture (recovery) was calculated using the Eq. (3):

$$\text{Solid capture (\%)} = \frac{\text{solids in the feed} - \text{solids in the filtrate}}{\text{solids in the feed}} \times 100 \tag{3}$$

A Paar-Physica MCR-51 rheometer fitted with a parallel-plate geometry, with a measuring cell CP50 of 50 mm diameter and a gap of 1 mm, was used for determining the sludge yield stress. The rheological tests were conducted in the controlled shear rate mode with the shear rate being the control parameter. Rheological measurements were performed by decreasing the shear rate linearly from 700 s^{-1} to 100 s^{-1} to exclude data with secondary flows at high shear rates and low torque at low shear rates. Thirty data points were collected, and each point was measured for 5 seconds. This protocol was repeated three times for each sludge sample to ensure reproducibility of the measurements. The data were then fitted with the Bingham model to obtain the yield stress.

The sludge samples tested were collected on the linear screen just after rake number 6. Before this point, the sludge proved to be difficult to measure due to dilute nature with rapid separation of sludge flocs and water as the shear force was applied. Due to the nature of sludge, there is some initial structure that is broken down when sheared several times. The sample was run several times to obtain representative sets of curves from repeat runs of three fresh samples. The average of the yield stress of the highest and lowest curve was determined for each run as a comparative result. It is recommended that the structure of the flocs be interrogated in future in subsequent test runs using oscillation tests. For this work to determine the comparative trends, the analysis was deemed sufficient. A typical rheogram is shown in **Figure 3**.

3. Results and discussion

3.1 Feed, filtrate, and cake solids

The objective of these trial runs was to determine the operational factors of the belt filter press that contributes to efficient dewatering, indicated by the filtrate suspended solids and the percentage of solids in the cake. The rheological parameter describing the floc type produced by the specific polymer dosage rate, polymer concentration, the sludge feed rate, the belt speed, and the linear screen speed, with specific emphasis on determining the interaction that significantly affects the performance of the belt filter press. The factorial trial matrix with the responses is given in the Appendix. A summary of the feed solids concentration, the cake solids, and the filtrate suspended solids is shown in **Figure 4**. Cake solids of more than 14% were only obtained for one out of 31 runs.

3.2 Relationship between FSS and cake solids and yield stress

A power-law relationship was found between the filtrate suspended solids and the yield stress for the values obtained over the full range of the experimental results. Yield stress values between 1 and 5 Pa are sufficient to obtain FSS of between 0.9 and

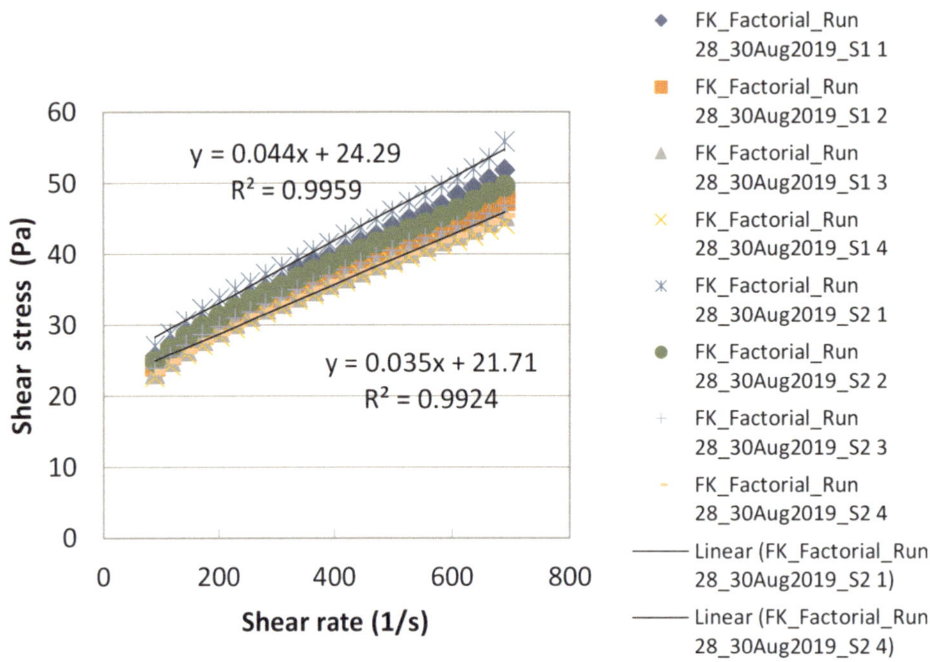

Figure 3.
Typical rheogram.

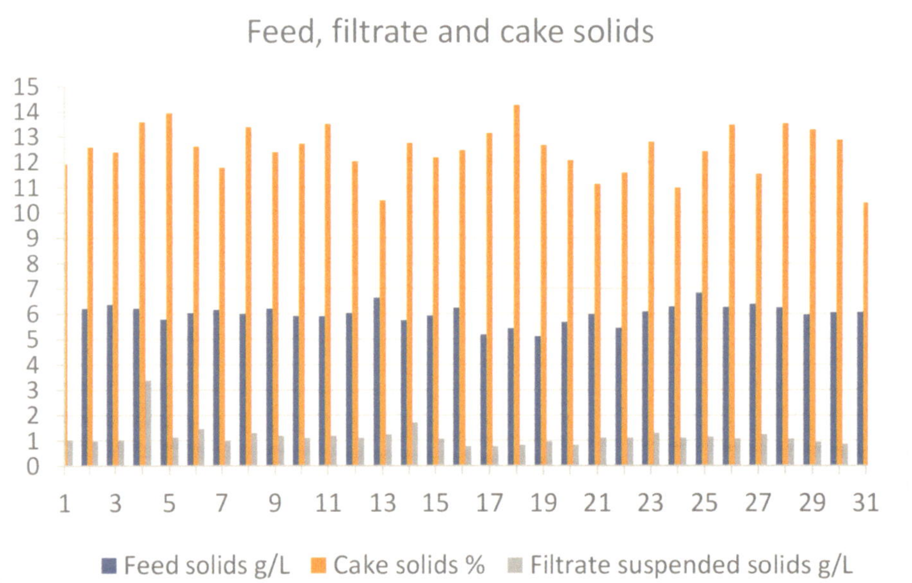

Figure 4.
Feed, filtrate, and cake solids results for all trial runs.

0.5 g/L. **Figure 5** is useful to demonstrate the relationship between the yield stress and the FSS, but it does not give an indication of the process conditions required to obtain these yield stress values. The FSS was less than 0.5 g/L for 58% of the trial run

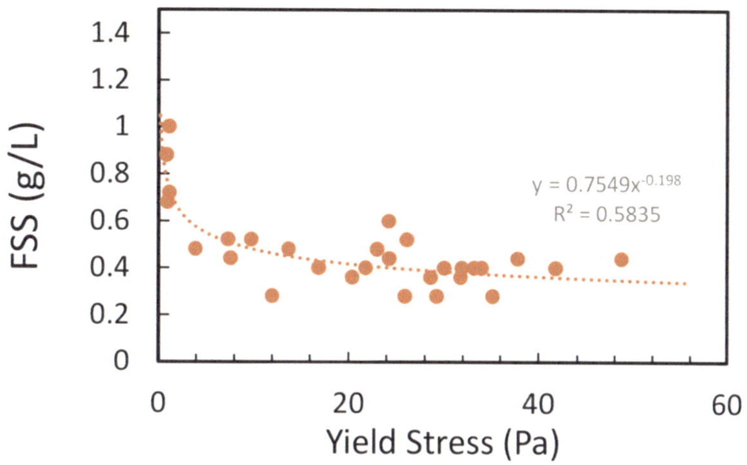

Figure 5.
Filtrate suspended solids as a function of yield stress.

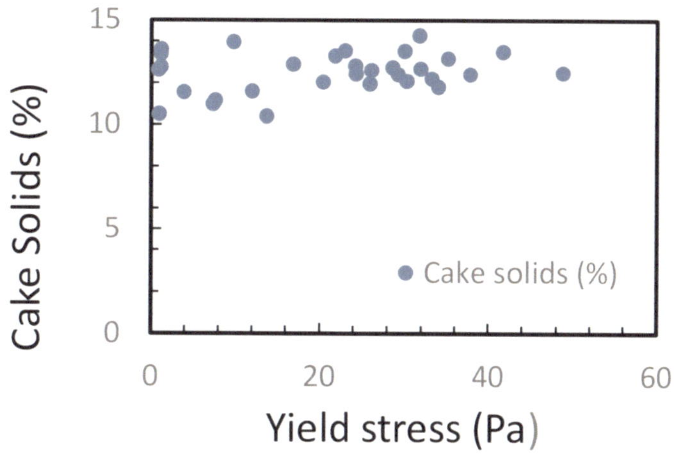

Figure 6.
Cake solids as a function of yield stress.

conditions. In contrast, there was no relationship found between the cake solids and the yield stress as shown in **Figure 6**.

3.3 The effect of process conditions on belt filter press performance

3.3.1 Filtrate suspended solids

The effect of process conditions on the filtrate suspended solids was investigated to determine the optimum process conditions. A split-plot design was used because of the number of variables as it also enabled the identification of process interactions that would normally not be seen when only one parameter was changed at a time. The filtrate suspended solids were measured at the outlet of the belt filter press. A sample was collected 20 minutes after the conditions were changed. The online FSS sensor was not responsive for the low readings obtained, and hence, a sample was collected, and the standard drying test was conducted as well as filtration through 0.45μm Millipore filter.

3.3.1.1 Analysis of variance

The analysis of variance (ANOVA) is presented in **Table 3**. A quadratic model was selected without any transformation, with a step-wise backward selection, a p-value criterion, and an alpha value of 0.1. However, based on the Box-Cox analysis, an inverse square root transformation was required. P-values less than 0.0500 indicate that model terms are significant. Values greater than 0.1000 indicate that the model terms are not significant. Only the sludge feed (C) and the belt speed (D) were significant with p-values equal to or less than 0.05. The polymer concentration (a), polymer dosing, and linear screen speed (E) were not significant, with a p-value of 0.99, 0.40, and 0.32, respectively. However, the interaction between polymer concentration (a) and sludge feed and belt speed and linear screen speed as well as B^2 was significant. In this case C, aC, aD, aE, CD, DE, B^2 are significant model terms with a, B, and E added to maintain hierarchy. The final fit statistics obtained is showing an R^2 value of 0.7415 and adjusted R^2 of 0.5919 and a C.V. of 13.42%. These could be improved if Run 4 is excluded, but we are certain of the results even though it seems out of range, it is expected from such low polymer dosing.

The final equation obtained to determine the contribution of each factor is given in Eq. (4) (coded), and the equation for the prediction of filtrate suspended solids is given in Eq. (5) (actual).

$$1/\sqrt{FSS} = 1.62 + 0.0007a + 0.0323B - 0.1352C + 0.0647D + 0.0371E + 0.1122\,aC + 0.1420aD - 0.1042DE - 0.1920B^2 \quad (4)$$

$$1/\sqrt{FSS} = -6.245 - 38.61a + 20.00B - 0.080C + 0.138D + 0.215E + 0.261aC + 0.570aD - 0.0046DE - 19.65B^2 \quad (5)$$

Source	Term df	Error df	F-value	p-value	
Whole-plot	1	3.53	0.0001	0.9937	not significant
a-Polymer concentration	1	3.53	0.0001	0.9937	
Subplot	8	18.60	5.34	0.0014	significant
B-Polymer dosing	1	17.85	0.7344	0.4028	
C-Sludge feed	1	18.09	12.29	0.0025	
D-Belt speed	1	19.17	2.48	0.1315	
E-Linear screen speed	1	18.05	1.04	0.3216	
aC	1	18.28	5.98	0.0248	
aD	1	19.13	9.24	0.0067	
DE	1	18.93	5.58	0.0290	
B^2	1	21.00	5.69	0.0265	

Table 3.
ANOVA for filtrate suspended solids.

3.3.1.2 Evaluation of the filtrate suspended model

The normal probability plot of the residuals is approximately linear, which shows that the model fits the data well as shown in **Figure 7**.

3.3.2 Cake solids

The resulting cake solids as a function of process conditions were investigated. The cake solids ranged from 10.39% to 14.26% over the full range of conditions used during the factorial trial. For the cake solids, it was found that an interaction exists between the polymer concentration and the sludge feed rate. Based on the statistical analysis (**Table 4**), the linear screen speed is a significant model term as well as the interaction between the polymer concentration and sludge feed, both of which had p-values less than 0.05. The terms a and C and B were added to maintain hierarchy. The statistical analysis of the model showed that the model was acceptable based on the linear plot of normal plot of the residuals, Box-Cox plot confirmed a Lambda of 1 and

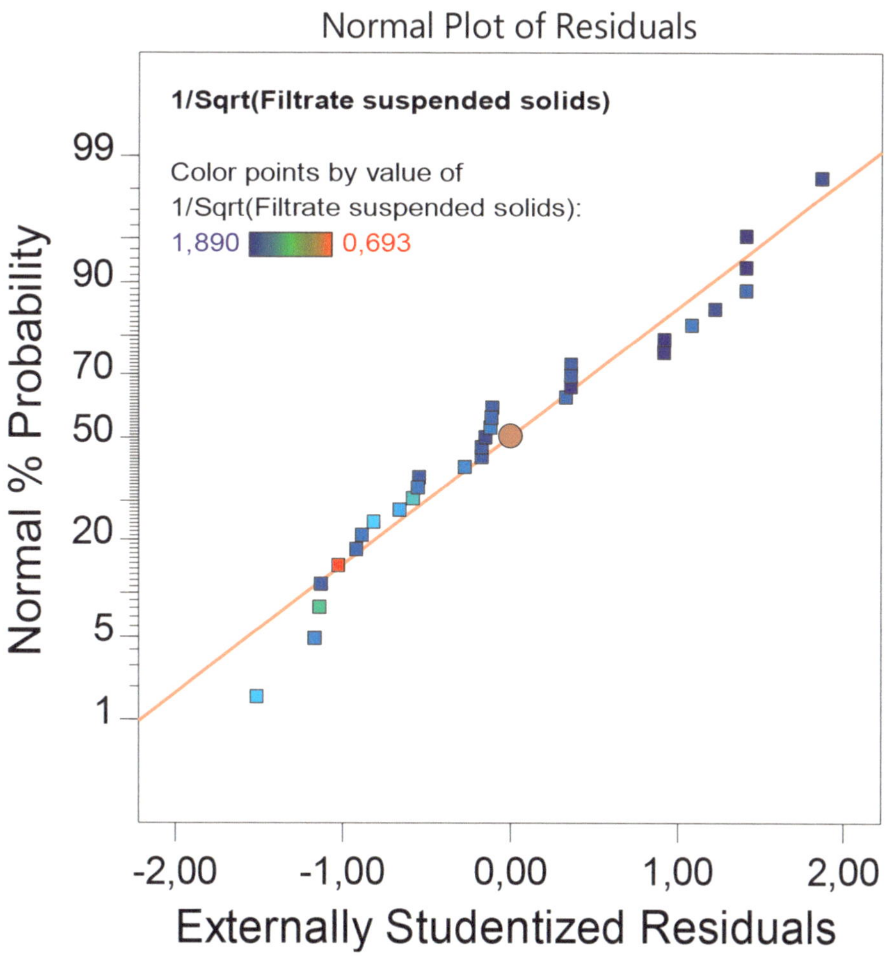

Figure 7.
Normal probability plot of residuals for filtrate suspended solids.

Source	Term df	Error df	F-value	p-value	
Whole-plot	1	25.00	1.11	0.3014	not significant
a-Polymer concentration	1	25.00	1.11	0.3014	
Subplot	4	25.00	3.87	0.0139	significant
B-Polymer dosing	1	25.00	2.99	0.0960	
C-Sludge feed	1	25.00	0.4113	0.5271	
E-Linear screen speed	1	25.00	4.36	0.0472	
aC	1	25.00	7.19	0.0128	

Table 4.
ANOVA for cake solids.

that no further transform of the data was necessary. It is interesting to note that the belt speed is not a statistical significant operational factor in the prediction of the cake solids. Although the diagnostics are good, the Adj.R^2 of 22.9% shows a very poor fit.

3.3.3 Yield stress

The process conditions affecting the yield stress were evaluated. The experimental yield stress values obtained during the test runs ranged from to 0.86 Pa to 48.70 Pa. No transformation of the data was required according to the Box-Cox theory. In this case, parameters B, C, aB, and BD were found to be significant at the 5% level as shown in **Table 5**. In the case of the yield stress, the linear screen speed is not significant, but there is an interaction between belt speed and linear screen speed. The adjusted R^2 is 0.78.

Eq. (6) shows the coded equation and Eq. (7) the actual equation.

Source	Term df	Error df	F-value	p-value	
Whole-plot	1	1.72	1.32	0.3849	not significant
a-Polymer concentration	1	1.72	1.32	0.3849	
Subplot	8	18.00	16.49	< 0.0001	significant
B-Polymer dosing	1	16.95	9.48	0.0068	
C-Sludge feed	1	17.52	85.60	< 0.0001	
D-Belt speed	1	20.65	0.6446	0.4312	
E-Linear screen speed	1	17.60	1.34	0.2627	
aB	1	16.76	5.44	0.0325	
BD	1	20.35	9.20	0.0065	
DE	1	19.10	3.45	0.0786	
D^2	1	18.78	3.44	0.0795	

Table 5.
ANOVA for yield stress.

$$\text{Yield stress} = 24.1843 + 2.24613a + 4.38B - 13.38C - 1.277D + 1.581E + 3.833\,aB - 5.554BD - 3.0768DE - 5.33D^2 \tag{6}$$

$$\text{Yield stress} = -848 - 333a + 334B - 1.35C + 30.5D + 5.84184E + 754aB - 10.6BD - 0.1223DE - 0.194D^2 \tag{7}$$

3.3.4 Solid capture

The experimental values obtained for solid capture ranged from 66.5 to 95.6%. The significant model terms are C, aC, aD, aE, CD, DE, and B^2 as shown in **Table 6**.

Eq. (8) shows the coded equation and Eq. (9) the actual equation.

$$\text{Solid capture} = 93.5726 + 1.2131a + 0.787295B - 2.380C - 1.369D - 0.608E + 2.82703aC + 3.24954aD + 1.78aE - 1.84CD - 2.34DE - 3.71B^2 \tag{8}$$

$$\text{Solid capture} = -31.33 - 1256.6a + 369.42B - 0.215C + 5.005D + 2.912E + 6.11aC + 12.36aD + 6.457aE - 0.035CD - 0.1032DE - 361.3B^2 \tag{9}$$

The normal probability plot (**Figure 8**) of the residuals is approximately linear. Removing run 4 from the analysis could improve the adjusted R^2 from 68% to 71%, but the assumption that Run 4 is due to experimental error and based on experience it is not. Such a change to improve the statistics will also result in significant factor changing from polymer dosing (B2) to linear screen speed (E2) in the final equation.

Source	Term df	Error df	F-value	p-value	
Whole-plot	1	2.80	1.38	0.3305	not significant
a-Polymer concentration	1	2.80	1.38	0.3305	
Subplot	10	16.40	7.81	0.0002	significant
B-Polymer dosing	1	15.99	1.42	0.2516	
C-Sludge feed	1	16.41	12.53	0.0026	
D-Belt speed	1	18.09	3.58	0.0745	
E-Linear screen speed	1	16.15	0.8575	0.3681	
aC	1	16.73	12.46	0.0026	
aD	1	17.84	15.99	0.0009	
aE	1	16.31	5.45	0.0326	
CD	1	16.11	5.55	0.0315	
DE	1	17.69	9.22	0.0072	
B^2	1	18.26	7.45	0.0137	

Table 6.
ANOVA for solid capture.

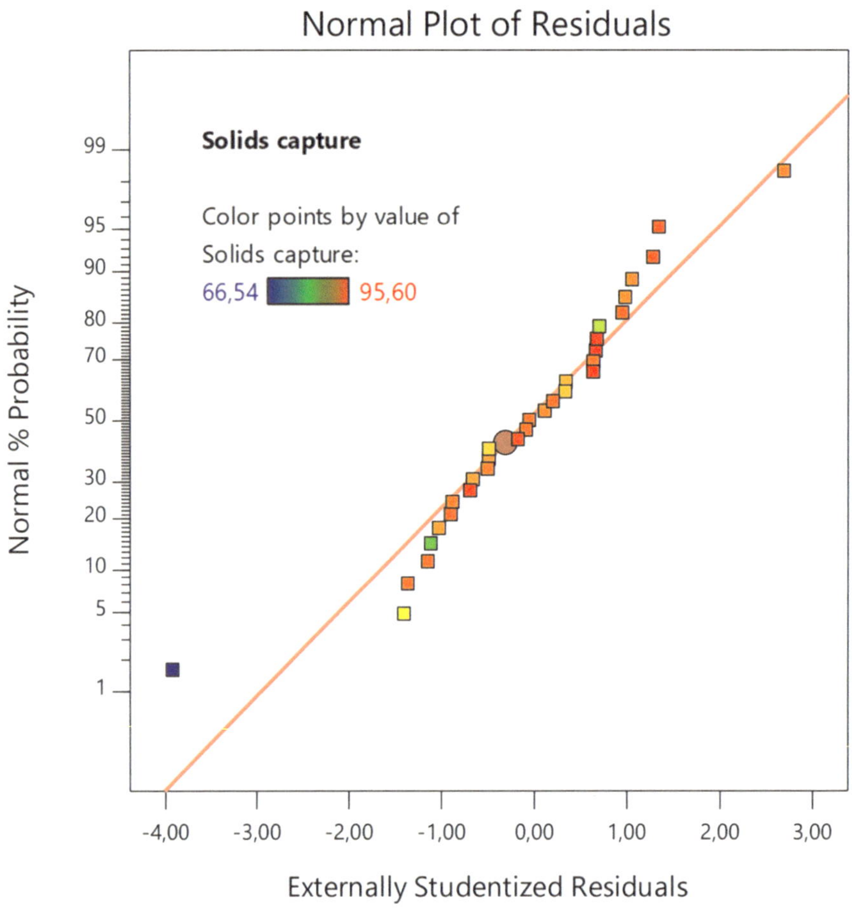

Figure 8.
Normal probability plot of residuals for solid capture.

4. Results and discussion

In order to understand the effect of the process conditions on belt filter press performance, 3D surface plots are utilized **Figure 9a** shows FSS as a function of sludge feed and polymer dosing at the lowest polymer concentration, belt speed, and linear screen speed. The filtrate suspended solids were all below 1 g/L. A minimum value of FSS is obtained at the maximum sludge flow rate and a medium polymer dosing rate due to process interaction. The situation remains the same if all the conditions are set at the maximum values as shown in **Figure 9b**.

When the polymer concentration is minimized with maximum belt and linear screen speed, the FSS is above 1 g/L. However, an acceptable FSS can be obtained by dosing the polymer at 0.5 m^3/hr, which is the midpoint. This interaction between polymer dosing and sludge flow rate is very useful to obtain acceptable FSS at high production rates as shown in **Figure 9c**. Furthermore, the amount of polymer usage can be reduced by decreasing the linear screen speed to the minimum and the sludge feed rate to just under the maximum at 59 m^3/hr; the resulting FSS will be below 1 g/L as shown in **Figure 9d**.

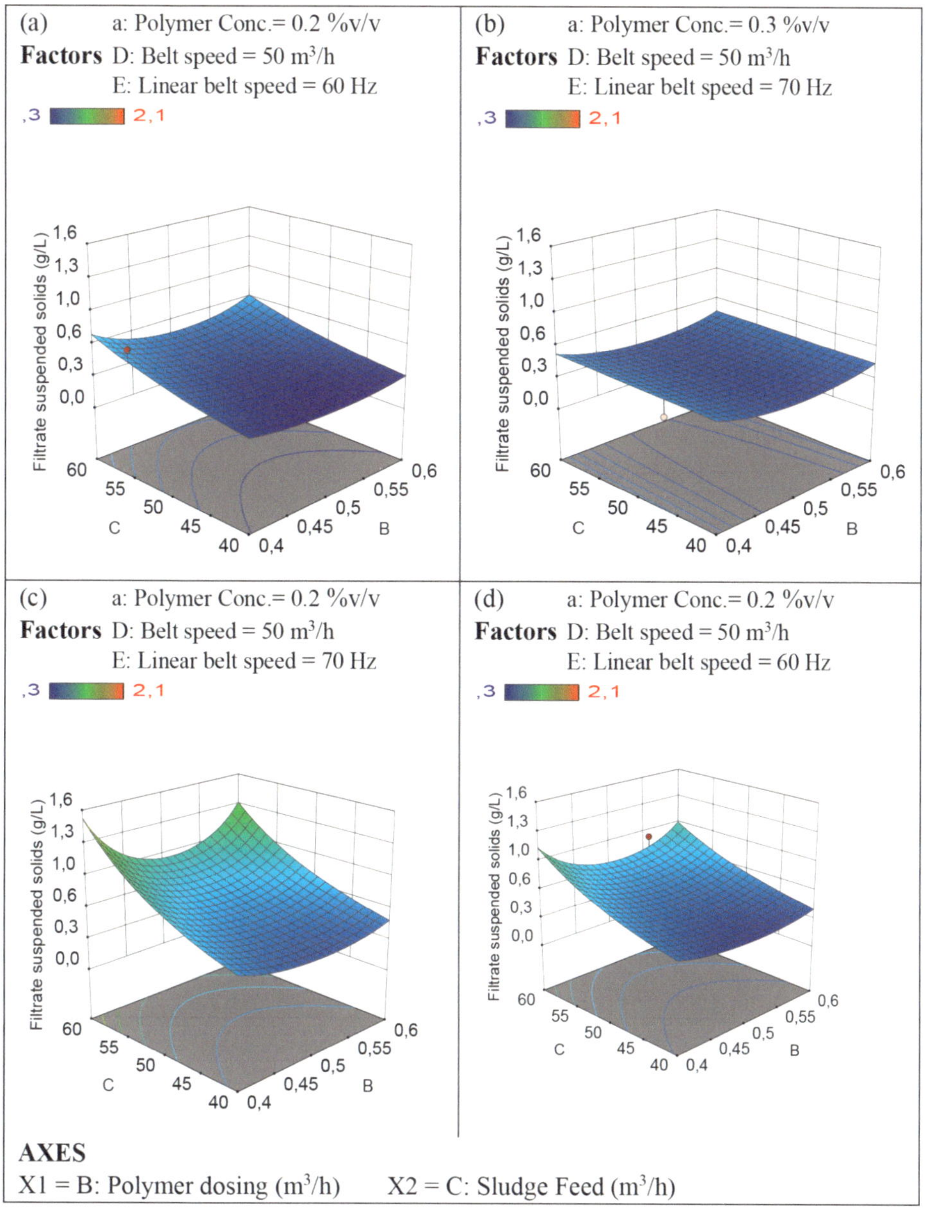

Figure 9.
3D surface plot of FSS as a function of sludge feed and polymer dosing.

To ascertain the performance of the filter cake, the prediction of cake solids is presented under the similar conditions as for the FSS. In contrast to the FSS, the cake solids increase linearly with increasing polymer dosage, with no minima or maxima observed at maximum sludge feed rate. **Figure 10a** shows that at the minimum settings for polymer concentration, belt and linear screen speed, the maximum cake solids of almost 14% can be obtained at the maximum polymer dosing rate and maximum sludge feed rate. Increasing the parameters has a detrimental effect on the cake solids, unlike the case of filtrate suspended solids, and a maximum of 13% cake solids are obtained at the minimum sludge feed rate and maximum polymer dosing as

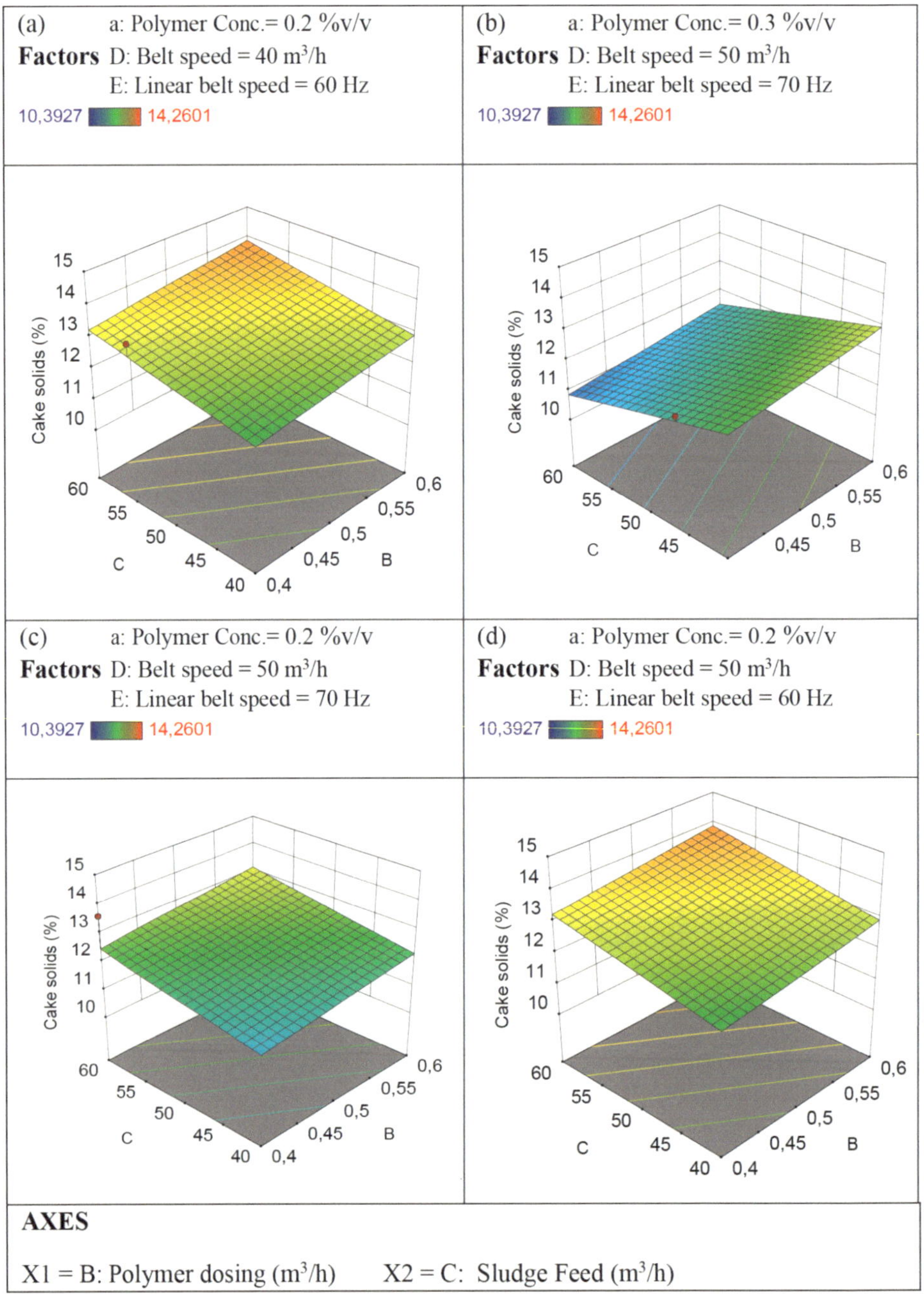

Figure 10.
3D surface plot of cake solids as a function of sludge feed and polymer dosing.

shown in **Figure 10b**. However, surprisingly, by minimizing the polymer concentration, production can be increased and maximum sludge feed rate and maximum polymer dosing with result in 13% cake solids. It should also be noted that the design point is higher than the prediction under these conditions as shown in **Figure 10c**. Similarly to the FSS, when reducing the linear screen speed, the cake solids can be improved by nearly 1% as seen in **Figure 10d**. Even though better FSS can be obtained

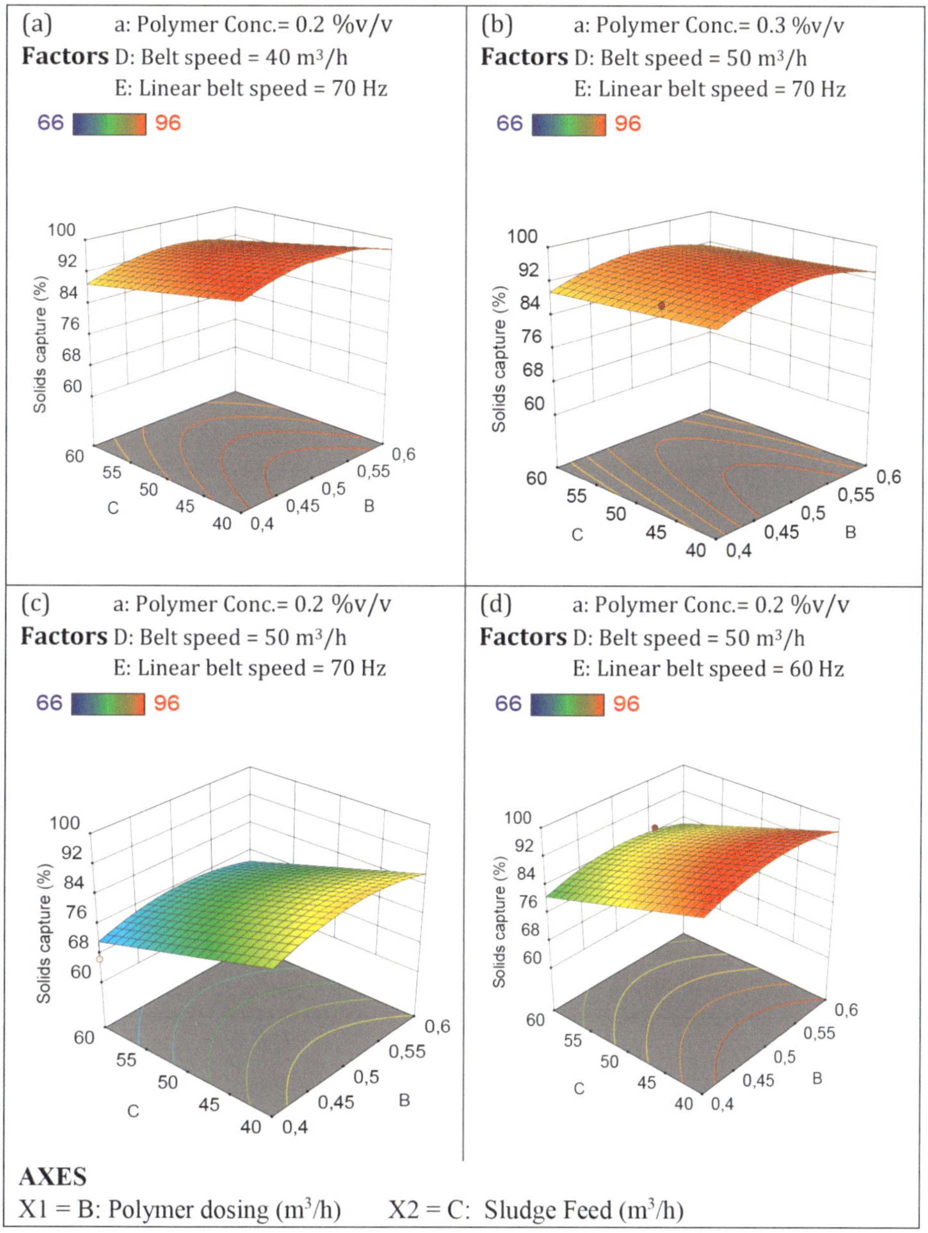

Figure 11.
3D surface plot of solid capture as a function of sludge feed and polymer dosing.

at the medium polymer dosing rate, the maximum polymer dosing rate is required for the maximum cake solids, and based on the prediction, the FSS will still be within the 1 g/L limit. A detailed study of polymer cost versus cake removal costs is needed to manage these limits to an optimum.

For the solid capture, similar graphs are presented in **Figure 11**. These are the inverse of FSS with a maximum obtained at the maximum sludge feed rate and the medium polymer dosing rate (**Figure 11a**). Running all conditions at maximum has

	Significant main effects	Interactions
Filtrate suspended solids	Sludge feed rate	Poly concentration * Sludge feed rate Poly concentration * Belt speed Belt speed * Linear screen speed
Cake solids	Linear screen speed	Poly concentration * Sludge feed rate
Yield stress	Polymer dosing Sludge feed rate	Poly concentration * Poly dosing rate Poly dosing rate * Belt speed Belt speed * Linear screen speed
Solids Capture	Sludge feed rate	Poly concentration * Sludge feed rate Poly concentration * Belt speed Poly concentration* Linear screen speed Sludge feed rate* Belt speed Belt speed * Linear screen speed

Table 7.
Summary of significant main factors and interactions.

limited impact on the performance of the belt filter press as shown in **Figure 11b**. Reducing the polymer concentration impacts the performance of the belt filter press negatively as the solid capture is reduced to less than 70% (**Figure 11c** compared with 90% under all minimum or all maximum conditions. Reducing the linear screen speed at the minimum polymer concentration improves the solids capture but only to mid- or low sludge feed rates as shown in **Figure 11d**, but it is ultimately the reduction of the belt speed at lower polymer concentration that will ensure maximum solid capture at high sludge flow rates (**Figure 11a**) at the mid-range polymer dosing rate.

A summary of the significant main factors and interactions is provided in **Table 7**. It shows that the polymer concentration is much more important than polymer dosing rate in interactions with the other conditions. Current practice in the plant is to keep the polymer concentration constant and to change polymer dosing rate. This work demonstrates that a control system that can incorporate changes to concentration is required for a fully automated polymer control system to reduce cost.

5. Conclusion

A factorial trial was conducted at a WWTW to establish correlations to predict the filter belt press performance as a function of process conditions. Correlations to predict the FSS, Cake solids, Yield stress, and Solid Capture were developed based on the factorial trial design. From the results obtained, it was found that a power-law relationship exists between FSS and the yield stress. There is no relationship between the yield stress and the cake solids. The cake solids are affected by the linear screen speed and the interaction between the polymer concentration and sludge feed. It is recommended that more work be done around the optimization of the cake solids based on this information. It is also the only parameter for which the linear screen is the most significant factor, and the belt speed is insignificant in this case. An important outcome from this work is that it shows that changes in polymer concentration rather than polymer dosing rate are more important in the control system. This is contrary to current practice where the polymer concentration is constant and only the polymer dosing rate is adjusted.

Acknowledgements

I would like to acknowledge the Technology Innovation Agency (TIA) South Africa and CPUT for funding this work. Further, I would like to acknowledge Richard du Toit for assistance with experimental work and the staff of the Wastewater Treatment Plant for assistance during the live scale trial work. Thanks are due to Dr D.W.Brown for assistance in reviewing this chapter.

Conflict of interest

The authors declare no conflict of interest.

Terminology used in this chapter

ADWF	Average Dry Weather Flow
ANOVA	Analysis of Variance
BBD	Box-Behnken Design
BFP	Belt Filter Press
EBPR	Enhanced Biological Phosphorus Removal
FSS	Filtrate Suspended Solids
MLSS	Mixed Liquor Suspended Solids
RAS	Return Activated Sludge Station
SCADA	Supervisory and Data Acquisition
SST	Secondary Settling Tanks
TTS	Total Suspended Solids
UCT	University of Cape Town
WAS	Waste Activated Sludge
WWTP	Municipal Wastewater Treatment Plant

A. Appendix: Box-Behnken experimental matrix and responses

Group/ Run	A % v/v	B m^3/h	C m^3/h	D Hz	E Hz	Image	Yield stress Pa	FSS g/L	Cake solids %	Solids capture %
1/1	0.25	0.50	50.00	45.00	65.00	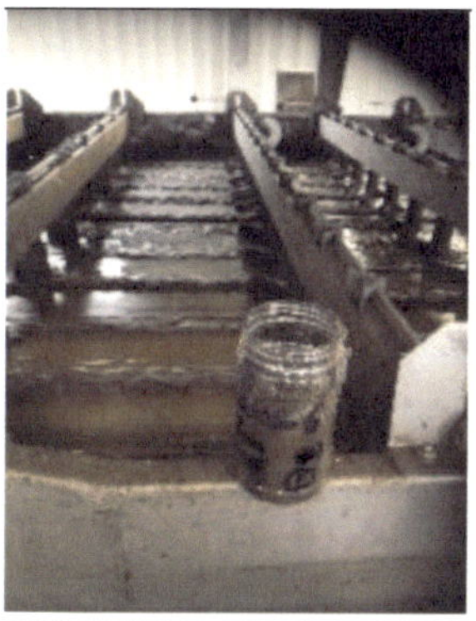	25.90	1.02	11.94	83.83
1/2	0.25	0.50	50.00	45.00	65.00		26.10	0.97	12.59	84.40
1/3	0.25	0.50	50.00	45.00	65.00		29.20	1.01	12.39	84.15

Group/ Run	A % v/v	B m^3/h	C m^3/h	D Hz	E Hz	Image	Yield stress Pa	FSS g/L	Cake solids %	Solids capture %
2/4	0.20	0.40	60.00	50.00	70.00	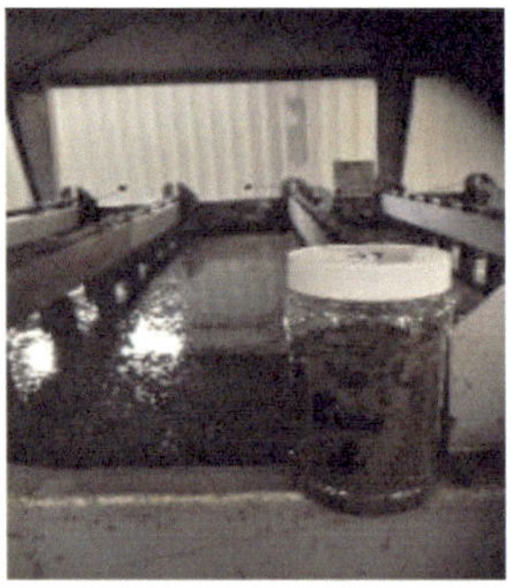	1.18	3.39	13.59	45.42
2/5	0.20	0.60	60.00	40.00	66.10	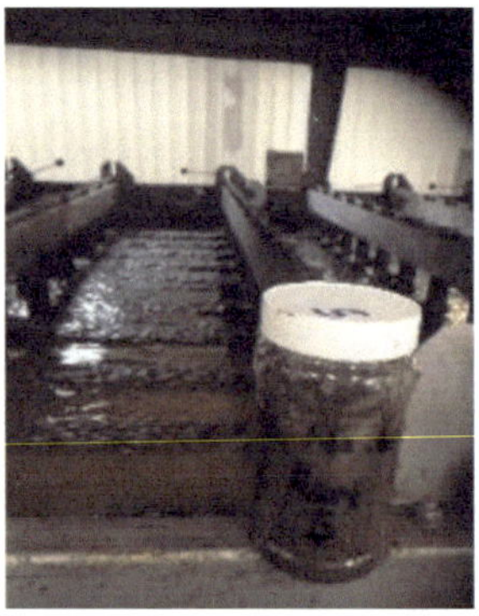	9.76	1.13	13.95	80.46
2/6	0.20	0.56	60.00	50.00	60.00	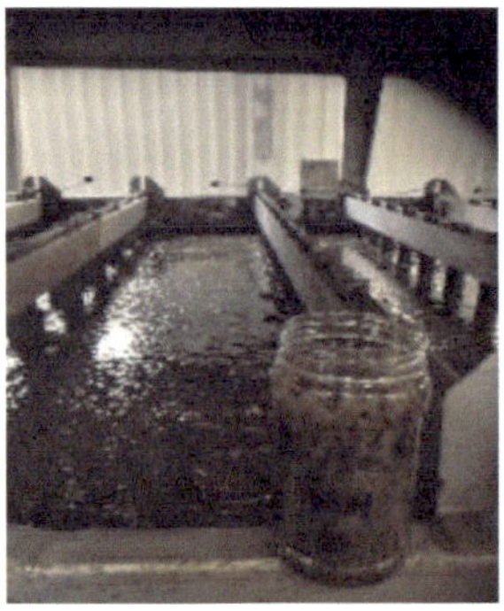	0.86	1.46	12.62	75.81
2/7	0.20	0.60	40.00	43.20	65.00	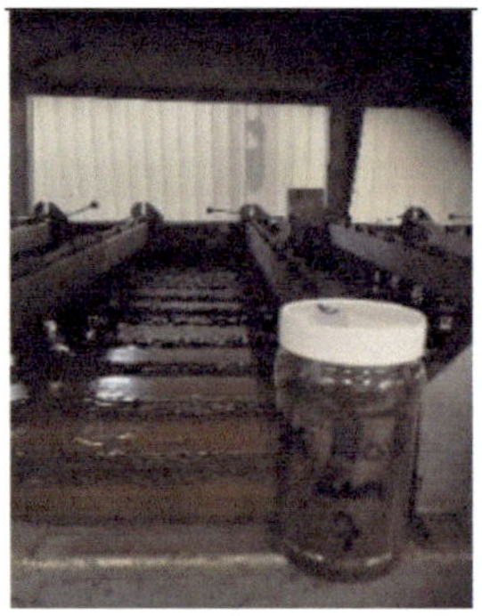	33.90	0.99	11.79	84.01

DOI: http://dx.doi.org/10.5772/intechopen.108978

Group/ Run	A % v/v	B m^3/h	C m^3/h	D Hz	E Hz	Image	Yield stress Pa	FSS g/L	Cake solids %	Solids capture %
2/8	0.20	0.40	55.00	40.00	60.00	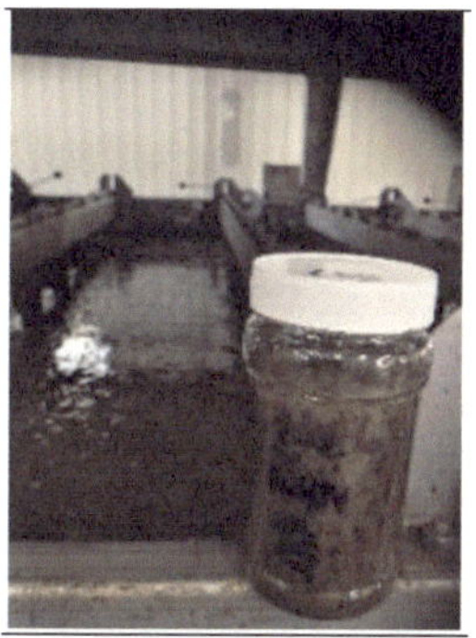	1.15	1.30	13.38	78.37
2/9	0.20	0.41	40.00	59.00	61.75	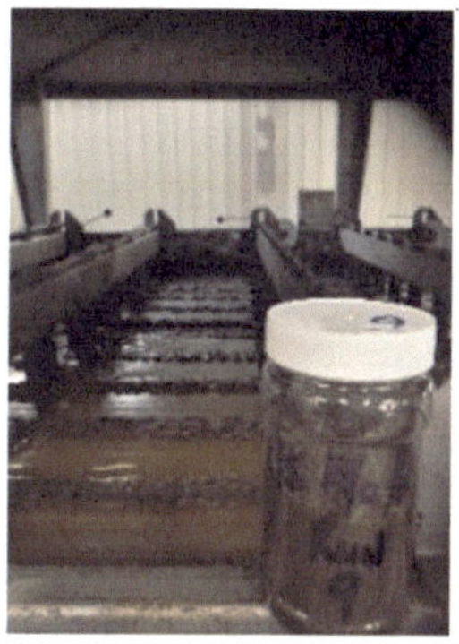	37.82	1.20	12.39	80.74
2/10	0.20	0.50	48.60	44.55	70.00	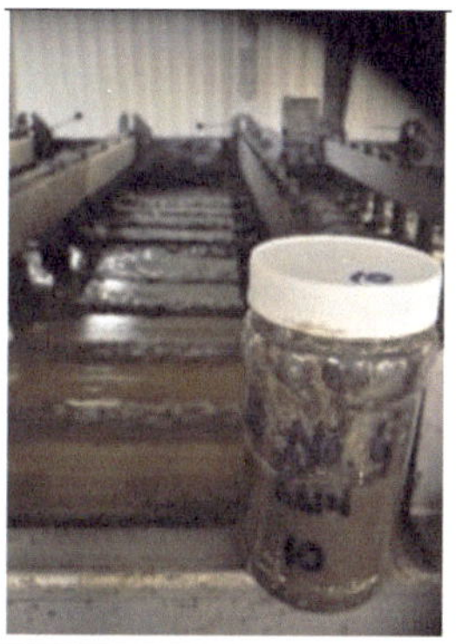	28.57	1.10	12.73	81.37
3/11	0.30	0.60	40.00	50.00	60.00	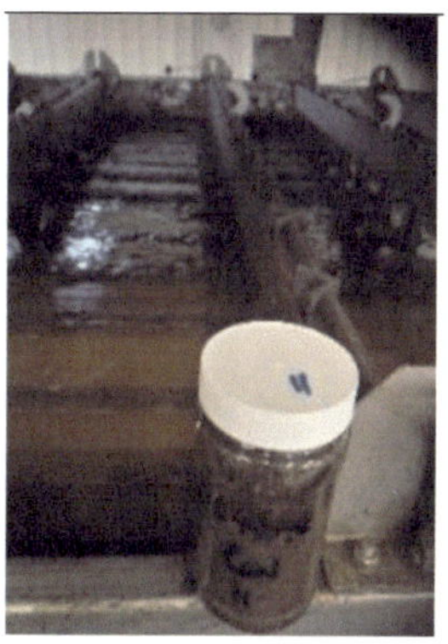	29.90	1.19	13.52	75.92

Group/ Run	A % v/v	B m^3/h	C m^3/h	D Hz	E Hz	Image	Yield stress Pa	FSS g/L	Cake solids %	Solids capture %
3/12	0.30	0.40	46.00	50.00	70.00	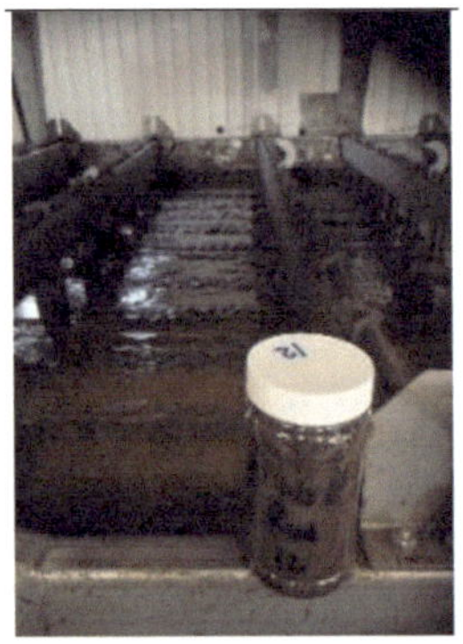	20.35	1.11	12.02	81.61
3/13	0.30	0.60	60.00	49.75	70.00	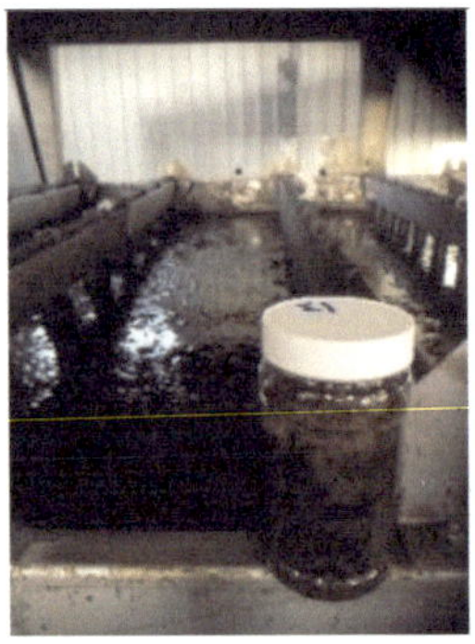	0.95	1.24	10.49	81.31
3/14	0.30	0.40	51.00	40.00	50.00	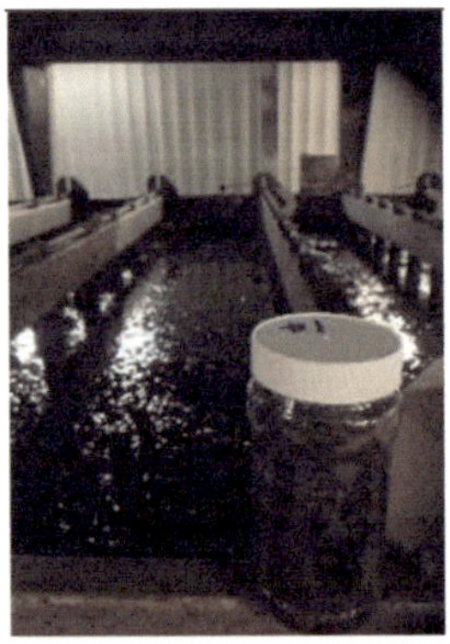	1.14	1.71	12.75	70.24
3/15	0.30	0.52	50.80	50.00	65.00	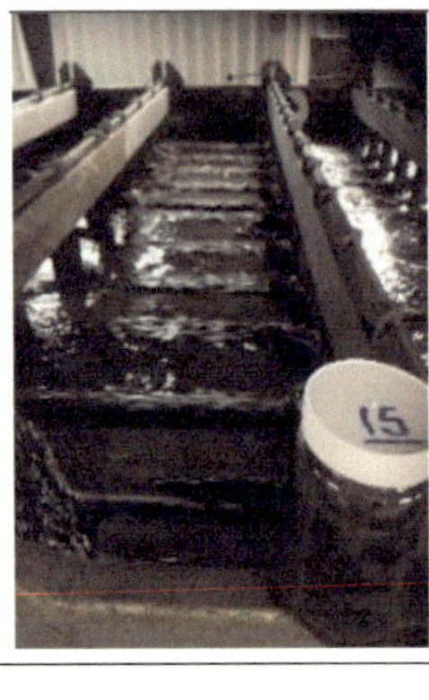	33.20	1.06	12.18	82.09

DOI: http://dx.doi.org/10.5772/intechopen.108978

Group/ Run	A % v/v	B m^3/h	C m^3/h	D Hz	E Hz	Image	Yield stress Pa	FSS g/L	Cake solids %	Solids capture %
3/16	0.30	0.52	40.00	44.85	70.00	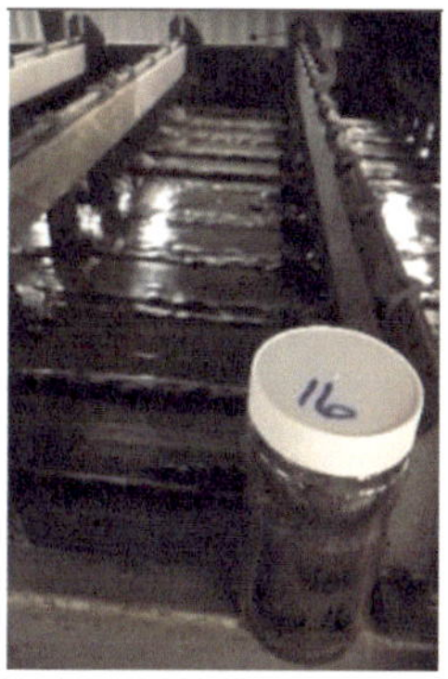	48.70	0.77	12.46	87.60
4/17	0.24	0.54	40.00	40.00	60.00	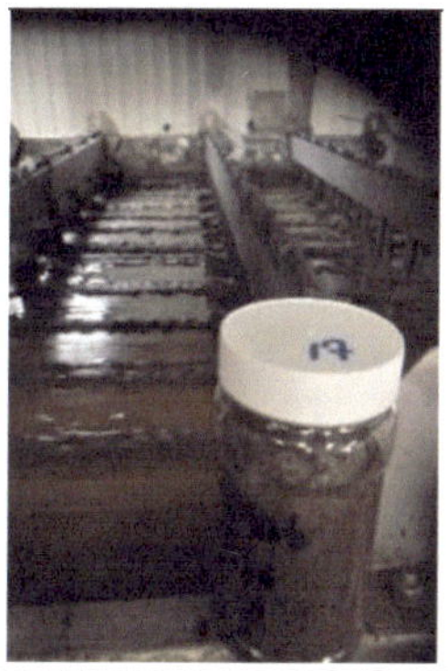	35.16	0.78	13.15	85.04
4/18	0.24	0.60	50.20	46.40	60.00	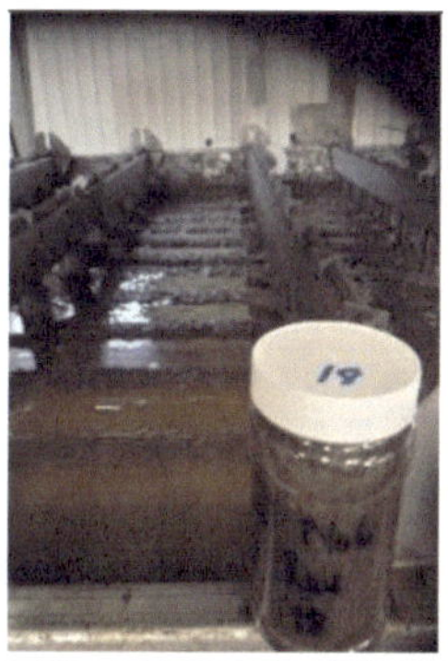	31.72	0.83	14.26	84.81
4/19	0.24	0.60	40.00	50.00	70.00	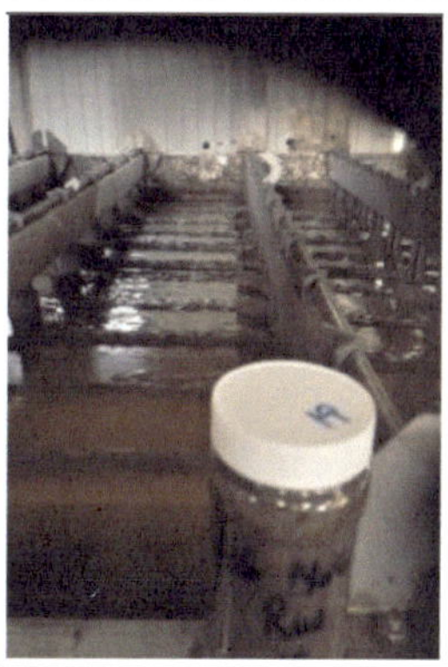	31.86	0.96	12.67	81.24

Group/ Run	A % v/v	B m³/h	C m³/h	D Hz	E Hz	Image	Yield stress Pa	FSS g/L	Cake solids %	Solids capture %
4/20	0.24	0.40	40.00	40.00	70.00	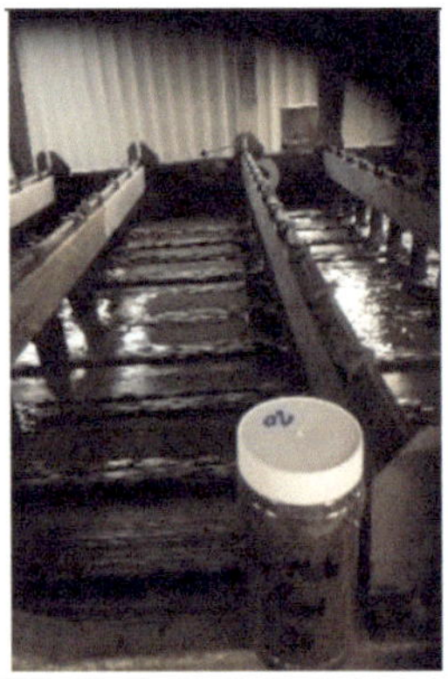	30.24	0.82	12.07	85.55
4/21	0.24	0.40	60.00	45.10	64.43	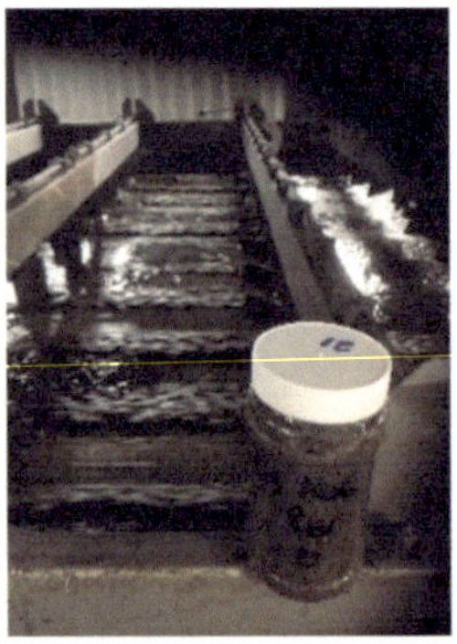	7.59	1.11	11.14	81.42
4/22	0.24	0.51	60.00	40.00	70.00	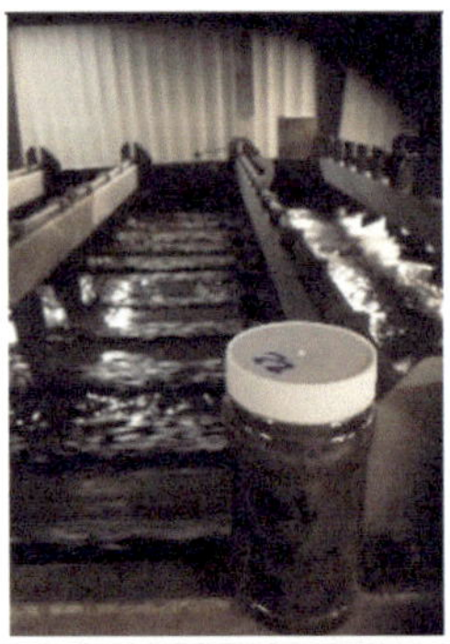	11.99	1.11	11.58	79.55
5/23	0.30	0.40	40.00	45.40	60.00	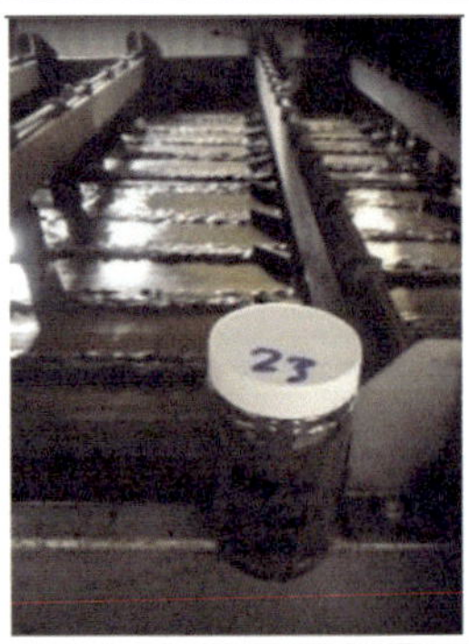	24.21	1.30	12.81	78.67

Group/ Run	A % v/v	B m^3/h	C m^3/h	D Hz	E Hz	Image	Yield stress Pa	FSS g/L	Cake solids %	Solids capture %
5/24	0.30	0.40	60.00	41.20	70.00	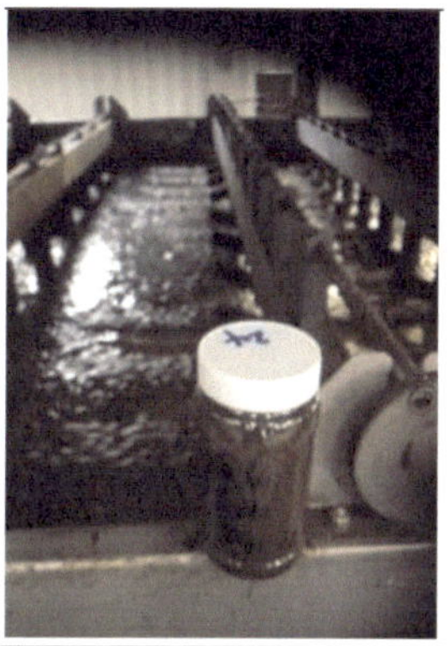	7.32	1.10	10.98	83.43
5/25	0.30	0.47	44.00	40.00	64.95	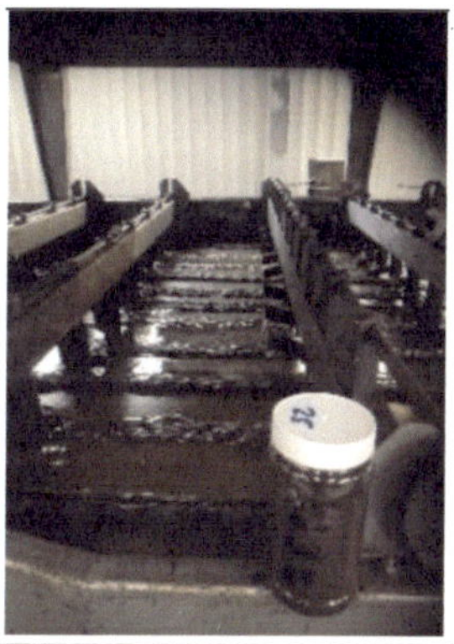	24.26	1.14	12.42	83.23
5/26	0.30	0.60	47.35	40.00	70.00	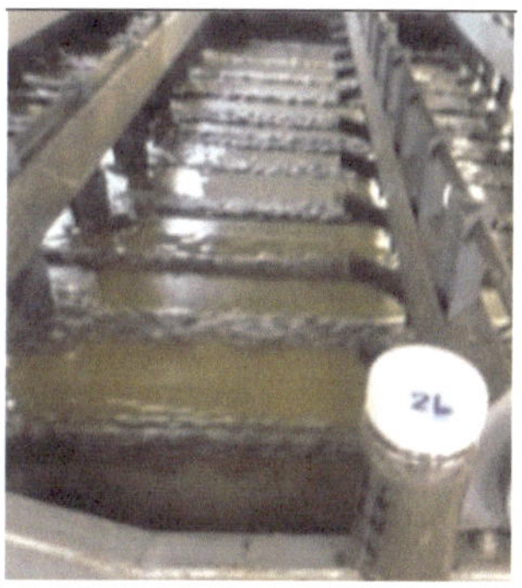	41.73	1.08	13.48	82.79
5/27	0.30	0.40	60.00	50.00	60.00	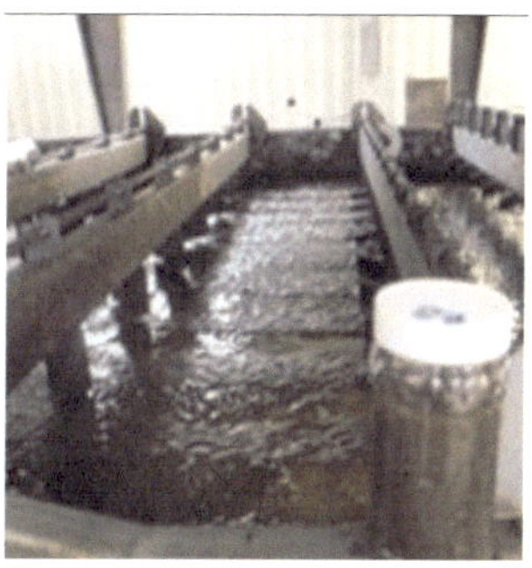	3.90	1.25	11.53	80.49

Group/ Run	A % v/v	B m^3/h	C m^3/h	D Hz	E Hz	Image	Yield stress Pa	FSS g/L	Cake solids %	Solids capture %
5/28	0.30	0.59	60.00	41.00	60.00	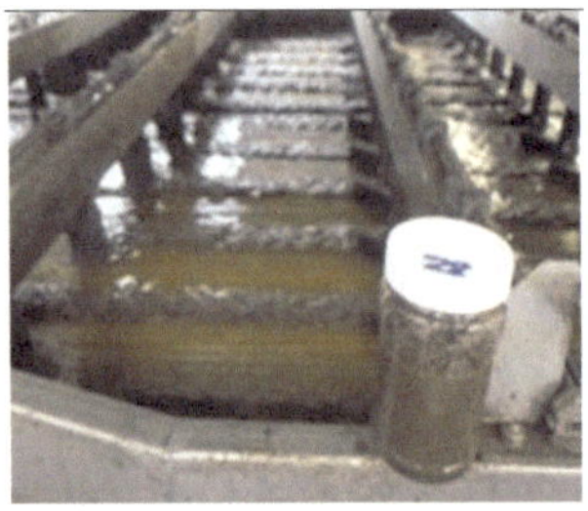	23.00	1.07	13.53	82.91
6/29	0.25	0.50	50.00	45.00	65.00	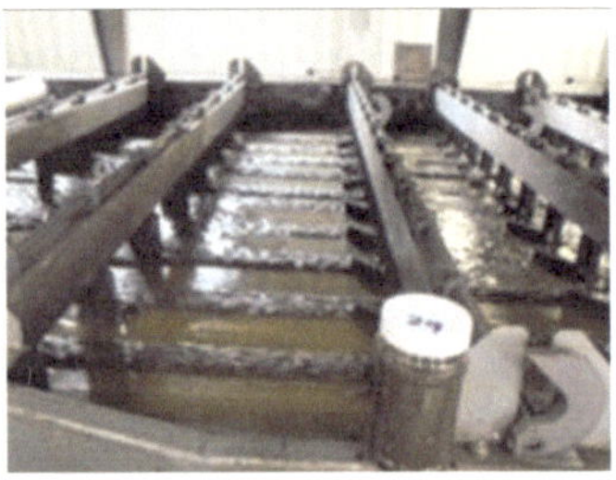	21.79	0.94	13.29	84.23
6/30	0.25	0.50	50.00	45.00	65.00	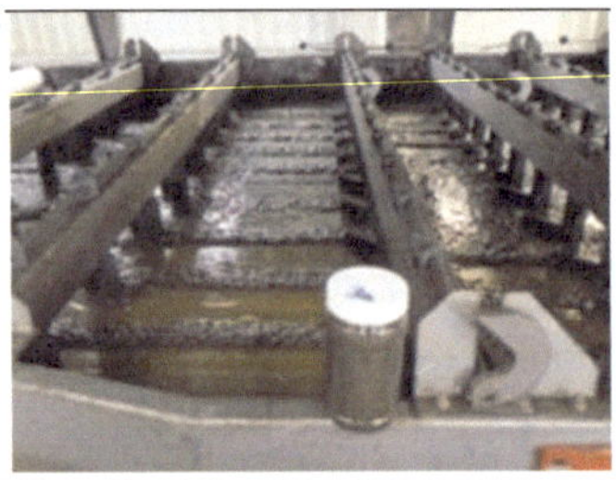	16.87	0.87	12.89	85.69
6/31	0.25	0.50	50.00	45.00	65.00	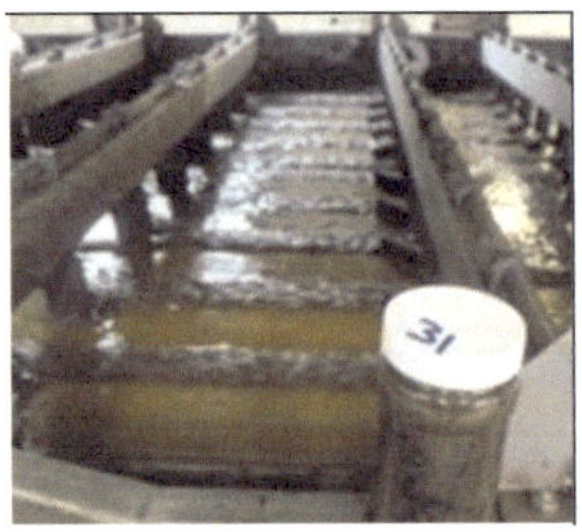	13.74	1.12	10.39	81.58

Author details

Veruscha Fester[1]* and Rössle Werner[2]

1 Flow Process and Rheology Centre, Cape Peninsula University of Technology, Cape Town, South Africa

2 Wastewater Branch, Bulk Services Department, Water and Sanitation Directorate, City of Cape Town, South Africa

*Address all correspondence to: festerv@cput.ac.za

References

[1] Goncalves RF, Luduvice M, von Sperling M. Sludge Treatment and Disposal. New Delhi: IWA Publishing; 2007

[2] U.S. EPA. Biosolids Technology Fact Sheet: Belt Filter Press. Washington, DC: U.S. EPA; 2000

[3] Judd, S. Belt filter presses for sludge dewatering. Sludge Processing. 2020. Available from: https://www.sludgeprocessing.com/sludge-dewatering/belt-filter-press/ [Accessed: September 14, 2022]

[4] Johnson G, Buchanan GG, Newkirk DD. Optimizing Belt Filter Press Dewatering at the Skinner Filtration Plant. American Water Works Association; John Wiley & Sons Publishers; 1992

[5] Kholisa B, Fester VG, Haldenwang R. Prediction of filtrate suspended solids and solids capture based on operating parameters for belt filter press. Chemical Engineering Research and Design. 2018; **134**:268-276

Section 6

Applications

Chapter 10

Review of Slurry Bed Reactor for Carbon One Chemistry

Fanhui Meng and Muhammad Asif Nawaz

Abstract

The slurry bed reactor has many advantages, which make it very suitable for gas-to-liquid processes, especially for the highly exothermic reactions. This chapter reviews three types of slurry bed reactors and their comparisons, including the mechanically stirred slurry reactor, bubble column slurry reactor and three-phase fluidized bed reactor. The application of the slurry bed reactors in carbon one (C_1) chemistry for syngas conversion to different valuable chemicals is presented, which includes four typical exothermic reactions, that is, the Fischer-Tropsch synthesis to oil, methanol synthesis, dimethyl ether synthesis and synthetic natural gas synthesis. The operation parameters and performance of slurry bed reactor, fixed bed reactor and fluidized bed reactor are compared while discussing the reasons of catalyst deactivation. Since, the development trend of slurry bed reactor for C_1 chemistry is finally proposed.

Keywords: slurry bed reactor, carbon one chemistry, syngas conversion, metal catalyst, deactivation

1. Introduction

The slurry bed reactors are gas-liquid-solid three-phase reactors, which are commonly used in many industrial processes [1, 2]. The research of slurry bed reactors can be traced back to the Second World War, where the most studied and the earliest application process is the low-temperature Fischer-Tropsch synthesis (FTS) to oil. The catalytic reactions in slurry bed reactors are highly complicated due to the presence of multi-phase mass transfer, intraparticle diffusion, adsorption, surface reaction and desorption of products [3, 4]. The difficulty in separating the catalyst and handling of the slurry limits the application of slurry reactors in continuous processes. However, the slurry bed reactors possess many advantages, such as the low investment cost and simple construction, high heat exchange efficiency, online catalyst addition and withdrawal [5]. Moreover, the catalyst consumption per unit product is only 30% of the fixed bed reactor, and the total amount of required catalyst for the slurry bed reactor can be greatly reduced, which make it very suitable for gas-to-liquid processes [6].

In this review, the difference in three types of slurry bed reactors is compared, including the mechanically stirred slurry reactor, bubble column slurry reactor and three-phase fluidized bed reactor. The second part shows the application of slurry bed reactors for C_1 chemistry, discussing the four typical exothermic reactions for syngas conversion to different valuable chemicals. The third part introduces the comparison between slurry bed, fixed bed, and fluidized bed reactors. The fourth part discusses the catalyst deactivation for syngas conversion in slurry bed reactors, which mainly includes the catalysts sintering, carbon deposition and effects of water on catalyst structure. While, the last part demonstrates the development trend of slurry bed reactors for carbon one chemistry.

2. Classification and comparison of slurry bed reactors

According to the way of catalyst particles suspending in the slurry bed, the slurry bed reactors can be divided into three categories, i.e., mechanically agitated slurry reactor, bubble column slurry reactor, and three-phase fluidized bed reactor. **Figure 1** shows these three types of reactors [7, 8].

2.1 Mechanically agitated slurry reactor

The mechanically agitated slurry reactors are commonly used in many chemical processes, such as the hydrogenation of unsaturated oils and nitro compounds. It has the advantages of high mass and heat transfer efficiency, which are best suited for laboratory kinetic studies. And it is because the catalyst particles are small in the reactor, the diffusion resistance in the particles is very low, and the utilization rate of the catalyst is very high. The disadvantages are the high power required for stirring, the presence of significant liquid back-mixing, and the difficulty of catalyst separation in continuous operation. The commonly used agitator in the reactor is a turbine-type radial flow agitator, and there is an optimal ratio of paddle to vessel diameter. To keep the catalyst particles suspended evenly, the number of the baffles should be 4 in most cases and the size is 1/10 ~ 1/12 of the container diameter. Moreover, the use of baffles

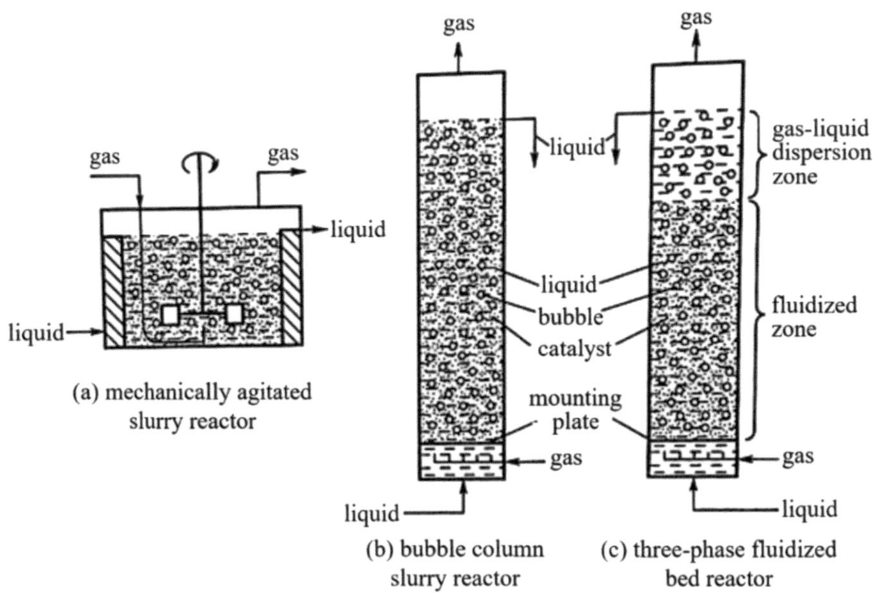

Figure 1.
Three different types of slurry bed reactors [7].

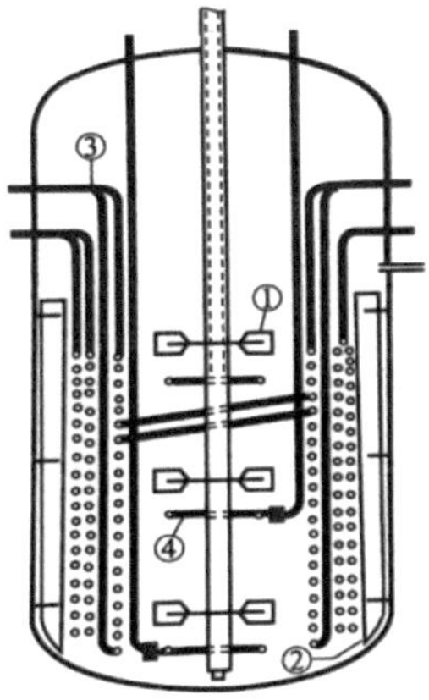

Figure 2.
Slurry bed reactor with multiple paddles [7]. 1. Paddle, 2. baffle, 3. cooling or heating coils, 4. annular pipes for supplying H_2.

could provide a proper gas distribution and avoid the formation of vortex on the surface of the liquid. Generally, the gas inlet should be as close to the paddle as possible, using an annular sparger rather than a single nozzle. The width of the sparger should be about 0.8 times of the paddle diameter. **Figure 2** shows the slurry bed reactor with multiple paddles, which is commonly used for the hydrogenation of unsaturated oils [7]. To reduce the back mixing in continuous operation, the horizontal inlets are provided at various locations in the reactor.

2.2 Bubble column slurry reactor

In a bubble column slurry reactor, the dispersion of the feed gas takes place through a deep pool of inert liquid in which the catalyst particles are suspended, and the momentum is transferred to the inert liquid by the movement of the bubbles. The operation is usually implemented in the columns with a height-to-diameter ratio of 4 to 10. For the conversion of liquid reactants, the operation can be semi-batch or continuously. The advantages of this type of reactor are that there are no moving parts, no need to seal the stirrer, less floor space and low power consumption compared to stirred reactors. Its main disadvantage is that the liquid phase has considerable back-mixing, which needs to overcome a large pressure drop, and when the height-diameter ratio is higher than 10, the gas-liquid interface area will be decreased quite rapidly. The bubble column slurry reactors have been used in many industrial processes, such as FTS to hydrocarbons, and the production of caprolactam, etc. **Figure 3(a)** shows a continuous bubble column slurry reactor with solid-liquid separation [7]. In another type of bubble column slurry reactor, the catalyst and liquid are circulated by using external pumps, and the catalyst can be operated at higher loads, either counter-current or co-current. The schematic diagram is shown in **Figure 3(b)**.

2.3 Three-phase fluidized bed reactor

In a three-phase fluidized bed reactor, the catalyst particles are primarily fluidized by the liquid, while the gas stream flows co-currently in the form of intermittent bubbles. An important difference between the three-phase fluidized bed reactor and

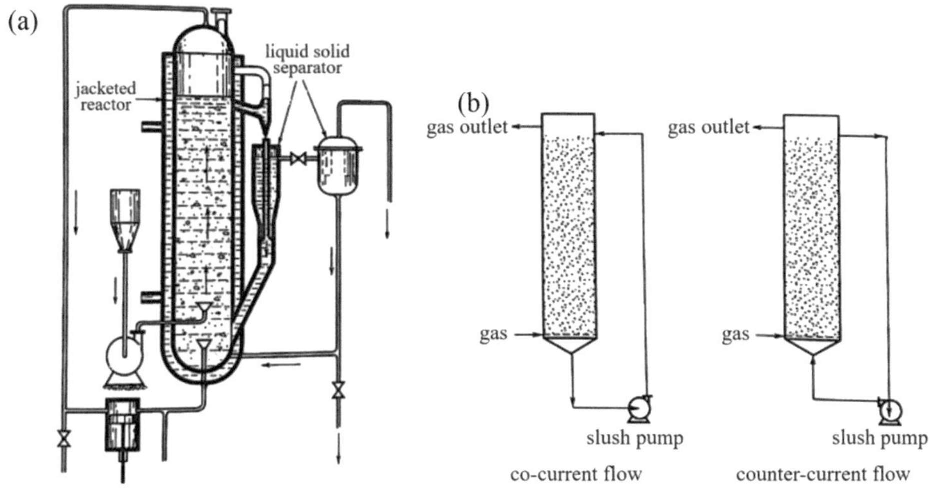

Figure 3.
(a) Schematic diagram of continuous bubble column slurry reactor, (b) schematic diagram of a bubble column slurry reactor circulating with a pump [7].

the bubble column slurry reactor is that the former transfers momentum through the movement of liquid, while the latter transfers momentum through the movement of the bubbles. Moreover, the relatively large catalyst particles can be used in three-phase fluidized bed reactors, which makes it suitable for continuous operation due to easy separation of catalyst particles from the liquid. The main industrial application of three-phase fluidized reactor is the hydrogenation of petroleum, including the hydrodesulfurization, hydrocracking to produce olefins, and the partial oxidation to produce aromatics. The three-phase fluidized bed reactors are generally operated in co-current flow, but in some cases, they can also be operated in counter-current flow (the liquid flows down while the gas flows up), such as when the density of catalyst particles (ion exchange resin) is lower than that of the liquid. In the industry, the particles are kept fluidized with internal circulation of the liquid, which can be accomplished by using a pump. This makes it possible to fluidize large catalyst particles. If the internal circulation is not used, the single-pass conversion rate will be too low due to the excessive liquid flow rate used.

2.4 Comparison of three types of slurry reactors

1. The catalyst particles in the mechanically stirred slurry reactor are suspended by the mechanical stirring of paddles, which shows high heat transfer and mass transfer efficiency. However, the power required for mechanical stirring is the largest, and the sealing problem of the stirrer needs to be considered. In addition, the wear of the catalyst during the mechanical stirring process is probably the most significant.

2. The catalyst particles in bubble column slurry reactor are suspended by the gas bubbling; however, the relatively small particles result in the difficulty in catalyst separation.

3. The catalyst suspension in three-phase fluidized bed reactor is the result of combination of the bubble movement and the co-current liquid flow. The main

difference between a fluidized bed and a bubbling bed is that the suspension of the particles for the former is the result of liquid flow, thus, the relatively large catalyst particles can be used, which benefits the catalyst separation. Due to the absence of moving parts, the design of bubble columns and three-phase fluidized bed reactors is simpler than that of mechanically stirred reactors.

3. Slurry bed reactors for carbon one chemistry

3.1 Fischer-Tropsch synthesis

FTS has been practiced on a large scale by Sasol in South Africa since the mid-1950s in tubular fixed-bed reactors and circulating fluidized-bed reactors using iron catalysts. The commercial scale conventional bubbling fluidized-bed reactor and slurry bubble column reactor (SBCR) were placed on stream by Sasol in 1989 and 1993, respectively. At present, the multi-tubular fixed bed reactor, fluidized bed reactor, gas-liquid-solid slurry reactor, and microchannel reactor are used for FTS. The reactor type and the operating conditions are the governing factors in controlling the product distribution with chain growth probability, catalyst activity, and product selectivity during FTS [9, 10]. The multi-tubular fixed bed reactor and slurry reactor are used for the low-temperature process, while the circulating fluidized bed reactor, fixed fluidized bed rector, and microchannel reactor are used for the high-temperature process. The high-temperature process yields large amounts of olefins, a lower boiling range, and very good gasoline while producing the substantial amounts of oxygenates. The low temperature process yields much more paraffin and linear products and can be adjusted to very high wax selectivity. The primary diesel cut and wax cracking products can give excellent diesel fuels. The very linear primary gasoline fraction needs further treatment to attain a good octane number. Olefin and oxygenate levels for the low-temperature process are lower than those for the high-temperature process.

3.1.1 Fixed bed reactor

The fixed bed reactor for FTS, such as the Arge reactor at Sasol with 12 m height and 0.5 m diameter, consists of a shell containing 2050 tubes packed with Fe-based catalyst that produced the 600–900 bbl/day/reactor [11]. Where, the heat generated in highly exothermic synthesis reaction of 220°C reaction temperature, and 25–45 bar pressure was used for the generation of steam on the shell side of the reactor. Similarly, some other reactors using Co-based catalyst were also introduced at Bintulu Malaysia, Las Raffan, Qatar, and the Pearl GtL facility which resulted the rate of 3000–140,000 bbl/day with 85–95% C_5^+ selectivity [12]. Despite the robust nature and high productivity, the fixed-bed multi tubular reactors contain the disadvantages of design complexity, high cost, low catalyst utilization, high pressure drops, and insufficient heat removal due to poor heat conductivity [13].

3.1.2 Fluidized bed reactor

Fluidized-bed reactors being deployed for the high temperature FT process of entire gas phase, have been designed to comparatively improve the efficiency of fixed-bed reactors in terms of superior heat transfer and temperature control during highly exothermic FT reactions; avoiding intraparticle diffusion, pressure drop and the reaction rate and the better mixing of catalyst particles while giving high production capacity [14]. However, it finds some limitations of difficulty in scale-up for causing the agglomeration and blockage of the fluidization and containing a high risk of attrition and heavy product deposition on catalyst, while requiring the special equipment (cyclones) for catalyst separation. Since, the technical and economic problems of the industrial scale reactor, discouraged their application in 1956 by Hydrocol and later by SASOL in 1980s [15].

3.1.3 Microchannel reactor

The recent advancement in terms of a new type of reactor—the microchannel reactor, which consist of a large number of parallel channels with diameters <1 mm and with the catalyst on a thin layer inside the channel walls. It has been demonstrated in different studies that the large temperature gradients in the furnace-heated conventional fixed-bed reactor can be avoided in the microchannel reactor under the same operating conditions, achieving the best catalyst utilization and thus a high productivity for the large transfer surface area with high heat transfer coefficient between the bed and wall [9]. However, the main challenges of the difficulty in changing the catalyst and high cost of scaling up several microchannel reactors to be operated in parallel, still avoided its commercial FT plant.

3.1.4 Slurry reactor

To replace the fixed bed reactor for the low-temperature FT process, the Sasol slurry reactor was developed. In 1993, a single slurry reactor with 5 m in diameter and 22 m in height realized the industrial production for FTS. Compared with the other reactors, the slurry reactors for FTS are less expensive to construct, maintain and operate [16]. It was reported that the capital cost required for a large-scale slurry reactor was less than 40% of that needed for an equivalent multi-tubular fixed bed reactor: The catalyst usage of the slurry reactor is about a third of that of the fixed bed reactor with a promise of even better performance, due to the catalyst's effectiveness and the higher average temperature used in the slurry reactor. Krishna and Sie compared the several reactor types for the FTS process and concluded that the slurry reactor was the best reactor type for large-scale plants [17].

The adopted catalysts for FTS in slurry bed reactors are commonly the iron-based or cobalt-based catalysts [18]. Parts of FTS using slurry bed reactors are listed in **Table 1**. The most common FTS catalysts have been usually regarded as Fe-based and Co-based catalysts, in which Fe-based catalyst have been synthesized by precipitation method [19]. While, the FTS process being carried out by cobalt-based catalysts were usually suspended in inert liquid [13], by impregnation method using Al_2O_3, SiO_2 or TiO_2 as support, with the Co loading of 10–30% (wt.). Sasol has developed cobalt-based catalyst SAC 2-100SB and applied in slurry bed reactor for FTS, providing this Co catalyst to two sets of natural gas-based synthetic oil production plants in Nigeria and Qatar. The Co catalyst show stable catalytic activity; however, it is only used for low-temperature FTS due to the high price of cobalt.

The pure iron catalysts are easily worn and deactivated in FTS, which needs to enhance the catalytic activity, selectivity, and stability by introduction of additives (electronic additives and structural additives). Fe/Cu/K catalyst is one of the most successful industrial catalysts for low-temperature FTS (200–250°C) [20]. The precipitated iron-based catalyst prepared by Sasol in South Africa exhibits

Company	Location	Capacity/(kt·a^{-1})	Catalyst	Reactor
Institute of Coal Chemistry, Chinese Academy of Sciences/ Synfuels China	Taiyuan, Shanxi	1.0–1.5	LTFT Fe	Slurry
			HTFT Fe	
	Ordos, Inner Mongolia	160	HTFT Fe	Slurry
	Luan, Shanxi	1600	HTFT Fe	Slurry
	Luan, Shanxi	7.5	LTFT Co	Fixed bed
YangKuang group	Thengzhou, Shandong	5	LTFT Fe	Slurry
	Thengzhou, Shandong	5	HTFT Fe	Fluidized bed
SINOPEC group	Zhenhai, Zhejiang	3	LTFT Co	Fixed bed
Shenhua group	Shanghai	0.08	LTFT Fe	Slurry
	Ordos, Inner Mongolia	180	LTFT Fe	Slurry
Rentech	US	0.5	LTFT Fe	Slurry
Syntroleum	Tulsa, US	3.5	LTFT Co	Slurry
Exxon-Mobil	Baton Rouge, US	10	LTFT Co	Slurry
Conoco-Phillips	Ponca, US	20	LTFT Co	Slurry
BP	Nikiski, US	15	LTFT Co	Fixed bed
Statoil/PetroSA	Mossel Bay, South Africa	50	LTFT Co	Slurry

LTFT: low temperature Fischer-Tropsch; HTFT: high temperature Fischer-Tropsch.

Table 1.
Installations for FTS with slurry reactors [18].

high activity, selectivity, and stability, and it has been industrialized. Subsequently, Synfuels China Technology Co., Ltd. proposed a high-temperature FTS in a slurry bed reactor (260–290°C), which greatly improve the steam pressure generated by the FTS reaction and significantly enhance the overall energy utilization efficiency of the FTS process. And based on the development of industrial iron-based catalyst for high-temperature FTS reaction, a complete set for high-temperature FTS process and product processing technologies were developed.

3.2 Methanol synthesis

The syngas conversion to methanol is a strongly exothermic reaction ($CO + 2H_2 = CH_3OH$, $\Delta H^{\Theta}_{298K} = -90.37$ kJ/mol). Inspired by the FTS in a slurry bed reactor, a liquid-phase methanol synthesis was first proposed in 1975. Compared with the gas-solid phase fixed-bed reactor, the gas-liquid-solid three-phase methanol synthesis selected long-chain hydrocarbons with high heat capacity and thermal conductivity liquid inert medium to remove the reaction heat, which makes the catalyst bed operated at a uniform temperature and easy to control. The slurry methanol synthesis can use the feed gas with high CO concentration to improve the single-pass conversion of CO, and the outlet methanol concentration is as high as

15–20%; moreover, there will be no local overheating and excessive temperature rise in catalyst bed [21].

In early studies, the catalysts applied in slurry methanol synthesis were mainly commercial fixed-bed CuZnAl catalysts [22]. In recent years, the slurry methanol catalysts have been intensively studied [23]. It is found that that the precipitation sequence of CuZnAl catalyst affected the catalytic performance. The catalyst prepared by precipitation of Al first and then co-precipitation of Cu and Al exhibit the highest activity and stability; the precipitation and aging temperature can not only affect the phase composition of CuZnAl catalyst precursor, but also affect its crystallinity. In addition, the introduction of microwave radiation heating can make the copper-based catalyst particles size smaller and more uniform, and the strengthened synergistic effect between copper and zinc is beneficial to improve the catalytic activity and stability.

3.3 DME synthesis

In 1991, a 10 t/d pilot-scale plant for synthesizing DME from syngas in a slurry bed was developed by Air Products and Chemicals, Inc., and Cu-based methanol synthesis catalysts and methanol dehydration catalysts γ-Al_2O_3 were adopted. Taiyuan University of Technology, Tsinghua University and Shanxi Coal Chemical Institute of Chinese Academy of Sciences have also done leading research work on slurry bed for DME synthesis. The catalyst for the one-step synthesis of dimethyl ether in the synthesis gas slurry bed is similar to the one-step catalyst in the fixed bed, which includes a methanol synthesis catalyst and a methanol dehydration catalyst. The methanol synthesis catalyst generally adopts CuZnAl catalyst or modified CuZnAl catalyst, and the catalyst for methanol dehydration generally adopts γ-Al_2O_3, zeolite, etc. **Table 2** summarizes the progress of DME synthesis in a slurry-bed reactor [24]. It can be seen that JFE (formally NKK) Corporation produced DME while Air Products Chemicals produced DME and methanol.

3.4 Synthetic natural gas synthesis

Slurry bed reactor is suitable for the strongly exothermic methanation reactions ($3H_2 + CO = CH_4 + H_2O$, $\Delta H^{\ominus}_{298K} = -206$ kJ/mol) [25]. The Chemical Systems Inc.

	JFE	Air Products	Tsinghua University
H_2/CO ratio	1	0.7	1
Catalysts		CuZnAl+γ-Al_2O_3	LP201 + TH16
Operating pressure, MPa	5	5–10	4.35–4.6
Temperature, °C	260	250–280	255–265
CO conversion, %	40	22	54–63
Selectivity, %	90	40–90	89–95
Reactor type	slurry bubble column	slurry bubble column	slurry airlift reactor
Reactor diameter, m	15	15.2	21.6
Reactor height, m	0.55	0.475	0.6
Design scale, t/d	5	10	10

Table 2.
Comparison of industrialization Technology of Dimethyl Ether Production in slurry bed [24].

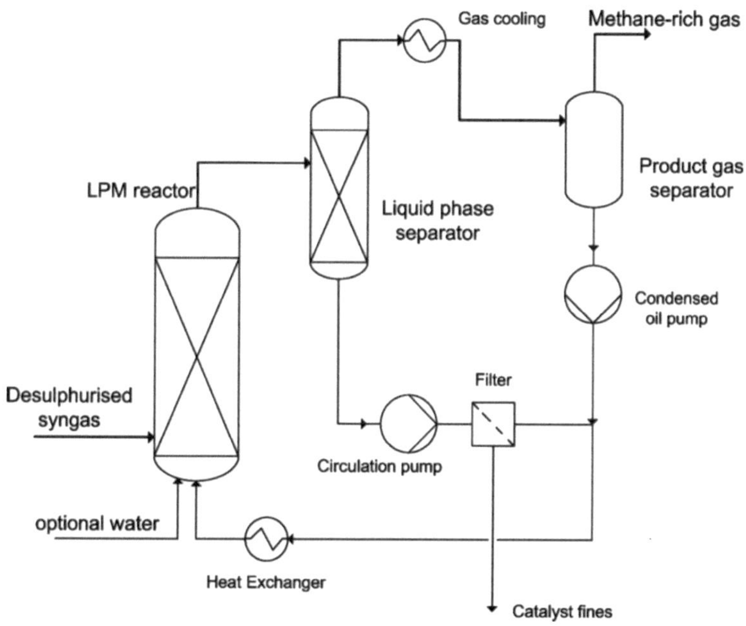

Figure 4.
Liquid phase methanation concept, adapted from [26].

(United States) developed a liquid-phase methanation process [26], as shown in **Figure 4**. The syngas produced in a coal gasifier was introduced into the catalytic liquid phase methanation reactor (LPM) along with a circulating process liquid (mineral oil), which absorbs the heat of reaction. The product gas was separated in a liquid phase separator and in a product gas separator. The process liquid was pumped through a filter to remove any catalyst fines and recirculated back to the LPM reactor. After a methanation reaction time for more than 300 h, the results showed low conversion and high catalyst loss, and thus the LPM-project was terminated in November 1981.

Taiyuan University of Technology and SEDIN Engineering Co., Ltd. have jointly developed a slurry-bed process for syngas methanation [27], as shown in **Figure 5**. The generated methanation gas together with the catalyst and the liquid-phase components enters through a gas-liquid separator, where the gas-phase product was condensed to produce synthetic natural gas, the liquid-phase product is mixed with fresh catalyst in the storage tank and added into the slurry bed methanation reactor to preheat the fresh catalyst. Due to the excellent heat transfer performance of the slurry bed, the adaptability of the feed gas for methanation of slurry bed is stronger, and the content of CO in feed gas can be adjusted within a wide range of 2–30%. The results show that the CO conversion for methanation reached 96% at the reaction temperature of 280°C in a slurry bed reactor.

For industrial fixed-bed methanation technology, the commercial catalysts are Ni-based catalyst, which is due to its cheap and excellent catalytic activity at high temperatures. However, the traditional industrial Ni-based catalysts exhibit poor catalytic performance in slurry bed reactors [28]. By optimizing the preparation method and conditions [29], adding additives, a slurry bed methanation catalyst with a high CO or CO_2 conversion of more than 99.5% can be obtained.

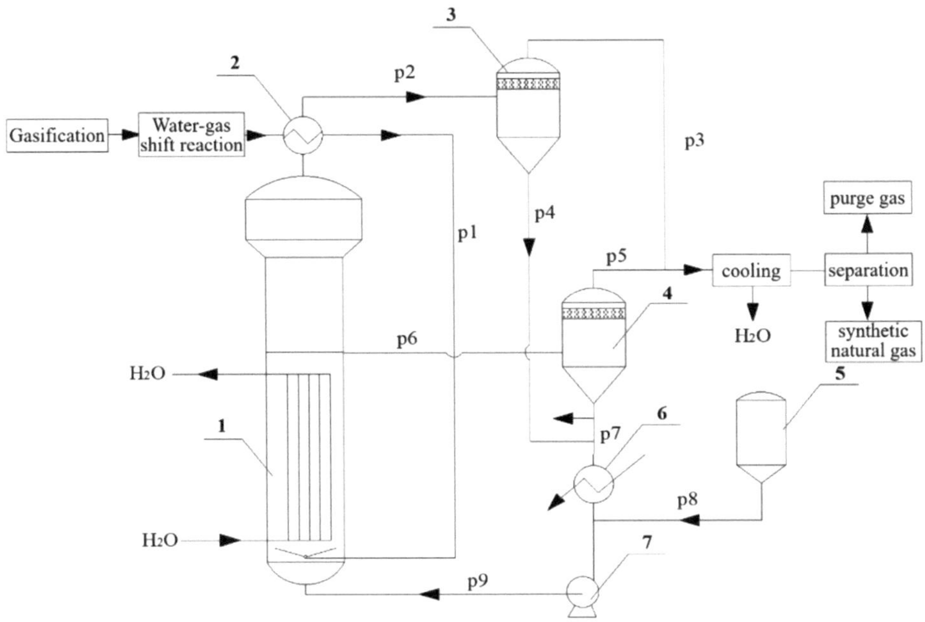

Figure 5.
Flow diagram of slurry-bed methanation for coal to synthetic natural gas. 1. Methanation reactor, 2. heat exchanger, 3. gas-liquid separator I, 4. gas-liquid separator II, 5. fresh catalyst storage tank, 6. heat exchanger II, 7. circulation pump, p1-p9 pipeline [27].

4. Comparison of fixed bed, circulating fluidized bed and slurry bed reactors for FTS

A schematic diagram for a common fixed bed reactor is shown in **Figure 6(a)**. A gas sparger at the reactor inlet is used to remove the initial kinetic energy of the gas stream. A certain gas space is left between the catalyst bed and the gas sparger for fluid buffering and uniform mixing. The packing (e.g., ceramic balls) spreads on the upper part of the bed can further make the stream enter the catalyst bed in a more uniform state. The small and uniform particle size of catalyst makes the resistance of each part of catalyst bed the same to enhance the reaction efficiency. After reacting in the catalyst channels, the unreacted syngas and the formed products leave the catalyst bed and reactor and release a large amount of heat. There is 1 ~ 2 thermocouple inserted in the reactor to monitor the temperature parameters of each section of the catalyst bed in time.

Fluidized bed reactors possess high heat transfer efficiency. Generally, the fluidized bed reactors are classified to circulating fluidized bed reactor and fixed fluidized bed reactor, as shown in **Figure 6(b and c)**. The feed gas is used as the power source to drive the catalyst, which is suitable for the strong exothermic reactions by using the intermediate heat exchange device to remove the reaction heat in time. However, the device structure of circulating fluidized bed reactor is complex, the investment and maintenance cost are high; Moreover, the reactor is difficult to operate and enlarge. In view of the limitations and defects of circulating fluidized bed reactor, a fixed fluidized bed reactor was designed by Sasol Corporation in 1995 and named as Sasol Advanced Synthnol reactor. Since the diameter of the fixed fluidized bed reactor can be much larger than that of circulating fluidized bed reactor, the space for

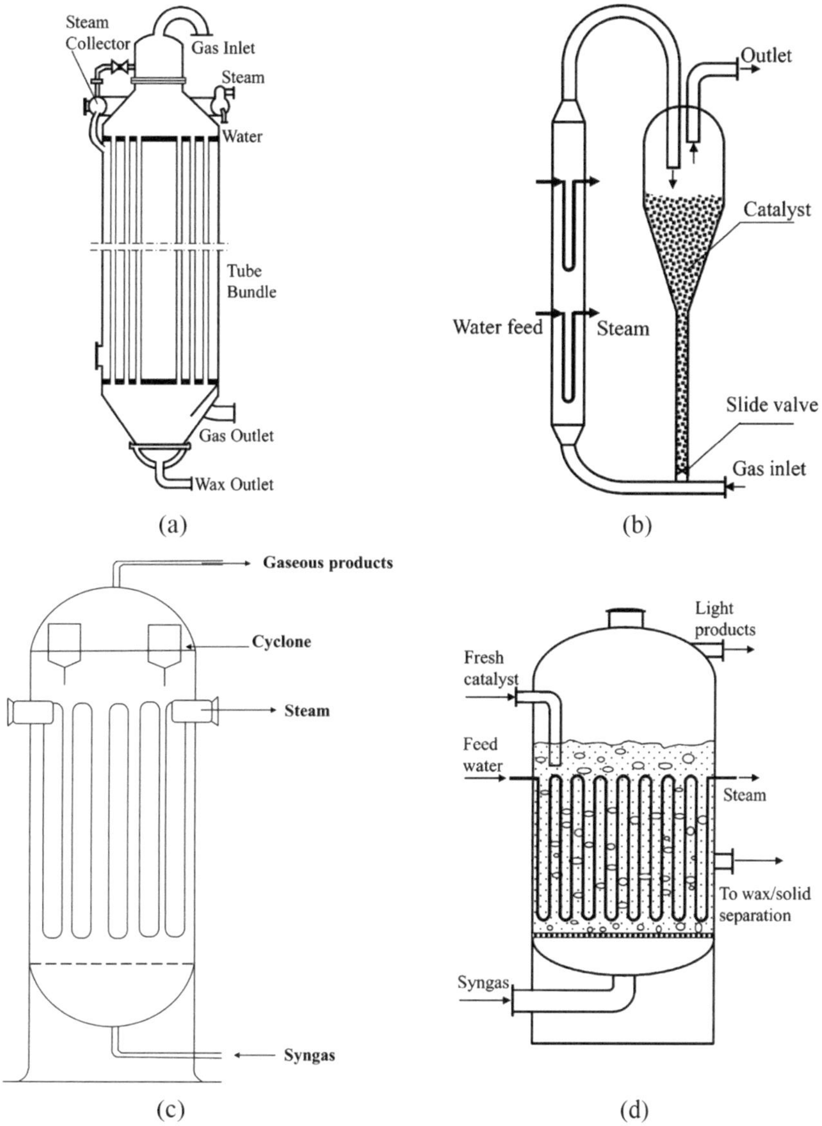

Figure 6.
Reactor types used for FTS. (a) Fixed bed reactor. (b) Circulating fluidized bed reactor. (c) Fixed fluidized bed reactor (d) slurry bubble column reactor [2].

installing the cooling plate is increased by more than 50%, which benefits to improve the CO conversion. However, the entrainment and attrition of the catalyst during the fluidization process is still very serious, which makes the fluidized bed methanation process is not practical for the expensive catalysts.

Since the heat transfer in the slurry bed reactor is more efficient than that in the fixed bed reactor, the temperature control is relatively easy. Therefore, the temperature of the catalyst active site in the slurry bed reactor could be uniform, which could avoid the formation of hot spots in the catalyst bed. In a continuous operation of the slurry bed reactor, the biggest difficulty and obstacle is the separation of fine catalyst, while in a fixed bed there is no such problem. However, the replacement of

Characteristic	Fixed bed	Circulating fluidized bed	Fixed fluidized bed	Slurry bed
Heat exchange rate or heat dissipation	slow	medium ~ high	high	high
Heat conduction in the system	bad	good	good	good
Reactor diameter limits	~8 cm	none	none	none
Pressure drop at high gas velocity	low	medium	high	medium ~ high
Gas phase residence time distribution	narrow	narrow	wide	narrow ~ wide
Axial mixing of the gas phase	low	low	high	low ~ medium
Axial mixing of catalysts	none	low	high	low ~ medium
Catalyst weight percentage/%	55 ~ 70	1 ~ 10	30 ~ 60	<30
Particle size of solid phase/ mm	1.5	0.01 ~ 0.5	0.003 ~ 1	0.1 ~ 1
Catalyst regeneration and replacement	intermittent	continuous	continuous	continuous
Catalyst loss	none	2% ~ 4%	wearred, cannot be recycled	low

Table 3.
Key parameters and performance comparison of different reactors [27].

the catalysts in a slurry bed reactor is easier than in a fixed bed reaction. If the catalyst needs to be removed and withdrew frequently in a process, the fixed bed reactor may not be appropriate, it is because that the replacement of the catalyst usually requires to stop and remove the reaction.

The key parameters and catalytic methanation performance of different reactors [27] are compared and summarized in **Table 3**. It can be seen that the heat exchange rate of fluidized bed and slurry bed reactor is significantly higher than that of fixed bed reactor, indicating that the fluidized bed or slurry bed reactor is very suitable for the strong exothermic reaction. However, the cost of fluidized bed reactor is high, the catalyst entrainment and wear are serious, and the catalyst cannot be recovered, which limits the application of large-scale production.

5. The deactivation of slurry bed catalyst

Dealing with the catalyst deactivation in a slurry bed reactor is a challenging phenomenon [30]. The detailed mechanistic insights in realizing the origin of the deactivation are much more complex, for the simultaneous involvement of various factors. Where, the most common factors could be relied on the S and/or N_2-containing compounds in the feed gas; the oxidation of the active metal (Co) components; strong metal-support interaction resulting into the hard to reduce species of silicates, aluminates; sintering, attrition, and carbon deposition on the nano-crystallites particles [31]. Since, these aforementioned factors of catalyst deactivation are mainly dependent on the type of reactor to be employed, the nature of the support, and the partial pressure of H_2O that can be further explained as follows.

5.1 Sulfur and nitrogen containing poisons

In carbon one chemical reactions, the poisons that may cause severe damage to the catalyst must be removed from the feed gas prior to the reaction, as these are independent of the catalyst nature to be used and operating conditions of the reactions. Since, the sensitive nature of cobalt-based catalysts to the sulfur content (<10 ppb) needs more attention of the additional gas cleaning steps for being expensive than Fe and also for its higher activity and a longer life time. In here, the different adsorption phenomena of the sulfur containing compounds (organic, inorganic) is more important for physically blocking the sites after being strongly adsorbed on the catalytic active sites, where one adsorbed S atom could deactivate the more than two Co atoms in a Co/Al_2O_3 catalyst. In a CO-rich syngas conversion to methanol reaction, the iron carbonyl, nickel carbonyl and carbonyl sulfide are severe catalyst poisons, which must be removed from the feed gas to avoid the catalyst deactivation [32]. Since, the removal of H_2S as the probe molecule and the nitrogen compounds such as NH_3, HCN (<50 ppb) are the crucial steps in gas purification, as they could lead to the severe damaging effect on the catalyst reducibility, activity, and selectivity.

5.2 Sintering

Besides the poisoning, the catalyst could also be deactivated due to the catalyst sintering at high temperature. Sintering is a common phenomenon of deactivation in metal catalysis, that is usually based on the minimization of surface energy of the crystallites. Sintering is usually accelerated by the high temperature and the partial pressure of water vapor; however, it can be controlled by interactions with the metal support. There are two empirical rules for the effect of temperature on highly dispersed metal crystallites: [1] When the temperature reaches $0.3T_m$ (called Hüttig temperature, T_m is the melting point), the migration of particles on the catalyst surface will occur [2]. When the temperature reaches $0.5T_m$ (Tammann temperature), the particle migration within the lattice phase will occur. For the methanol synthesis catalyst CuZnAl, the melting point of metallic Cu is 1358 K, and its Hüttig temperature is 407 K, and its Tammann temperature is 679 K; while the operation temperature of CuZnAl catalyst is generally at 480–553 K. Though the operation temperature is much lower than the Tammann temperature, it is higher than the Hüttig temperature, which inevitably resulted in the catalyst sintering and thus deactivated the catalyst. Lewnard et al. [33] investigated the stability test on CuZnAl catalyst, and obtained that the activation energy for catalyst deactivation is 91.3 kJ/mol. These activation energy data all demonstrate that catalyst sintering is an important reason for the deactivation of methanol synthesis catalyst in a gas-liquid-solid three-phase slurry bed.

5.3 Carbon deposition

Generally, the slurry bed reactor needs to be operated at the temperatures lower than 350°C due to the limitation of boiling point of mineral oil. Even at this low temperature, there are still some carbon deposited on the catalyst surface. For example, the result of CO methanation in a slurry-bed reactor over the Ni-Al_2O_3 catalyst [34] shows that, the catalytic activity of Ni-Al_2O_3 catalysts decreased slowly after a reaction time of 450 h. The thermogravimetric analysis and microscopic morphology results show the carbon deposition on catalyst surface, which was attributed to the amorphous carbon. The carbon deposition occupies the surface of the catalyst and covers the active sites, resulting in a decrease in Ni metal surface area and thus reduce the methanation activity. The regeneration of the spent catalyst shows that the catalyst carbon deposit can be removed by calcination in the air, and the catalyst structure and catalytic performance can be recovered.

5.4 Effects of water on catalyst structure

The reoxidation of Co metal active sites usually occurs when the oxygen atom of CO is eliminated mainly as H_2O (either from surface oxygen or OH species) during the FTS, where the influence of water contents in terms of its higher partial pressure than that of H_2 and CO become more crucial at high CO conversion. Since, the effect of water contents on the catalyst deactivation is mainly adopted from the possible reoxidation of the surface depending on the operating conditions, presence of different promoters (Pt, Mn, Zn, Mg, etc.), nature of the support (Al_2O_3, SiO_2, TiO_2) to be used, dispersion of metal components, and on the size of the pores of the support. For the methanol synthesis from syngas in a slurry-bed reactor over Cu-based catalysts, the addition of water in the reaction shows that too much H_2O accelerates the growth of grain and agglomeration of Cu-based catalyst, and a certain degree of carbon deposition, which leads to a fast catalyst deactivation, as shown in **Figure** 7 [35].

For the syngas to DME in a slurry bed reactor, the methanol dehydrated and formed DME in the reaction, if the generated water cannot be removed in time, the pores of the catalyst will be blocked and the reaction performance will be affected [36]. If the partial pressure of CO_2 in the feed gas is high, more $ZnCO_3$ will be appeared on the surface of CuZnAl catalyst, which is due to that the solubility of $ZnCO_3$ in water is several times higher than that of ZnO. Therefore, the leaching of Zn in the presence of water is one of the important reasons for the rapid deactivation of CuZnAl catalyst [37]. In addition, in the methanation reaction, the presence of water reacts with the γ-Al_2O_3 support of Ni-Al_2O_3 catalyst and thus formed AlOOH, which is one of the reasons for the deactivation of Ni-Al_2O_3 methanation catalyst.

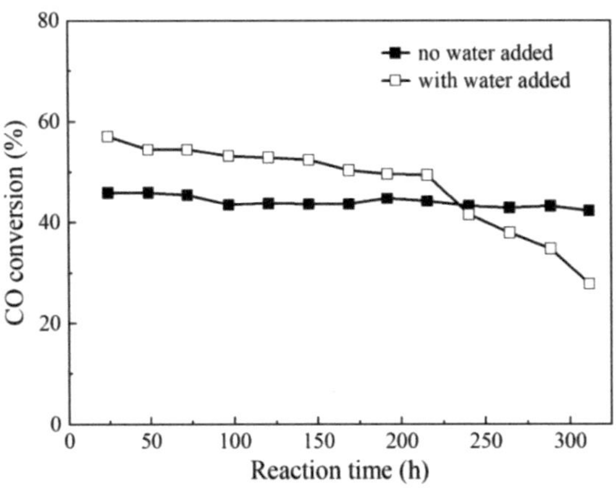

Figure 7.
Effect of H_2O on CO conversion for methanol synthesis [35].

5.5 Attrition of catalyst particles

One of the serious concerns of catalyst deactivation is the catalyst attrition by mixed particle fragmentation or surface abrasion, for breaking the particles into various fragments. It is a common phenomenon in fluidized or slurry bed reactors, where the interparticle collisions and bed-to-wall impacts cause the high mechanical stresses to catalyst bed particles, thus resulting the loss of valuable material, generation of fine particles, and the degradation of catalyst efficiency [38]. Usually, it is a time-dependent process that may systematically change with time, being more severe in the start of reaction and tends to a constant value of the nonsteady-state attrition rate with time. However, different strategies can be applied for increasing the attrition resistance and catalytic performance and decreasing the fraction of fines by spray-dried Fe-based FTS catalysts in a stirred-tank slurry reactor.

6. Current developments in slurry bed reactor for C_1 chemistry

Since, in a relative comparison it can be demonstrated that, the slurry bed reactors show the advantages of high efficiency of mass transfer and heat transfer, uniform reaction temperature, online replacement catalyst and low investment costs as compared to that of fixed-bed/fluidized-bed reactors [3, 6]. However, the industrialization process of the slurry bed reactor is relatively slow, it is because the enlargement of slurry bed reactor can only be achieved by increasing the diameter of the reactor, and the flow behavior in a large-scale industrial slurry bed is extremely complex under the working conditions of high temperature and high pressure. The blockage of the reactor distributor, uneven gas distribution led to the unstable operation state, which puts forward higher requirements for the rapid heat transfer of the slurry reactor [4, 39].

The process intensification is one of the methods to improve performance or solve problems in slurry bed reactors. The development of new high-efficiency internal components, the optimization of performance based on the existing internal components, and the coupling arrangement of multiple internal components can enhance the mixing and mass/heat transfer in slurry bed reactors [40]. Now, the research in slurry bed reactor mainly focuses on the fluid mechanics such as gas holdup, bubble size distribution, internal mass transfer, and heat transfer characteristics. Some or all the above problems can be solved by introduction of suitable internals into the reactor; however, the critical internals are difficult to obtain in published reports. Therefore, the structural optimization and function enhancement technology of internal components has become a challenging hot issue in the process of slurry bed design and scale-up [41]. Moreover, though the research of particle size on the effect of gas-liquid flow behavior in slurry bed reactors has been carried out earlier, however, these results in different reports are often inconsistent, which is due to the complexity of the gas-liquid-solid three-phase system, and in most cases, the influence mechanism of catalyst particles is based on analysis and prediction, without direct and sufficient proofs. Therefore, the research on the effect of particles is always the focus of attention and research.

7. Conclusions

Since, the comparative analysis of three different types slurry bed reactors, has been well discussed in the first part of this review while revealing the application of slurry bed reactors for C_1 chemistry, along with the four typical exothermic reactions for syngas conversion to different valuable chemicals. Similarly, the comparison between slurry bed, fixed bed, and fluidized bed reactors in second part also emphasized the catalyst deactivation for syngas conversion in slurry bed reactors, including the catalysts sintering, carbon deposition, effects of water on catalyst structure and the catalyst attrition by mixed particle fragmentation. While, the current development trend of slurry bed reactors for C_1 chemistry in the last part demonstrates the optimization of the reactor structure, higher active catalysts, and improvement of process conditions that could promote the development of slurry bed reactor. Since, the various techno economic aspects of slurry bed reactor make it very suitable for gas-to-liquid processes, especially for the highly exothermic reactions in C_1 chemistry for different valuable chemicals.

Acknowledgements

This work was financially supported by the Natural Science Foundation of Shanxi Province (202103021224073, 201801D121056). The authors would like to thank Liping Wang, Baozhen Li, Lina Wang, Zhiyuan Gong, Qian Wang, and Pengfei Ding from Taiyuan University of Technology for the help in finding and collecting the information.

Conflict of interest

The authors declare no conflict of interest.

Author details

Fanhui Meng[1*] and Muhammad Asif Nawaz[2,3]

1 State Key Laboratory of Clean and Efficient Coal Utilization, Taiyuan University of Technology, Taiyuan, China

2 State Key Laboratory of Chemical Engineering, East China University of Science and Technology, Shanghai, China

3 Department of Inorganic Chemistry and Materials Sciences Institute, University of Seville-CSIC, Seville, Spain

*Address all correspondence to: mengfanhui@tyut.edu.cn

References

[1] Chaudhari RV, Ramachandran PA. Three phase slurry reactors. AIChE Journal. 1980;**26**:177-201. DOI: 10.1002/aic.690260202

[2] Wang T, Wang J, Jin Y. Slurry reactors for gas-to-liquid processes: A review. Industrial & Engineering Chemistry Research. 2007;**46**:5824-5847. DOI: 10.1021/ie070330t

[3] Reay D, Ramshaw C, Harvey A. Chapter 5 - reactors. In: Reay D, Ramshaw C, Harvey A, editors. Process Intensification. 2nd ed. Oxford: Butterworth-Heinemann; 2013. pp. 121-204. DOI: 10.1016/B978-0-08-098304-2.00005-5

[4] Sinnott R, Towler G. Chapter 15 - Design of reactors and mixers. In: Sinnott R, Towler G, editors. Chemical Engineering Design. 6th ed. Oxfordshire: Butterworth-Heinemann; 2020. pp. 1039-1146. DOI: 10.1016/B978-0-08-102599-4.00015-1

[5] Meng F, Li X, Li M, Cui X, Li Z. Catalytic performance of CO methanation over La-promoted Ni/Al_2O_3 catalyst in a slurry-bed reactor. Chemical Engineering Journal. 2017;**313**:1548-1555. DOI: 10.1016/j.cej.2016.11.038

[6] Cimenler U, Kuhn JN, Chapter 15 - Heterogeneous catalysts encapsulated in inorganic systems to enhance reaction performances for XTL processes. In: Sadjadi S, editor. Encapsulated Catalysts. London: Academic Press; 2017. pp. 505-524. DOI: 10.1016/B978-0-12-803836-9.00015-8

[7] Chen S, Sun Y. Catalytic Reactor Engineering. Beijing: Chemical Industrial Press; 2011. pp. 39-107

[8] Li S. Chapter 9 - Multiple-phase reactors. In: Li S, editor. Reaction Engineering. Boston: Butterworth-Heinemann; 2017. pp. 405-444. DOI: 10.1016/B978-0-12-410416-7.00009-4

[9] Rauch R, Kiennemann A, Sauciuc A. Chapter 12 - Fischer-Tropsch synthesis to biofuels (BtL process). In: Triantafyllidis KS, Lappas AA, Stöcker M, editors. The Role of Catalysis for the Sustainable Production of Bio-Fuels and Bio-Chemicals. Amsterdam: Elsevier; 2013. pp. 397-443

[10] Nawaz MA, Saif M, Li M, Song G, Zihao W, Liu D. Tailoring the synergistic dual-decoration of (Cu–Co) transition metal auxiliaries in Fe-oxide/zeolite composite catalyst for the direct conversion of syngas to aromatics. Catalysis Science & Technology. 2021;**11**:7992-8006. DOI: 10.1039/D1CY01717A

[11] Jager B, Espinoza R. Advances in low temperature Fischer-Tropsch synthesis. Catalysis Today. 1995;**23**:17-28. DOI: 10.1016/0920-5861(94)00136-P

[12] Leckel D. Hydroprocessing euro 4-type diesel from high-temperature Fischer–Tropsch vacuum gas oils. Energy & Fuels. 2009;**23**:38-45. DOI: 10.1021/ef800614p

[13] Schulz H. Short history and present trends of Fischer-Tropsch synthesis. Applied Catalysis A General. 1999;**186**:3-12. DOI: 10.1016/S0926-860X(99)00160-X

[14] Corsaro A, Wiltowski T, Honus DJ, S. Conversion of syngas to LPG and aromatics over commercial Fischer-Tropsch catalyst and HZSM-5 in a dual bed reactor. Petroleum Science & Technology. 2014;**32**:2497-2505

[15] Sie ST, Krishna R. Fundamentals and selection of advanced Fischer–Tropsch reactors. Applied Catalysis A: General. 1999;**186**:55-70. DOI: 10.1016/S0926-860X(99)00164-7

[16] Bukur DB, Lang X, Nowicki L. Comparative study of an iron Fischer–Tropsch catalyst performance in stirred tank slurry and fixed-bed reactors. Industrial & Engineering Chemistry Research. 2005;**44**:6038-6044. DOI: 10.1021/ie0492146

[17] Krishna R, Sie ST. Design and scale-up of the Fischer–Tropsch bubble column slurry reactor. Fuel Processing Technology. 2000;**64**:73-105. DOI: 10.1016/S0378-3820(99)00128-9

[18] Zhu J, Lv Y, Chang H. Progresses in the research of slurry reactor and catalysts for Fischer-Tropsch synthesis. Petrochemical Technology. 2012;**41**:597-602

[19] De Blasio C. Fischer–Tropsch (FT) synthesis to biofuels (BtL process). In: De Blasio C, editor. Fundamentals of Biofuels Engineering and Technology. Cham: Springer International Publishing; 2019. pp. 287-306

[20] Wu B, Bai L, Xiang H, Li Y-W, Zhang Z, Zhong B. An active iron catalyst containing sulfur for Fischer–Tropsch synthesis. Fuel. 2004;**83**:205-212. DOI: 10.1016/S0016-2361(03)00253-9

[21] Spencer MS. Methanol synthesis technology: By Sunggyu Lee. CRC Press, Boca Raton, 1990, 236. Chemical Engineering Science. 1991;**46**:2385. DOI: 10.1016/0009-2509(91)85141-J

[22] Cybulski A. Liquid-phase methanol synthesis: Catalysts, mechanism, kinetics, chemical equilibria, vapor-liquid equilibria, and modeling—A review. Catalysis Reviews. 1994;**36**:557-615. DOI: 10.1080/01614949408013929

[23] Salehi K, Jokar SM, Shariati J, Bahmani M, Sedghamiz MA, Rahimpour MR. Enhancement of CO conversion in a novel slurry bubble column reactor for methanol synthesis. Journal of Natural Gas Science and Engineering. 2014;**21**:170-183. DOI: 10.1016/j.jngse.2014.07.030

[24] Wang J, Ren F, Wang D, Jin Y. Research of DME synthesis in slurry reactor by one step process. Chemical Engineering of Oil & Gas. 2004;**33**:42-43

[25] Bhattacharjee S, Tierney JW, Shah YT. Thermal behavior of a slurry reactor: Application to synthesis gas conversion. Industrial & Engineering Chemistry Process Design and Development. 1986;**25**:117-126. DOI: 10.1021/i200032a018

[26] Kopyscinski J, Schildhauer TJ, Biollaz SMA. Production of synthetic natural gas (SNG) from coal and dry biomass: A technology review from 1950 to 2009. Fuel. 2010;**89**:1763-1783. DOI: 10.1016/j.fuel.2010.01.027

[27] Shen J. Coal Chemical Technology. Beijing: Chemical Industry Press; 2020. pp. 172-187

[28] Meng F, Song Y, Li X, Cheng Y, Li Z. Catalytic methanation performance in a low-temperature slurry-bed reactor over Ni–ZrO_2 catalyst: Effect of the preparation method. Journal of Sol-Gel Science and Technology. 2016;**80**:759-768. DOI: 10.1007/s10971-016-4139-4

[29] Zhang J, Bai Y, Zhang Q, Wang X, Zhang T, Tan Y, et al. Low-temperature methanation of syngas in slurry phase over Zr-doped Ni/γ-Al_2O_3 catalysts prepared using different methods. Fuel. 2014;**132**:211-218. DOI: 10.1016/j.fuel.2014.04.085

[30] Nawaz MA, Saif M, Li M, Song G, Zihao W, Chen C, et al. Elucidating the synergistic fabrication of dual embedded (χ-Fe_5C_2 + θ-Fe_3C) carbide nanocomposites in Na-FeCa@AC/HZSM-5 integrated catalyst for syngas conversion to aromatics. Fuel. 2022;**324**:124390. DOI: 10.1016/j.fuel.2022.124390

[31] Nawaz MA, Li M, Saif M, Song G, Wang Z, Liu D. Harnessing the synergistic interplay of Fischer-Tropsch synthesis (Fe-Co) bimetallic oxides in Na-FeMnCo/HZSM-5 composite catalyst for syngas conversion to aromatic hydrocarbons. ChemCatChem. 2021;**13**:1966-1980. DOI: 10.1002/cctc.202100024

[32] Roberts GW, Brown DM, Hsiung TH, Lewnard JJ. Catalyst poisoning during the synthesis of methanol in a slurry reactor. Chemical Engineering Science. 1990;**45**:2713-2720. DOI: 10.1016/0009-2509(90)80162-8

[33] Lewnard JJ, Hsiung TH. Temperature effects on catalyst activity in the liquid phase methanol process. Studies in Surface Science and Catalysis. 1988;**38**:141-152. DOI: 10.1016/S0167-2991(09)60651-0

[34] Ji K, Meng F, Xun J, Liu P, Zhang K, Li Z, et al. Carbon deposition behavior of Ni catalyst prepared by combustion method in slurry methanation reaction. Catalysts. 2019;**9**:570. DOI: 10.3390/catal9070570

[35] Wang D, Tan Y, Han Y, Noritatsu T. Study on deactivation of hybrid catalyst for dimethyl ether synthesis in slurry bed reactor. Journal of Fuel Chemistry and Technology. 2008;**36**:176-180

[36] Lee S, Lee BG, Kulik CJ. Post-reduction treatment of liquid phase methanol synthesis catalyst using carbon dioxide. Fuel Science and Technology International. 1991;**9**:977-998. DOI: 10.1080/08843759108942307

[37] Lee S, Sawant A, Rodrigues K, Kulik CJ. Effects of carbon dioxide and water on the methanol synthesis catalyst. Energy & Fuels. 1989;**3**:2-7. DOI: 10.1021/ef00013a001

[38] Bukur DB, Ma W-P, Carreto-Vazquez V, Nowicki L, Adeyiga AA. Attrition resistance and catalytic performance of spray-dried iron Fischer-Tropsch catalysts in a stirred-tank slurry reactor. Industrial and Engineering Chemistry Research. 2004;**43**:1359-1365. DOI: 10.1021/ie034056o

[39] Towler G, Sinnott R. Chapter 15 - Design of reactors and mixers. In: Towler G, Sinnott R, editors. Chemical Engineering Design. 3rd ed. Oxfordshire: Butterworth-Heinemann; 2022. pp. 497-588. DOI: 10.1016/B978-0-12-821179-3.00015-7

[40] Ravi R. Chapter 2 - Flow characteristics of reactors—Flow modeling. In: Ravi R, Vinu R, Gummadi SN, editors. Coulson and Richardson's Chemical Engineering. 4th ed. Oxfordshire: Butterworth-Heinemann; 2017. pp. 103-160. DOI: 10.1016/B978-0-08-101096-9.00002-9

[41] Shao M, Li Y, Chen J, Zhang Y. Chapter Six - Mesoscale effects on product distribution of Fischer–Tropsch synthesis. In: Marin GB, Li J, editors. Advances in Chemical Engineering. Vol. 47. London: Academic Press; 2015. pp. 337-387. DOI: 10.1016/bs.ache.2015.10.002